Thyroid Eye Disease

Raymond S. Douglas • Allison N. McCoy
Shivani Gupta
Editors

Thyroid Eye Disease

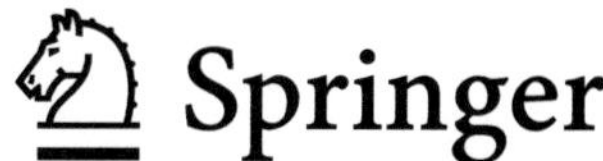

Editors
Dr. Raymond S. Douglas
Division of Eye Plastic, Orbital,
and Facial Cosmetic Surgery
Kellogg Eye Center
University of Michigan
Ann Arbor, MI, USA

Dr. Allison N. McCoy
Division of Eye Plastic, Orbital,
and Facial Cosmetic Surgery
Kellogg Eye Center
University of Michigan
Ann Arbor, MI, USA

Dr. Shivani Gupta
Division of Eye Plastic, Orbital,
and Facial Cosmetic Surgery
Kellogg Eye Center
University of Michigan
Ann Arbor, MI, USA

ISBN 978-1-4939-1745-7 ISBN 978-1-4939-1746-4 (eBook)
DOI 10.1007/978-1-4939-1746-4
Springer New York Heidelberg Dordrecht London

Library of Congress Control Number: 2014949863

Printed on acid-free paper

Springer is part of Springer Science+Business Media (www.springer.com)

Preface

Thyroid eye disease (TED) presents enormous challenges to our patients and to the physicians caring for them. The disease is heterogeneous and unpredictable, and most importantly it substantially impacts the quality of life of our patients. Based upon the input from a world community, we hope to provide the practitioner a resource to guide patients through this disease process. Each author has worked diligently toward this international endeavor, bridging the gaps of our knowledge for an international audience.

The textbook can be read in its entirety to give a perspective of the field or treated as a reference as clinical questions arise. Our goal is to deliver data-driven guidance and discreet approaches and suggestions useful for clinical decision making.

A multidisciplinary approach with the knowledge and acumen of many subspecialties was utilized to develop the textbook. Most authors practice at multidisciplinary centers such as ours at the University of Michigan, where the focus of the team is patient-centered. Multidisciplinary TED centers provide synergy among specialties, which prompts early intervention, refines quality of care, and improves outcomes. Each of the chapters reflects the contributions which become possible in a team-oriented approach.

Several advances have been made in the pathogenesis of the disease and hopefully these will result in new approaches and eventual cures. For the first time in decades, the advances of science are permeating into the clinical realm providing optimism for new treatment approaches.

The endocrinologic management of Graves' disease is critical for the health of our patients as is the ability to properly define TED; both of these are discussed in the initial chapters of the text. The role of nutrition, supplements, pregnancy, and the external environment in the disease process is under increasing scrutiny and may alter the long-term consequences of disease. Discussion of these topics will allow the clinician to adequately counsel patients.

TED is a vexing problem and debate still exists regarding the medical management of the process in addition to subsequent surgical rehabilitation. Input from experts around the world was critical to give proper perspective to this discussion and to give readers a framework with which to approach each patient.

Overcoming the psychological and functional impediments created by TED is paramount and discussed in detail. Specifically, rehabilitative surgery has evolved to offer most patients substantial improvement and can be individualized according to their needs.

Capturing the perspective of the world community was critical for this endeavor. Overcoming the remaining obstacles and working toward a cure is dependent upon this continued partnership.

Ann Arbor, MI, USA

Raymond S. Douglas
Allison N. McCoy
Shivani Gupta

Contents

Contributors

Sally L. Baxter, M.D., M.Sc. Department of Ophthalmology, Shiley Eye Center, University of California San Diego, La Jolla, CA, USA

Lucy Clarke Newcastle Eye Centre, Royal Victoria Infirmary, Newcastle upon Tyne, UK

Peter J. Dolman, M.D., F.R.C.S.C. Department of Ophthalmology, University of British Columbia, Vancouver, BC, Canada

Eye Care Centre, Section I, Vancouver, BC, Canada

Raymond S. Douglas, M.D., Ph.D. Division of Eye Plastic, Orbital, and Facial Cosmetic Surgery, Kellogg Eye Center, University of Michigan, Ann Arbor, MI, USA

Roman Farjardo, M.D. Division of Ophthalmic Plastic and Reconstructive Surgery, Department of Ophthalmology, Shiley Eye Center, University of California San Diego, La Jolla, CA, USA

Andrew G. Gianoukakis, M.D. Department of Medicine, Division of Endocrinology and Metabolism, Harbor-UCLA Medical Center, Torrance, CA, USA

Robert A. Goldberg, M.D. Orbital and Ophthalmic Plastic Surgery, Jules Stein Eye Institute, Los Angeles, CA, USA

Shivani Gupta, M.D., M.P.H. Division of Eye Plastic, Orbital, and Facial Cosmetic Surgery, Kellogg Eye Center, University of Michigan, Ann Arbor, MI, USA

Rebecca A. Hicks, M.D. Department of Pediatrics, Division of Endocrinology and Metabolism, Harbor-UCLA Medical Center, Torrance, CA, USA

Teeranun Jirajariyavej, M.D. Department of Medicine, Division of Endocrinology and Metabolism, Harbor-UCLA Medical Center, Torrance, CA, USA

Bokkwan Jun, M.D., Ph.D. Division of Neuro-Ophthalmology, Department of Ophthalmology, Wilmer Eye Institute, The Johns Hopkins Hospital, Johns Hopkins University School of Medicine, Baltimore, MD, USA

George J. Kahaly, M.D., Ph.D., Medicine and Endocrinology/Metabolism, Gutenberg University Medical Center, Mainz, Germany

Don O. Kikkawa, M.D., F.A.C.S. Division of Ophthalmic Plastic and Reconstructive Surgery, Department of Ophthalmology, Shiley Eye Center, University of California San Diego, La Jolla, CA, USA

Bobby S. Korn, M.D., Ph.D., F.A.C.S. Division of Ophthalmic Plastic and Reconstructive Surgery, UCSD Department of Ophthalmology, Shiley Eye Center, University of California San Diego, La Jolla, CA, USA

Claudio Marcocci Department of Clinical and Experimental Medicine, University of Pisa, Pisa, Italy

Allison N. McCoy, M.D., Ph.D. Division of Eye Plastic, Orbital, and Facial Cosmetic Surgery, Kellogg Eye Center, University of Michigan, Ann Arbor, MI, USA

Francesca Menconi Department of Clinical and Experimental Medicine, University of Pisa, Pisa, Italy

Petros Perros, B.Sc., M.B.B.S., M.D., F.R.C.P. Department of Endocrinology, Royal Victoria Infirmary, Newcastle upon Tyne, UK

Fatemeh Rajaii, M.D., Ph.D. Division of Eye Plastic, Orbital, and Facial Cosmetic Surgery, Kellogg Eye Center, University of Michigan, Ann Arbor, MI, USA

Daniel B. Rootman, M.Sc., M.D. Orbital and Ophthalmic Plastic Surgery, Jules Stein Eye Institute, Los Angeles, CA, USA

Mario Salvi, M.D. Department of Clinical Sciences and Community Health, Graves Orbitopathy Unit, Fondazione Ca'Granda IRCCS, University of Milan, Milan, Italy

Richard L. Scawn, M.B.B.S., F.R.C.Ophth. Division of Ophthalmic Plastic and Reconstructive Surgery, Department of Ophthalmology, Shiley Eye Center, University of California San Diego, La Jolla, CA, USA

Terry J. Smith, M.D. Department of Ophthalmology and Visual Sciences, Kellogg Eye Center, University of Michigan, Ann Arbor, MI, USA

Internal Medicine, University of Michigan Medical School, Ann Arbor, MI, USA

Prem S. Subramanian, M.D., Ph.D. Department of Ophthalmology, Neurology, and Neurosurgery, The Johns Hopkins Hospital, Johns Hopkins University School of Medicine, Baltimore, MD, USA

Wilmar M. Wiersinga, M.D., Ph.D. Department of Endocrinology & Metabolism, Academic Medical Center, University of Amsterdam, Amsterdam, The Netherlands

Jennifer K. Yee, M.D. Department of Pediatrics, Division of Endocrinology and Metabolism, Harbor-UCLA Medical Center, Torrance, CA, USA

1 Diagnosis and Endocrine Management of Graves' Disease

George J. Kahaly

Introduction and Pathogenesis

Thyrotoxicosis is defined as the state of thyroid hormone excess and is synonymous with hyperthyroidism, which is the result of excessive thyroid function. Hyperthyroidism is a common disorder affecting about 1–2 % of women and 0.2–0.5 % of men. The major etiologies of thyrotoxicosis are hyperthyroidism caused by Graves' disease (GD), toxic multinodular goiter, and toxic adenomas. GD accounts for 60–80 % of thyrotoxicosis, though the prevalence varies among populations, depending mainly on iodine intake [1]. GD occurs more often in women than in men with a female:male ratio of 5:1 and a population prevalence of 1–2 % [2]. The disorder rarely begins before adolescence and typically occurs between 20 and 50 years of age, though it also occurs in the elderly [3].

GD is an autoimmune thyroid disorder characterized by the infiltration of immune effector cells and thyroid-antigen-specific T cells into the thyroid and TSH receptor (TSHR) expressing tissues, with the production of autoantibodies to well-defined thyroidal antigens such as thyroid peroxidase, thyroglobulin, and the TSHR. A genetic determinant to the susceptibility to GD is suspected because of familial clustering of the disease [4, 5], a high sibling recurrence risk, the familial occurrence of thyroid autoantibodies and concurrent autoimmune diseases [6, 7], and the 30 % concordance in disease status between identical twins [8, 9]. Smoking and other lifestyle factors also increase the risk for Graves' hyperthyroidism [10]. The TSHR expressed on the plasma membrane of thyroid epithelial cells is central to the regulation of thyroid growth and function. However, it is also expressed on a variety of other tissues, including adipocytes and bone cells. The TSHR is the major autoantigen in the autoimmune hyperthyroidism of GD where T cells and autoantibodies are directed at the TSHR antigen. Stimulatory autoantibodies in GD activate TSHR on thyroid follicular cells, leading to thyroid hyperplasia and unregulated thyroid hormone production and secretion [11].

The close clinical relationship between Graves' hyperthyroidism and Graves' orbitopathy or thyroid eye disease (TED) has suggested that immunoreactivity against TSHR present in both the thyroid and orbit underlies both conditions [12]. A prerequisite for involvement of TSHR as an autoantigen in TED is that it be expressed in affected orbital tissues [13]. Numerous studies have demonstrated that TSHR mRNA and protein are present in TED. Further, TSHR expression has been shown to be higher in orbital fat from patients with TED compared with normal orbital adipose tissues. Also, in individual

G.J. Kahaly, M.D., Ph.D. (✉)
Medicine and Endocrinology/Metabolism,
Gutenberg University Medical Center,
Mainz 55101, Germany
e-mail: Kahaly@ukmainz.de

R.S. Douglas et al. (eds.), *Thyroid Eye Disease*,
DOI 10.1007/978-1-4939-1746-4_1, © Springer Science+Business Media New York 2015

patients with TED, a positive correlation exists between TSHR mRNA levels in orbital connective tissue specimens and clinical disease activity [14]. The extrathyroidal manifestations of GD, i.e., TED and dermopathy, are due to immunologically mediated activation of fibroblasts in the extraocular muscles and skin, with accumulation of glycosaminoglycans, leading to the trapping of water and edema [15]. Later, fibrosis becomes prominent. The fibroblast activation is caused by proinflammatory cytokines derived from locally infiltrating T cells and macrophages [16].

Clinical Spectrum

Signs and symptoms include features that are common to any cause of thyrotoxicosis (Table 1.1) as well as those specific for GD [17]. The clinical presentation depends on the severity of thyrotoxicosis, the duration of the disease, individual susceptibility to excess thyroid hormone, and the age of the patient. In the elderly, features of thyrotoxicosis may be subtle or masked, and patients may present mainly with fatigue and weight loss, leading to apathetic hyperthyroidism. Thyrotoxicosis may cause unexplained weight loss, despite an enhanced appetite, and is due to the increased metabolic rate (Table 1.2). Weight gain occurs in 5–10 % of patients, however, as a result of increased food intake. Other prominent features include hyperactivity, nervousness, and irritability, ultimately leading to a sense of easy fatiguability in some patients. Insomnia and impaired concentration are common; apathetic thyrotoxicosis may be mistaken for depression in the elderly [18].

In GD the thyroid is usually diffusely enlarged to two to three times its normal size. The consistency is firm, but less so than in multinodular goiter. There may be a thrill or bruit due to the increased vascularity of the gland and the hyperdynamic circulation. The most common cardiovascular manifestation is sinus tachycardia, often associated with palpitations and sometimes due to supraventricular tachycardia. The high cardiac output produces a bounding pulse, widened pulse pressure, and an aortic systolic murmur, and can lead to worsening of angina or heart failure in the elderly or those with preexisting heart disease [19]. Atrial fibrillation is more common in patients >50 years. Treatment of the thyrotoxic state alone reverts atrial fibrillation to normal

Table 1.1 Causes and differential diagnosis of hyperthyroidism

Primary hyperthyroidism
• Graves' disease
• Toxic multinodular goiter
• Toxic adenoma
• Amiodarone, iodine excess
• Ingestion of excess thyroid hormone (thyrotoxicosis factitia) or thyroid tissue
• Subacute thyroiditis
• Silent thyroiditis
• Activating mutation of the TSH receptor (autosomal dominant)
• Struma ovarii
• Functioning thyroid carcinoma metastases
Secondary hyperthyroidism
• TSH-secreting pituitary adenoma
• Thyroid hormone resistance syndrome
• Chorionic gonadotropin-secreting tumors
• Gestational thyrotoxicosis

Table 1.2 Signs and symptoms of Graves' hyperthyroidism

Symptoms
• Hyperactivity, irritability
• Heat intolerance and sweating
• Palpitations
• Dysphoria
• Fatigue and weakness
• Weight loss with increased appetite
• Diarrhea
• Polyuria
• Oligomenorrhea, loss of libido
Signs
• Tachycardia
• Atrial fibrillation in the elderly
• Tremor
• Goiter
• Warm, moist skin
• Muscle weakness, proximal myopathy
• Lid retraction or lag
• Exophthalmos
• Gynecomastia

sinus rhythm in fewer than half of patients, suggesting the existence of an underlying cardiac problem in the remainder.

The skin is usually warm and moist, and the patient typically reports sweating and heat intolerance, particularly during warm weather. Palmar erythema, onycholysis, and less commonly, pruritus, urticaria, and diffuse hyperpigmentation may be evident. Hair texture may become fine, and a diffuse alopecia occurs in up to 40 % of patients, persisting for months after restoration of euthyroidism. Fine tremor is a very frequent finding, best elicited by asking patients to stretch out the fingers and feeling the fingertips with the palm. Common neurologic manifestations include hyperreflexia, muscle wasting, and proximal myopathy without fasciculation. Chorea is a rare feature. Thyrotoxicosis is sometimes associated with a form of hypokalemic periodic paralysis; this disorder is particularly common in Asian males with thyrotoxicosis. Gastrointestinal transit time is decreased, leading to increased stool frequency, often with diarrhea and occasionally mild steatorrhea. Women frequently experience oligomenorrhea or amenorrhea; in men there may be impaired sexual function and, rarely, gynecomastia. The direct effect of thyroid hormones on bone resorption leads to osteopenia in long-standing thyrotoxicosis; mild hypercalcemia occurs in up to 20 % of patients, but hypercalciuria is more common. There is a small increase in fracture rate in patients with a previous history of thyrotoxicosis.

Extrathyroidal Manifestations

Lid retraction, causing a staring appearance, can occur in any form of thyrotoxicosis and is the result of sympathetic overactivity. However, GD is associated with specific eye signs that comprise TAO. This condition may occur in the absence of GD in 10 % of patients. Most of these individuals have autoimmune hypothyroidism or thyroid antibodies. The onset of TAO occurs within the year before or after the diagnosis of thyrotoxicosis in 75 % of patients but can sometimes precede or follow thyrotoxicosis by several years, accounting for some cases of euthyroid TED. Many patients with GD have little clinical evidence of TED. However, the enlarged extraocular muscles typical of the disease can be detected in almost all patients when investigated by ultrasound or computed tomography (CT) imaging of the orbits [20]. Unilateral signs are found in up to 10 % of patients.

The earliest manifestations of TED are a sensation of grittiness, eye discomfort, and excess tearing. About a third of patients have proptosis, best detected by visualization of the sclera between the lower border of the iris and the lower eyelid, with the eyes in the primary position. Proptosis can be measured using an exophthalmometer. In severe cases, proptosis may cause corneal exposure and damage, especially if the lids fail to close during sleep. Periorbital edema, scleral injection, and chemosis are also frequent. In 5–10 % of patients, the muscle swelling is so severe that diplopia results, typically but not exclusively when the patient looks up and laterally. Muscle swelling may also cause compression of the optic nerve at the apex of the orbit, leading to optic nerve swelling, visual field defects, and if left untreated, permanent loss of vision.

Clinical features of TED vary from a mild grittiness of the eyes to severe diplopia, disfiguring proptosis, and loss of vision. There is a natural tendency towards spontaneous improvement: the spontaneous course depicts an active phase, which slowly abates after which an inactive phase ensues [21]. The most common signs of TED are eyelid retraction (90 %), soft tissue involvement (80 %), proptosis (50–60 %), dry eye syndrome (50 %), motility disorders (40 %), optic neuropathy (3–5 %), and superior limbic keratitis (2 %) [17]. The autoimmune process leads to an accumulation of collagen and hydrophilic glycosaminoglycans within the orbit. Inflammatory changes of the eyelids cause visible edema and erythema. If extraocular muscles are affected motility disorders may occur. Patients with motility disturbances, severe and active disease have a severely impaired health-related quality of life [22].

Many scoring systems have been used to gauge the extent and severity of the orbital changes in GD. The NOSPECS scheme [23, 24] includes six classes of eye changes. TED is classified as severe if corneal involvement, severe proptosis, constant diplopia, or optic neuropathy is present [25]. Evaluating the activity of TED is required to choose the most effective and stage adjusted therapy. TED is active when inflammatory signs such as redness and swelling predominate and there are progressive changes in objective measurements such as exophthalmos, eyelid position, and motility. Several groups have tried to develop methods to assess activity of TED. These include purely clinical assessments (clinical activity score, CAS [26]), laboratory measurements (cytokines, glycosaminoglycan excretion, TSHR stimulating autoantibodies or TSAb [27]), and imaging techniques [20]. Clinical evaluation of the CAS together with measurement of TSAb serum levels is helpful to document disease activity.

General ophthalmic assessment should include examination of anterior and posterior eye segment, applanation tonometry, Hertel exophthalmometry, and motility tests. Additionally, the observer classifies whether there is optic disc edema or disc pallor and records whether choroidal folds are present. In addition to fundus exam, relative afferent pupillary defects, visual field defects, color vision abnormalities, visually evoked potentials, and visual acuity are tested to determine whether optic neuropathy is present. Cigarette smoking can profoundly influence the occurrence and the course of TED [28], and also impairs its response to conservative treatment [29]. Accordingly, patients should be strongly urged to stop smoking, as refraining from smoking favorably influences the course of TED. Also, emotional distress and stressful life events are risk factors for TED and should therefore be minimized [30, 31].

Graves' Dermopathy and Graves' Acropachy

Graves' dermopathy is characterized by a localized thickening of the skin (mostly in the pretibial area), whereas in Graves' acropachy there is digital clubbing, thickening of the skin of the digits, and sometimes periostitis of the distal bones [32]. While TED usually precedes dermopathy, acropachy appears around the same time or subsequent to dermopathy. Dermopathy and acropachy may be regarded as markers of severe TED. The rate of orbital decompression surgery is significantly higher in TED patients who suffered from dermopathy. Also, patients with dermopathy have higher TSAb serum levels compared with those with Graves' thyroidal disease only [33]. It is recommended to rule out other skin diseases if Graves' dermopathy without eye involvement is present. Topical local steroid therapy may help [34]; however, severe skin involvement requires long-term management with high doses of IV steroids. Patients with systemic involvement, i.e., Graves' dermopathy and/or acropachy, are best managed in a multidisciplinary Graves' center with a joint thyroid eye clinic during the active phase of the disease.

Laboratory Evaluation and Thyroid Imaging

In GD, below-normal to suppressed levels of baseline serum TSH, normal to elevated serum levels of T4, elevated serum levels of T3 and of TSHR autoantibodies, as well as a diffusely enlarged, heterogeneous, hypervascular thyroid gland (increased Doppler flow in the ultrasound evaluation of the neck) confirm diagnosis of GD [1, 35, 36]. In 2–5 % of patients and more commonly in areas of borderline iodine intake, only T3 is increased (T3 toxicosis). The converse state of T4 toxicosis, with elevated total and free T4 and normal T3 levels, is occasionally seen when hyperthyroidism is induced by excess iodine, providing surplus substrate for thyroid hormone synthesis. Associated abnormalities that may cause diagnostic confusion in thyrotoxicosis include elevation of bilirubin, liver enzymes, and ferritin. Microcytic anemia and thrombocytopenia occur less often.

The Clinical Relevance of Anti-TSHR Antibodies

Currently, two different methods of assessing autoantibodies directed against the TSHR are used. The TSHR binding inhibitory immunoglobulin (TBII) assay detects antibodies that inhibit the binding of TSH to purified or recombinant TSHR. It thus measures both thyroid stimulating (TSAb) and thyroid blocking (TBAb) antibodies that target the receptor. During the entire pregnancy of patients with GD, circulating anti-TSHR-autoantibodies can pass to the baby and cause either neonatal autoimmune thyrotoxicosis (functionally stimulating autoantibodies) or hypothyroidism (blocking autoantibodies). The second method is a cell-based reporter bioassay that can distinguish between TSHR-stimulating, -neutral (binding), and -blocking autoantibodies through their effect on cyclic adenosine monophosphate (cAMP) production in a cell line stably transfected with the receptor [27, 37–39]. The levels of TSAb closely correlate with activity and severity of TED [33], and in approximately 50 % of the cases also are of prognostic value regarding the course of the disease [40].

The commercially available TBII tests that are used to measure the binding of sera to TSHR display high sensitivity and specificity for TSHR autoantibodies, but unfortunately do not measure the functional activity of immunoglobulins and do not distinguish between stimulatory, blocking, and neutral activity [35]. In contrast, anti-TSHR bioassays offer the following advantages: (1) the biological activity of specific immunoglobulins is directly assessed on a fully functional TSHR holoreceptor expressed on intact live cells, a platform that is easily adaptable and tailored to detect antibodies of specific function; (2) the bioassay measures the specific function of autoantibody that highly correlates with Graves' activity; (3) the monitoring of TSAb levels and TSAb titers add another dimension to the assessment of TED severity in individual patients.

Differential Diagnosis

Diagnosis of GD is straightforward in a patient with biochemically confirmed thyrotoxicosis, diffuse goiter on palpation, associated TED, positive TSHR antibodies, and often a personal or family history of autoimmune disorders [1, 2]. For patients with thyrotoxicosis who lack these features, the most reliable diagnostic methods are ultrasound evaluation [36] of the neck looking for a hypervascular gland and/or a radionuclide scan of the thyroid, which will distinguish the diffuse, high uptake of Graves' disease from nodular thyroid disease, destructive thyroiditis, ectopic thyroid tissue, and factitious thyrotoxicosis. In secondary hyperthyroidism due to a TSH-secreting pituitary tumor, there is also a diffuse goiter. The presence of a non-suppressed TSH level and the finding of a pituitary tumor on CT or magnetic resonance imaging (MRI) scan readily identify such patients [20]. While MRI is helpful in the differential diagnosis of proptosis, though computed tomography (CT) of the orbits remains the mainstay of radiographic imaging in the evaluation of patients with known TED for assessment of orbital tissue expansion and bony anatomy in preparation for surgical intervention [41]. Clinical features of thyrotoxicosis can mimic certain aspects of other disorders including panic attacks, mania, pheochromocytoma, and the weight loss associated with malignancy. The diagnosis of thyrotoxicosis can be easily excluded if the TSH level is normal. A normal TSH also excludes GD as a cause of diffuse goiter.

Clinical Course of Graves' Disease

Clinical features generally worsen without treatment; mortality was 10–30 % before the introduction of satisfactory therapy. Some patients with mild GD experience spontaneous relapses and remissions. Rarely, there may be fluctuation between hypo- and hyperthyroidism due to changes in the functional activity of TSHR antibodies. About 15 % of patients who enter remission after conservative treatment develop hypothyroidism 10–15 years later as a result of the destructive autoimmune process. The clinical course of TED does not follow that of the thyroid disease. TED typically worsens over the initial 3–6 months, followed by a plateau phase over the next 12–18 months, with spontaneous improvement, particularly in the soft tissue changes. However, the course is more fulminant in up to 5 % of patients, requiring intervention in the acute phase if there is optic nerve compression or corneal ulceration. Diplopia may appear late in the disease due to fibrosis of the extraocular muscles. Radioiodine (RAI) treatment for hyperthyroidism worsens the eye disease [42] in approximately 15–20 % of patients (foremost smokers). Antithyroid drugs and/or surgery have no adverse effects on the clinical course of TED [43]. Dermopathy, when it occurs, usually appears 1–2 years after the development of Graves' hyperthyroidism; it may improve spontaneously.

Management of Graves' Disease

The hyperthyroidism of GD is treated by reducing thyroid hormone synthesis, using antithyroid drugs (anti-TDs), or by reducing the amount of thyroid tissue with RAI treatment or near-total thyroidectomy [44–46]. Anti-TDs are the predominant therapy in many centers in Europe and Japan, whereas RAI is more often the first line of treatment in North America [47]. These differences reflect the fact that no single approach is optimal and that patients may require multiple treatments to achieve remission. The main anti-TDs are the thionamides, such as propylthiouracil (PTU), carbimazole, and the active metabolite of the latter, methimazole (MZ). Carbimazole is not an active substance; it has to be decarboxylated to MZ in the liver. Thionamides are the most widely used anti-TD [48]. They inhibit the coupling of iodothyronines and hence the biosynthesis of thyroid hormones. All inhibit the function of thyro-peroxidase, reducing oxidation and organification of iodide (Table 1.3). Anti-TDs are indicated as a first-line treatment of GD, particularly in younger subjects, and for short-term treatment of GD before RAI therapy or thyroidectomy [49]. Anti-TDs also reduce thyroid antibody levels, and they appear to enhance rates of remission. PTU inhibits deiodination of T4:T3 [50]. However, this effect is of minor benefit, except in the most severe thyrotoxicosis, and is offset by the much shorter half-life of this drug compared to MZ (Table 1.4). There are many variations of anti-TD regimens. The initial dose

Table 1.3 Mechanism of action of antithyroid drugs

- Intrathyroidal inhibition of:
  - Iodine oxidation/organification
  - Iodotyrosine coupling
  - Thyroglobulin biosynthesis
  - Follicular cell growth
- Extrathyroidal inhibition of T4/T3 conversion (Propylthiouracil)

Table 1.4 Pharmacology and pharmacokinetics of antithyroid drugs

	Methimazole	Propylthiouracil
Absorption	Rapid	Rapid
Bioavailability (%)	~100	~100
Peak serum level (min)	60–120	60
Serum half-life	6–8 h	90 min
Thyroidal concentration	5×10^{-5} mol/L	Unknown
Thyroidal turnover	Slow	Moderate
Duration of action (h)	>24	8–12
Serum protein binding	Nil	>75
Crosses placenta	++	+
Levels in breast milk	++	+
Volume of distribution (L)	40	20
Extraction	Renal	Renal
Metabolism during illness		
Renal	Nil	Nil
Liver	Prolonged	Nil
Potency	10–50	1
Normalization T3/T4	6	12 weeks
Adverse events (AE, %)	15	20
Agranulocytosis (%)	0.6	1.8
Cross-reaction of AE (%)	13.8	15.2
Compliance	High	Fair
Costs	Low	Moderate

of MZ is usually 10–15 mg every 12 h, but once-daily dosing is possible after euthyroidism is restored. PTU is given at a dose of 100–200 mg every 6–8 h, and divided doses are usually given throughout the course. Lower doses of each drug may suffice in areas of low iodine intake. The starting dose of anti-TD drugs can be gradually reduced (titration regimen) as thyrotoxicosis improves. Alternatively, high doses may be given combined with levothyroxine supplementation (block and replace regimen) to avoid drug-induced hypothyroidism. Initial reports suggesting superior remission rates with the block-replace regimen have not been reproduced in several other trials [44, 47]. The titration regimen is often preferred to minimize the dose of anti-TD and provide an index of treatment response. Thyroid function tests and clinical manifestations are reviewed 3–4 weeks after starting treatment, and the dose is titrated based on free T4 levels. Most patients do not achieve euthyroidism until 6–8 weeks after treatment is initiated. TSH levels often remain suppressed for several months and therefore do not provide a sensitive index of treatment response. The usual daily maintenance doses of anti-TD in the titration regimen are 2.5–10 mg of MZ and 50–100 mg of PTU.

Maximum remission rates (up to 50 % in some populations) are achieved by 18–24 months. Relapse is most likely within the first 6 months after anti-TD withdrawal but may occur years later. For unclear reasons, remission rates appear to vary in different geographic regions. Patients with severe hyperthyroidism and large goiters are most likely to relapse when treatment stops, but outcome is difficult to predict. All patients should be followed closely for relapse during the first year after treatment and at least annually thereafter [44–47].

The common side effects of anti-TDs (Table 1.5) are rash, urticaria, fever, and arthralgia (1–5 % of patients). These may resolve spontaneously or after substituting an alternative anti-TD [48]. Rare but major side effects include hepatitis, an SLE-like syndrome, and, most importantly, agranulocytosis (i.e., neutrophil count <500/mL), which occurs in 0.1–0.5 % of patients, and which can be treated by granulocyte colony stimulation factor. PTU-associated hepatotoxicity may cause liver failure and death, foremost in children. PTU should therefore be avoided in pediatric patients unless the patient is intolerant of MZ and no other treatment options are available. MZ can also induce hepatotoxicity, but the effects are usually milder, limited to cholestasis [52]. It is essential that anti-TDs are stopped and not restarted if a patient develops major side effects. Patients should be given written instructions regarding the symptoms of possible agranulocytosis (e.g., sore throat, fever, mouth ulcers) and the need to stop treatment pending a complete blood count to confirm that agranulocytosis is not present. The use of routine hematological and liver function tests is not useful. Most physicians do not prospectively monitor blood counts, as the onset of agranulocytosis is abrupt [48, 49].

Table 1.5 Adverse events of antithyroid drugs

Common (1–5 %)
• Skin rash
• Urticaria
• Arthralgia
• Fever
• Transient mild leukopenia
Rare (0.2–0.5 %)
• Gastrointestinal
• Abnormalities of taste and smell
• Agranulocytosis
Very rare
• Aplastic anemia (Propylthiouracil, PTU)
• Thrombocytopenia (PTU)
• Vasculitis, Lupus-like (PTU)
• Hepatitis (PTU)
• Hypoglycemia (anti-insulin Abs), PTU
• Cholestatic jaundice (Methimazole)

Propranolol (20–40 mg every 6 h) or longer acting beta blockers, such as atenolol, may be useful to control adrenergic symptoms such as palpitations and tremor, especially in the early stages before anti-TDs take effect. High doses of propranolol (40 mg four times daily) also contribute to inhibit peripheral conversion of T4 to T3. Anticoagulation with warfarin should be considered in all patients with atrial fibrillation. If digoxin is used, increased doses are often needed in the thyrotoxic state [44–47].

Pregnancy, Postpartum Period, and Childhood. Both MZ and PTU may be used during pregnancy and lactation although they both cross the placenta [51]. Many studies at term showed no difference between the two drugs in suppressing fetal thyroid function [52]. However, current guidelines recommend PTU during the first trimester then a switch to MZ for the remaining pregnancy [44]. The drug chosen should be given at the lowest possible dose (but not higher than 10–15 mg MZ or 100–150 mg PTU daily) to maintain maternal-free T4 and free T3 in the high normal range. In general, this will ensure euthyroidism in the fetus since free T4 levels in mother serum are correlated with free T4 levels, as assessed in cord blood. Furthermore, low doses of thionamides (up to 15 mg MZ or 150 mg PTU), given daily to the hyperthyroid mother during breast-feeding do not affect thyroid function in the infant. The titration regimen of anti-TD should be used to manage GD in pregnancy, as blocking doses of these drugs produce fetal hypothyroidism. PTU is usually used because of relatively low transplacental transfer and its ability to block T4:T3 conversion. Also, MZ has been associated with rare cases of fetal aplasia cutis. The lowest effective dose of PTU should be given, and it is often possible to stop treatment in the last trimester since TSH-R antibodies tend to decline in pregnancy. Nonetheless, the transplacental transfer of these antibodies rarely causes fetal thyrotoxicosis or neonatal thyrotoxicosis. Poor intrauterine growth, a fetal heart rate of 160 beats/min, and high levels of maternal TSH-R antibodies should suggest this complication. Anti-TD given to the mother can be used to treat the fetus and may be needed for 1–3 months after delivery, until the maternal antibodies disappear from the baby's circulation. The postpartum period is a time of major risk for relapse of GD. Breast-feeding is safe with low doses of anti-TD.

GD in children is best managed with anti-TD (MZ), often given as a prolonged course of the titration regimen [53]. Due to the reported PTU-induced liver failure in children [54], this compound is now avoided in the medical management of hyperthyroid children with GD. Surgery may be indicated for severe disease. RAI can also be used in children, though most experts defer this treatment until adolescence or later.

Alternative antithyroid drugs: Potassium perchlorate is rarely utilized as the sole antithyroid agent, but its use in combination with MZ may improve the outcome of therapy in iodine-induced thyrotoxicosis. The dose is 0.5–1 g daily for less than 30 days. Prolonged use may cause adverse effects (renal failure, gastrointestinal symptoms, etc.). Lithium carbonate inhibits thyroidal secretion of T4 and T3 and is especially helpful in severe thyrotoxicosis. It is not a first-line therapy and its adverse effects (nausea, vomiting, and arrhythmias) are largely dependent on serum lithium concentration [44, 47].

RAI causes progressive destruction of thyroid cells and can be used as initial treatment or for relapses after a trial of anti-TD [44–47]. There is a small risk of thyrotoxic crisis after RAI, which can be avoided by pretreatment with anti-TD for at least a month before RAI. Antecedent treatment with anti-TD should be considered in all elderly patients, or in those with cardiac problems, to deplete thyroid hormone stores before administration of RAI. Anti-TD must be stopped 3–5 days before RAI administration to achieve optimum iodine uptake. Certain radiation safety precautions are necessary in the first few days after RAI treatment, but the exact guidelines vary depending on local protocols. In general, patients need to avoid close, prolonged contact with children and pregnant women for several days because of possible transmission of residual isotope and excessive exposure to radiation emanating from the gland. Rarely there may be mild pain due to radiation thyroiditis 1–2 weeks after treatment. Hyperthyroidism can persist for 2–3 months before RAI takes full effect. For this reason, adrenergic blockers or anti-TDs can be used to control symptoms during this interval. Persistent hyperthyroidism can be treated with a second dose of RAI, usually 6 months after the first dose. The risk of hypothyroidism after RAI depends on the dosage but is at least 10–20 % in the first year and 5 % per year thereafter. Patients should be informed of this possibility before treatment and require close follow-up during the first year and annual thyroid function testing thereafter.

Pregnancy and breast-feeding are absolute contraindications to RAI treatment, but patients can conceive safely 6–12 months after treatment. The presence of TED requires caution, and American guidelines [44] advocate the use of prednisone, 40 mg/day, at the time of RAI treatment, tapered over 2–3 months to prevent exacerbation of TED [44–46]. The overall risk of cancer after RAI treatment in adults is not increased, but many physicians avoid RAI in children and adolescents because of the theoretical risks of malignancy.

Thyroidectomy is an option for patients who relapse after anti-TD and prefer this treatment to RAI [44–47]. Some experts recommend surgery in young individuals, particularly when the goiter is very large. Careful control of thyrotoxicosis with anti-TD, followed by potassium iodide orally is needed prior to surgery to avoid thyrotoxic crisis and to reduce the vascularity of the gland. The major complications of surgery (i.e., bleeding, laryngeal edema, hypoparathyroidism, and damage to the recurrent laryngeal nerves) are unusual when the procedure is performed by highly experienced surgeons. Recurrence rates in the best series are 2 %, but the rate of hypothyroidism is only slightly less than that following RAI treatment.

References

1. Brent GA. Clinical practice. Graves' disease. N Engl J Med. 2008;358(24):2594–605.
2. Vanderpump MP, Tunbridge WM, French GM. The incidence of thyroid disorders in the community; a twenty year follow-up. Clin Endocrinol. 1995;43:55–68.
3. Pearce SHS. Graves' disease. In: Weetman AP, editor. Autoimmune diseases in endocrinology. Humana: Totowa; 2008. p. 117–35.
4. Dittmar M, Libich C, Brenzel T, Kahaly GJ. Increased familial clustering of autoimmune thyroid diseases. Horm Metab Res. 2011;43:200–4.
5. Dultz G, Matheis N, Dittmar M, Bender K, Kahaly GJ. CTLA-4 CT60 polymorphism in thyroid and polyglandular autoimmunity. Horm Metab Res. 2009; 41(6):426–9.
6. Teufel A, Weinmann A, Kahaly GJ, Centner C, Piendl A, Wörns M, Lohse AW, Galle PR, Kanzler S. Concurrent autoimmune diseases in patients with autoimmune hepatitis. Clin Gastroenterol. 2010;44(3):208–13.
7. Boelaert K, Newby PR, Simmonds MJ, Holder RL, Carr-Smith JD, Heward JM, Manji N, Allahabadia A, Armitage M, Chatterjee KV, Lazarus JH, Pearce SH, Vaidya B, Gough SC, Franklyn JA. Prevalence and relative risk of other autoimmune diseases in subjects with autoimmune thyroid disease. Am J Med. 2010; 123(2):183.e1–9.
8. Vaidya B, Kendall-Taylor P, Pearce SHS. The genetics of autoimmune thyroid disease. J Clin Endocrinol Metab. 2002;87:5385–97.
9. Brix TH, Kyvik KO, Christensen K, Hegedus L. Evidence for a major role of heredity in Graves' disease: a population-based study of two Danish twin cohorts. J Clin Endocrinol Metab. 2001;86:930–4.
10. Holm IA, Manson JE, Michels KB, Alexander EK, Willet WC, Utiger RD. Smoking and other lifestyle factors and the risk of Graves' hyperthyroidism. Arch Intern Med. 2005;165:1606–11.
11. Weetman AP. Determinants of autoimmune thyroid disease. Nat Immunol. 2001;2:769–70.
12. Lazarus J, Marino M. Orbit-thyroid relationship. In: Wiersinga WM, Kahaly GJ, editors. Graves' orbitopathy—a multidisciplinary approach—questions and answers. 2nd revised ed. Basel: Karger; 2010. p. 26–32.
13. Kahaly GJ. The thyrocyte-fibrocyte link: closing the loop in the pathogenesis of Graves' disease? J Clin Endocrinol Metab. 2010;95(1):62–5.
14. Bahn RS. Graves' opthalmopathy. N Engl J Med. 2010;362(8):726–38.
15. Orgiazzi J, Ludgate M. Pathogenesis. In: Wiersinga WM, Kahaly GJ, editors. Graves' orbitopathy—a multidisciplinary approach—questions and answers. 2nd revised ed. Basel: Karger; 2010. p. 40–56.
16. Kahaly GJ, Shimony O, Gellman YN, Lytton SD, Eshkar-Sebban L, Rosenblum N, Refaeli E, Kassem S, Ilany J, Naor D. Regulatory T-cells in graves' orbitopathy: baseline findings and immunomodulation by anti-T lymphocyte globulin. J Clin Endocrinol Metab. 2011;96(2):422–9.
17. Bartalena L, Tanda ML. Clinical practice. Graves' ophthalmopathy. N Engl J Med. 2009;360(10):994–1001.
18. Boelaert K, Torlinska B, Holder RL, Franklyn JA. Older subjects with hyperthyroidism present with a paucity of symptoms and signs: a large cross-sectional study. J Clin Endocrinol Metab. 2010;95(6):2715–26.
19. Biondi B, Kahaly GJ. Cardiovascular involvement in patients with different causes of hyperthyroidism. Nat Rev Endocrinol. 2010;6(8):431–43.
20. Kahaly GJ. Imaging in thyroid-associated orbitopathy. Eur J Endocrinol. 2001;145(2):107–18.
21. Hales IB, Rundle FF. Ocular changes in Graves' disease. A long-term follow-up study. Q J Med. 1960;29: 113–26.
22. Ponto KA, Kahaly GJ. Quality of life in patients suffering from thyroid orbitopathy. Pediatr Endocrinol Rev. 2010;7 Suppl 2:245–9.
23. Werner SC. Modification of the classification of the eye changes in Graves' disease. Am J Ophthalmol. 1977;83(5):725–7.
24. Dickinson AJ. Clinical manifestation. In: Wiersinga WM, Kahaly GJ, editors. Graves' orbitopathy—a

multidisciplinary approach—questions and answers. 2nd revised ed. Basel: Karger; 2010. p. 1–25.
25. Bartalena L, Baldeschi L, Dickinson AJ, Eckstein A, Kendall-Taylor P, Marcocci C, Mourits MP, Perros P, Boboridis K, Boschi A, Currò N, Daumerie C, Kahaly GJ, Krassas G, Lane CM, Lazarus JH, Marinò M, Nardi M, Neoh C, Orgiazzi J, Pearce S, Pinchera A, Pitz S, Salvi M, Sivelli P, Stahl M, von Arx G, Wiersinga WM. Consensus statement of the European group on Graves' orbitopathy (EUGOGO) on management of Graves' orbitopathy. Thyroid. 2008;18(3):333–46.
26. Mourits MP, Koornneef L, Wiersinga WM, Prummel MF, Berghout A, van der Gaag R. Clinical criteria for the assessment of disease activity in Graves' ophthalmopathy: a novel approach. Br J Ophthalmol. 1989; 73(8):639–44.
27. Lytton SD, Ponto KA, Kanitz M, Matheis N, Kohn LD, Kahaly GJ. A novel thyroid stimulating immunoglobulin bioassay is a functional indicator of activity and severity of Graves' orbitopathy. J Clin Endocrinol Metab. 2010;95(5):2123–31.
28. Bartalena L, Martino E, Marcocci C, Bogazzi F, Panicucci M, Velluzzi F, Loviselli A, Pinchera A. More on smoking habits and Graves' ophthalmopathy. J Endocrinol Invest. 1989;12(10):733–7.
29. Bartalena L, Marcocci C, Tanda ML, Manetti L, Dell'Unto E, Bartolomei MP, Nardi M, Martino E, Pinchera A. Cigarette smoking and treatment outcomes in Graves' ophthalmopathy. Ann Intern Med. 1998;129(8):632–5.
30. Winsa B, Adami HO, Bergström R, Gamstedt A, Dahlberg PA, Adamson U, Jansson R, Karlsson A. Stressful life events and Graves' disease. Lancet. 1991;338(8781):1475–9.
31. Yoshiuchi K, Kumano H, Nomura S, Yoshimura H, Ito K, Kanaji Y, Kuboki T, Suematsu H. Psychosocial factors influencing the short-term outcome of antithyroid drug therapy in Graves' disease. Psychosom Med. 1998;60(5):592–6.
32. Fatourechi V, Bartley GB, Eghbali-Fatourechi GZ, Powell CC, Ahmed DD, Garrity JA. Graves' dermopathy and acropachy are markers of severe Graves' ophthalmopathy. Thyroid. 2003;13(12):1141–4.
33. Gerding MN, van der Meer JW, Broenink M, Bakker O, Wiersinga WM, Prummel MF. Association of thyrotrophin receptor antibodies with the clinical features of Graves' ophthalmopathy. Clin Endocrinol (Oxf). 2000;52(3):267–71.
34. Schwartz KM, Fatourechi V, Ahmed DD, Pond GR. Dermopathy of Graves' disease (pretibial myxedema): long-term outcome. J Clin Endocrinol Metab. 2002;87(2):438–46.
35. Grebe SK, Kahaly GJ. Laboratory testing in hyperthyroidism. Am J Med. 2012;125(9):S2.
36. Sipos JA, Kahaly GJ. Imaging of thyrotoxicosis. Am J Med. 2012;125(9):S1–2.
37. Lytton SD, Li Y, Olivo PD, Kohn LD, Kahaly GJ. Novel chimeric thyroid-stimulating hormone-receptor bioassay for thyroid-stimulating immunoglobulins. Clin Exp Immunol. 2010;162(3):438–46.
38. Kamijo K, Murayama H, Uzu T, Togashi K, Kahaly GJ. A novel bioreporter assay for thyrotropin receptor antibodies using a chimeric thyrotropin receptor (mc4) is more useful in differentiation of Graves' disease from painless thyroiditis than conventional thyrotropin-stimulating antibody assay using porcine thyroid cells. Thyroid. 2010;20(8):851–6.
39. Lytton SD, Kahaly GJ. Bioassays for TSH-receptor autoantibodies: an update. Autoimmun Rev. 2010;10(2): 116–22.
40. Eckstein AK, Plicht M, Lax H, Neuhäuser M, Mann K, Lederbogen S, Heckmann C, Esser J, Morgenthaler NG. Thyrotropin receptor autoantibodies are independent risk factors for Graves' ophthalmopathy and help to predict severity and outcome of the disease. J Clin Endocrinol Metab. 2006;91(9):3464–70.
41. Mourits MP. Diagnosis and differential diagnosis of graves' orbitopathy. In: Wiersinga WM, Kahaly GJ, editors. Graves' orbitopathy—a multidisciplinary approach—questions and answers. 2nd revised ed. Basel: Karger; 2010. p. 66–76.
42. Ponto KA, Zang S, Kahaly GJ. The tale of radioiodine and Graves' orbitopathy. Thyroid. 2010;20(7):785–93.
43. Marcocci C, Pinchera A. Thyroid treatment. In: Wiersinga WM, Kahaly GJ, editors. Graves' orbitopathy—a multidisciplinary approach—questions and answers. 2nd revised edition. Basel: Karger; 2010. p. 100–110.
44. Bahn RS, Burch HB, Cooper DS, Garber JR, Greenlee MC, Klein I, Laurberg P, McDougall IR, Montori VM, Rivkees SA, Ross DS, Sosa JA, Stan MN. Hyperthyroidism and other causes of thyrotoxicosis: management guidelines of the American Thyroid Association and American Association of Clinical Endocrinologists. Thyroid. 2011;21(6):593–646.
45. Kahaly GJ, Bartalena L, Hegedus L. The American Thyroid Association/American Association of Clinical Endocrinologists guidelines for hyperthyroidism and other causes of thyrotoxicosis: a European perspective. Thyroid. 2011;21(6):585–91.
46. Pearce EN, Hennessey JV, McDermott MT. New American Thyroid Association and American Association of Clinical Endocrinologists guidelines for thyrotoxicosis and other forms of hyperthyroidism: significant progress for the clinician and a guide to future research. Thyroid. 2011;21(6):573–6.
47. Bartalena L. Diagnosis and management of Graves' disease: a global overview. Nat Rev Endocrinol. 2013. doi:10.1038/nrendo.2013.193.
48. Cooper DS. Antithyroid drugs. N Engl J Med. 2005; 352(9):905–17.
49. Cooper DS. Antithyroid drugs in the management of patients with Graves' disease: an evidence-based approach to therapeutic controversies. J Clin Endocrinol Metab. 2003;88(8):3474–81.
50. Emiliano AB, Governale L, Parks M, Cooper DS. Shifts in propylthiouracil and methimazole prescribing practices: antithyroid drug use in the United States from 1991 to 2008. J Clin Endocrinol Metab. 2010;95(5):2227–33.

51. Stagnaro-Green A, Abalovich M, Alexander E, Azizi F, Mestman J, Negro R, Nixon A, Pearce EN, Soldin OP, Sullivan S, Wiersinga W, American Thyroid Association Taskforce on Thyroid Disease During Pregnancy and Postpartum. Guidelines of the American Thyroid Association for the diagnosis and management of thyroid disease during pregnancy and postpartum. Thyroid. 2011;21(10):1081–125.
52. Rivkees SA, Szarfman A. Dissimilar hepatotoxicity profiles of propylthiouracil and methimazole in children. J Clin Endocrinol Metab. 2010;95(7):3260–7.
53. Rivkees SA. Pediatric Graves' disease: controversies in management. Horm Res Paediatr. 2010;74(5):305–11.
54. Rivkees SA, Mattison DR. Ending propylthiouracil-induced liver failure in children. N Engl J Med. 2009;360(15):1574–5.

Natural History of Thyroid Eye Disease

2

Peter J. Dolman

Introduction

Thyroid eye disease (TED) is an autoimmune inflammatory disorder affecting orbital fat, extraocular muscles, and lacrimal gland, resulting in tissue expansion from glycosaminoglycan deposition and edema, and in some cases fibrosis from collagen production [1, 2].

Most individuals develop primarily fat expansion with eyelid retraction, proptosis, and ocular exposure (Fig. 2.1). In a third of affected individuals, more serious manifestations may result from significant extraocular muscle involvement, including periocular soft tissue erythema and edema, restricted ocular motility and double vision, and occasionally vision loss from compressive optic neuropathy, CON (Fig. 2.2) [3]. This spectrum of ocular findings is graded as "disease severity."

The more severe form of TED follows a biphasic course, with a progressive or active phase lasting up to 18 months, followed by a stable or inactive phase. The plot of orbital disease severity against time is called Rundle's curve (Fig. 2.3), and a steeper slope in the active phase reflects a more acute onset with the possibility of more serious sequelae [4–6]. During the early active phase, immunomodulators and radiotherapy may be offered with the hope of limiting the destructive consequences of the immune cascade [7, 8]. Once the disease has stabilized, surgery may be considered to improve orbital comfort, cosmesis, and function. Surgery is sometimes necessary during the active phase to prevent visual loss from CON or severe corneal exposure. The stages of the disease are graded as "clinical activity."

Although TED is self-limited, it may cause permanent cosmetic disfigurement and functional visual impairment, and has been shown to impact quality of life more than chronic lung disease or diabetes mellitus [9]. Understanding the natural history of this disease helps in earlier diagnosis, in identifying those at risk for serious disease consequences, and in choosing appropriate therapy.

Incidence, Epidemiology, and Relationship to Other Autoimmune Disorders

TED is the most common orbital disease in the Americas and Europe, with an annual incidence in females of approximately 14 per 100,000 and approximately one-fifth of that for males [10]. It occurs in all races and ages and is most prevalent between the second and sixth decades [11].

Portions of this chapter were previously published in: Dolman PJ, Evaluating Graves Orbitopathy. *Best Pract Res Clin Endocrinol Metab.* 2012 Jun;26(3):229–48 (Elsevier Limited).

P.J. Dolman, M.D., F.R.C.S.C. (✉)
Department of Ophthalmology, University of British Columbia, Vancouver, BC, Canada

Eye Care Centre, Section I, 2550 Willow Street, Vancouver, BC, Canada V5Z 3N9
e-mail: peterdolman@hotmail.com

R.S. Douglas et al. (eds.), *Thyroid Eye Disease*,
DOI 10.1007/978-1-4939-1746-4_2, © Springer Science+Business Media New York 2015

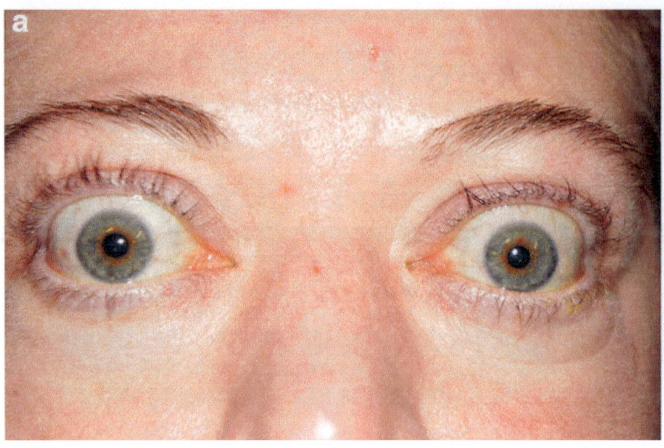

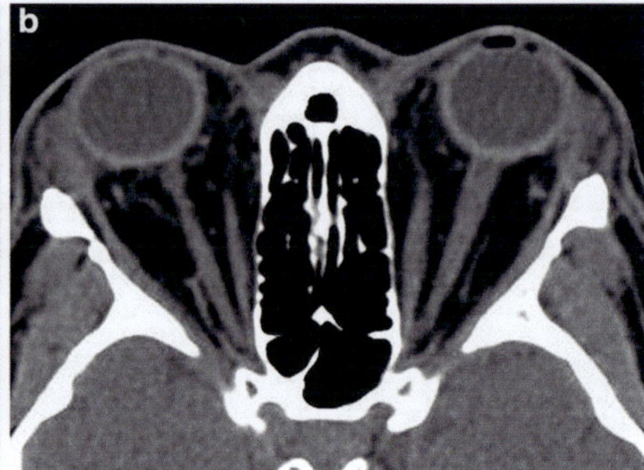

Fig. 2.1 (**a**) Young female with proptosis and bilateral upper lid retraction and lacrimal gland prolapse. (**b**) Axial computerized tomography (CT) scan of same patient showing marked proptosis from fat expansion but minimal muscle enlargement. Lacrimal glands are displaced beyond lateral rim

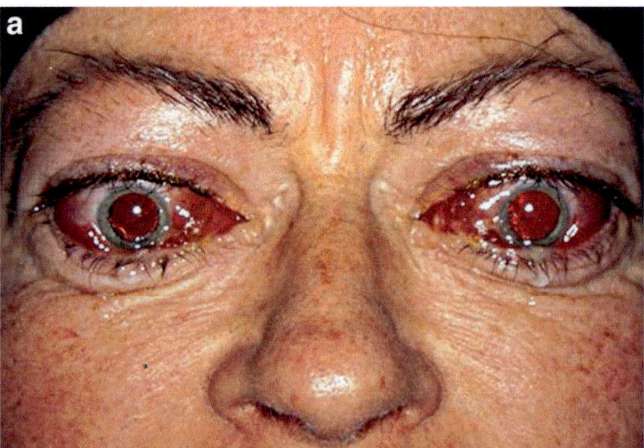

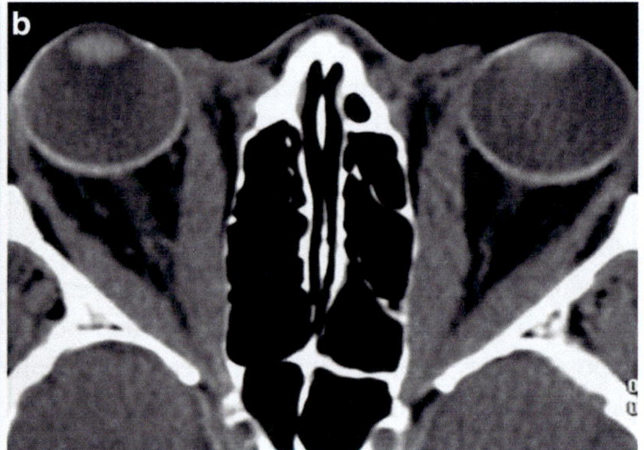

Fig. 2.2 (**a**) Older woman showing features of periorbital inflammation with restricted ocular movements and compressive optic neuropathy (CON). (**b**) Axial CT scan of same patient shows enlargement of muscles with proptosis and apical crowding

TED is strongly associated with autoimmune thyroid diseases such as Graves' disease (90 %) or Hashimoto's thyroiditis (3 %). Autoantibodies are believed to target common receptors such as TSH-R or IGF1-R within the thyroid gland, orbital fibroblasts, and skin [1, 10, 11]. Ninety percent of patients with orbitopathy have a current or past history of abnormal systemic thyroid hormone levels (usually hyperthyroid), while others may develop abnormal levels in the future. Between 25 and 50 % of patients with immune thyroid diseases develop orbital involvement, and of those, up to one third may develop more severe consequences as mentioned above [12–14]. Graves' dermopathy (pretibial myxedema) and acropachy/clubbing of fingers may occur in 5–10 % of patients [15].

Clinical Features

Appearance and Exposure Changes

Over 80 % of patients with TED develop upper eyelid retraction, often with an insidious onset that is first noticed by others [2]. The "thyroid stare" has a characteristic lateral flare that fluctuates with emotion or fixation giving the patient an angry look. It is associated with lid lag on downgaze, apparent spasmodic lid overaction on

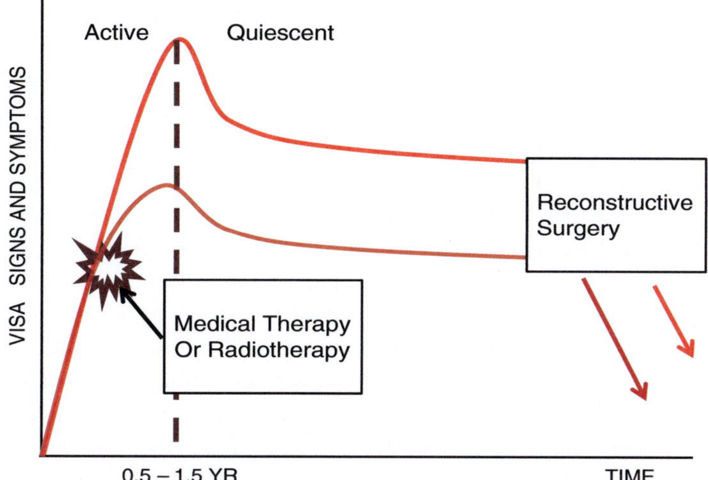

Fig. 2.3 Modified Rundle's curve shows biphasic course of thyroid eye disease. The active (inflammatory) phase is represented by progression in orbital symptoms and signs on the *Y* axis, typically lasting 0.5–1.5 years. This is followed by a stable phase, represented by a flattening of the curve. Immunosuppressive therapy (medication or radiotherapy) is offered during the active phase with the hope of reducing orbital sequellae, shown by a displacement of the upper untreated curve to the lower treated curve. Once the disease has stabilized, reconstructive therapy may be considered

upgaze, and incomplete lid closure while asleep (lagophthalmos). Proposed mechanisms include increased circulating catecholamines, overaction of the levator palpebrae superioris in conjunction with the superior rectus muscle to compensate for inferior rectus restriction, or inflammation with scarring of the levator muscle or aponeurosis [16].

Proptosis is the second most common finding in TED, resulting from expansion of the orbital fat and/or muscles. It may be less conspicuous in East Asians with tight eyelids limiting forward protrusion. Complete subluxation of the globe beyond the lids is a rare but troubling complication that may lead to visual loss if treatment is delayed. Prolapse of the orbital lacrimal gland may cause a tender fullness in the superotemporal orbital rim.

The lower lid margin typically rests at or slightly above the inferior limbus. Lower lid retraction is present when sclera is visible inferiorly and is associated with increasing proptosis.

Lid retraction is measured with a ruler from the pupillary light reflex to the lid margin and proptosis is measured with an exophthalmometer or from CT scan images.

The combination of lid retraction and proptosis increases corneal exposure and may lead to symptoms of irritation, grittiness, photophobia, secondary epiphora, and blurred vision. Signs of exposure are best assessed with the slit-lamp microscope and may include corneal epithelial erosions, frank abrasions or in severe cases, ulcerations and risk of perforation. The latter complications typically result from a combination of significant lagophthalmos and the absence of the normal protective Bell's phenomenon due to a tight inferior rectus muscle.

Periorbital Soft Tissue Inflammation and Congestion

Symptoms and signs of periorbital soft tissue inflammation or congestion include orbital ache at rest or with movement, conjunctival and caruncular injection and edema, eyelid redness and edema, and diurnal variation (worse with the head dependent after sleeping). Assessment is subjective although reliability can be improved using precise verbal descriptors or by reference to an atlas of standardized photographs [17].

Eyelid redness may be difficult to assess in darkly pigmented individuals, while lid edema may be confused with orbital fat prolapse. Orbital discomfort (at rest or with gaze) must be distinguished from ocular surface irritation, which is usually relieved by topical lubricants and anesthetics.

Various grading schemes have been described for each of these features: the simplest binary scale (present/absent) has good reproducibility, but is relatively insensitive at documenting change. Wider scoring systems may be more sensitive but have poorer concordance between observers.

These soft tissue changes may be an indicator of active inflammation but are also seen in patients with chronic congestion. Congestive features typically reflect significant involvement of orbital muscles, and thus should increase vigilance for more serious complications of the disease [2].

Restricted Ocular Motility and Strabismus

The extraocular muscles become clinically involved in only a third of patients with TED, more commonly in older individuals. Early evidence of involvement may include discomfort with ocular movement and injection over the muscle insertion sites [18]. During the active inflammatory phase, progressive restriction of motility develops, initially intermittent or in certain positions of gaze. Later in the course of disease, motility restriction may be related to secondary fibrosis.

The symptoms for strabismus are best graded using the Bahn-Gorman scale: 0 = no diplopia, I = intermittent diplopia (present with fatigue), II = inconstant diplopia (with vertical or horizontal gaze), III = constant diplopia in straight gaze, correctable with prisms, IV = constant diplopia, not correctable with prisms.

Ocular ductions can be graded from 0 to 45° in four directions using the Hirschberg principle: as the patient looks maximally in four cardinal positions, the observer points a bright light at the eyes and studies the light reflex on the surface of the eye. If the light reflex hits the edge of the pupil, the eye has rotated 15°, between the pupil edge and the limbus, 30° and at the limbus, 45°. This technique is as reliable as the "gold standard" Goldmann perimetry technique with a coefficient of reliability of 12° [19]. Strabismus can be measured objectively by prism alternate cover testing in different gaze directions.

A field of single binocular vision provides a plot of area where the patient sees single versus double because of ocular restriction. The patient keeps both eyes open and follows a specified light target on the Goldmann perimeter, indicating when the image splits into two.

Orbital CT imaging identifies which muscles are enlarged and with contrast may show increased enhancement in the fat surrounding effected muscles during the active phase [20]. In disease quiescent for many years, lucent zones are identified in the enlarged muscles, thought to be areas of hyaluronate deposition. T2-weighted MR scans may show enhancement of muscles thought to be due to edema during the active, inflammatory phase [21].

Compressive Optic Neuropathy

CON (also known as dysthyroid optic neuropathy, or DON, when relating specifically to TED) is a potentially reversible optic nerve dysfunction seen in 5–7 % of all cases of TED. Most cases are caused by direct compression of the nerve by swollen muscles in the narrow confines of the bony orbital apex, presumably impairing axoplasmic flow. In rare cases with severe fat expansion and axial proptosis, vision loss has been reported from optic nerve stretch [22].

Symptoms typically consist of desaturation of colors and blurring of central vision. This is usually confirmed on clinical examination, although a EUGOGO (European Group on Graves' Orbitopathy) survey of its members found that 20 % of patients with diagnosed CON had Snellen visual acuity better than 6/9 [23]. Color vision impairment is a particularly sensitive test for CON, best tested with HRR (Hardy Rand Rittler) pseudoisochromatic plates. An afferent pupillary defect is a specific sign of CON but is not detected in 50 % of patients because of symmetric loss of vision. Disc edema is also a specific sign when present, but is absent in over 40 % of patients with CON [23].

CON usually presents during the active phase of TED, since the onset of visual loss provokes the patient or clinician to investigate further. However, it may also develop insidiously, sometimes with little other clinical findings of TED. Most cases are associated with muscle enlargement, with resultant subjective diplopia and motility restriction. Congestive and inflammatory features are typically present, but may be subtle. Likewise, proptosis is not typically a striking finding associated with CON, and some argue that CON is associated with tight eyelids, limiting anterior decompression of the orbit. Patients who develop CON are more likely to be male, older, and diabetic compared with their non-CON counterparts.

Coronal CT scans demonstrate the enlarged extraocular muscles crowding the optic nerve at the orbital apex and causing effacement of the surrounding fat [24]. Ancillary tests include Humphrey visual field testing, which demonstrates paracentral scotomas or generalized reduction in sensitivity in 70 % of CON cases. Visually evoked potentials (VEP) show abnormal latency in 75 % of those with CON, but are not available in many centers [23].

In spite of these clinical findings and investigations, the diagnosis of CON may be uncertain in its early stages, necessitating close follow-up.

Grading Severity

Several classification systems have been devised to grade severity of these clinical manifestations.

Dr. Werner's "NO SPECS" classification, which clusters TED-related symptoms and signs roughly in order of presentation, provides a useful mnemonic for the different clinical features, and assigns a global severity score [25]. However, the grading system descriptors are imprecise and are often based on only one aspect of the domain, such as Snellen visual acuity for sight-threatening disease. Global ophthalmopathy scores also tend to bury the details about how the patient is specifically affected and provide insufficient information to document disease progression between visits. Finally, the NO SPECS classification does not assess clinical activity nor provide guidance for planning management.

The European Group on Graves' Orbitopathy (EUGOGO) grades TED from mild to very severe [26]. Mild disease has minimal eyelid swelling, lid retraction, or proptosis with little or no extraocular muscle dysfunction. Moderate to severe disease implies some form of active disease with or without ocular motility dysfunction with diplopia and inflammatory features interfering with the ability to function. It may also include significant proptosis >25 mm. In these cases, medical intervention might be considered. Very severe disease refers to sight-threatening conditions such as CON or corneal ulceration, often necessitating some form of surgical intervention. This classification separates the disease into management categories, but the moderate category is a heterogeneous group comprising individuals with soft tissue changes, motility disruption, or severe proptosis. Finally, there is an implied rank order for severity that may disagree with the patient's perception of their disease. For example, an individual with early CON might not even be aware of their color desaturation or mild central vision loss but would be categorized as severe, while another individual with marked restriction of ocular movement and bothersome diplopia would be rated as only moderately affected [2].

Clinical Activity

Rundle's Curve

Evaluating severity of orbital changes provides a snapshot of TED on a particular visit, but equally important are measures of how the disease is progressing over time, reflecting where it lies on Rundle's curve.

In cases with primarily fat expansion, the disease onset may be gradual and distinguishing active from quiescent phases may be difficult;

however, these cases often present in a stable phase when surgery can be offered on a non-urgent basis. Cases with muscle involvement tend to have a more obvious progression through the active and stable phases. The more acute the onset and rapid the deterioration in clinical findings, the greater the chance that more serious damage may occur, and consequently the greater the urgency for intervention. Inflammatory and congestive periocular changes are commonly noted during this progressive phase and can alert the clinician to disease activity.

Disease Duration and Progression

Individuals developing TED are keen observers of their condition and in more aggressive presentations can specify the date of symptom onset and whether their symptoms have been progressive (better or worse) or have stabilized. They can also report whether deterioration has been rapid or more indolent (the steepness of the slope of Rundle's curve), helping define the urgency of intervention. In general, immunosuppressive medical therapy and radiotherapy are likely to be most effective early in TED and when the disease is progressive, and a thorough history can identify such cases even on the first encounter.

Careful documentation of ophthalmic signs on each visit allows the clinician to determine onset and progression objectively. An observed change can only be considered significant if it is greater than the known coefficient of reliability for the measurement [21].

Clinical Activity Score

The Clinical Activity Score (CAS) was introduced in 1989 to help identify active TED patients who are likely to respond to immunosuppressive therapy [27]. It uses a binary scale with a single point given for seven periocular soft tissue inflammatory symptoms and signs as surrogate markers of disease activity. On follow-up visits, additional points are given for increased proptosis (2 mm or more), decreased ocular motility (8° or more), or decreased visual acuity over the previous 3 months. A total CAS score of 4 or higher has been shown to have an 80 % positive predictive value and a 64 % negative predictive value in predicting response to corticosteroid therapy.

Although the scale was devised to identify active disease, it increasingly is being used as a primary outcome in research on TED therapy, which may be inappropriate. First, the score value has not been shown to correlate with risk of developing significant complications such as TED-related strabismus or CON. Second, each clinical feature carries equal weight; for example, development of optic neuropathy carries no more impact than conjunctival redness. Third, each variable is scored in binary fashion, so positive or negative changes are documented only when they appear or resolve.

While these inflammatory periocular soft tissue changes may reflect underlying TED activity, the clinician should recognize that patients with low CAS scores may develop severe disease complications such as CON, and conversely, patients with high CAS scores may have long-standing congestive changes that are unresponsive to any immunotherapy, but that respond best to mechanical surgical decompression.

Laboratory and Imaging

Several potential markers for TED disease activity have been studied including urine and serum glycosaminoglycans (GAG) and serum thyrotropin (TSH) receptor antibodies [28]. Imaging techniques have attempted to assess vascularity around extraocular muscles with contrast CT scans, soft tissue edema on T2-weighted or STIR sequenced MRI scans, and inflammation using gallium or octreotide scintigraphy [29]. Facial thermography, PET scans, and Doppler ultrasonography have also recently been studied, but most of these ancillary tests seem less consistent than the clinical assessment tools described above.

Trial of Therapy

In some cases, determination of activity is uncertain based on borderline inflammatory changes and equivocal history of progression. A trial of therapy using a 3-day course of oral prednisolone 50 mg may determine whether clinical features show improvement, in which case more definitive therapy such as intravenous corticosteroids and/or radiotherapy might be considered.

VISA Classification

Overview

The VISA classification is a clinical recording form for office use that grades both clinical severity and activity based on both subjective and objective inputs. It separates the various clinical features of TED into four discrete parameters: V (vision threat, CON); I (inflammation, congestion); S (strabismus, motility restriction); A (appearance, exposure) [30].

The basic follow-up visit form (Table 2.1) is divided into four sections recording specific symptoms on the left and validated signs for each eye on the right. After each section is a progress row (better, same, worse) for both the patient's and clinician's impression of the overall change of that parameter since the last visit. The clinician determines progress on the basis of defined interval changes (i.e., 2 mm change in proptosis, 12° change in ocular ductions) rather than on global scores.

The layout is based on the natural order of the ocular examination and is intended to simplify data recording and possible later research data collation. Individual measurements may be omitted at the clinician's discretion.

The end of the form lists a summary grade for the severity and progress for each of the four disease parameters. The severity grades are used as a capsule summary for the patient but not for determining progression. Rather than grading TED severity based on a rank order of the four parameters, each feature is considered and graded independently.

Activity is determined on the basis of deterioration in any one of the four parameters. An elevated inflammatory score should raise concern that the extraocular muscles may be enlarged and that the disease may be active.

On the first visit, the date and rate of onset as well as historic progress of both the systemic and orbital symptoms are recorded, helping define characteristics of the disease activity. Additional questions also determine risk factors for more serious TED outcomes including smoking, family history, and diabetes. A 3-question Likert scale quality of life scale (TED-QOL) can be included as part of the form [31]. A downloadable first visit form (two pages) and follow-up form (one page) is available through the ITEDS website: www.thyroideyedisease.org.

Specific VISA Sections

V: Vision/CON

The focus of this section is to identify the presence of CON, with space provided for recording all relevant clinical features. As a summary grade, VISA lists CON as present or absent since therapy is usually offered if the condition is suspected. The severity and its response to therapy are reflected in the individual measurements for central and color vision as well as findings on visual fields, VEP, and imaging studies.

I: Inflammation/Congestion

VISA records features of orbital soft tissue inflammation or congestion as a separate parameter which can be graded and followed for progression. Symptoms include orbital ache at rest or with movement and diurnal variation while signs include injection and edema of the ocular surface or eyelid. These are summed to form a VISA Inflammatory Score based on the worst score for either eye or eyelid. This differs from CAS by widening the grade for chemosis and lid edema from 0 to 2. Unlike CAS, evidence of activity is based on a documented deterioration of the inflammatory score rather than an absolute value.

Table 2.1 VISA classification follow-up form

VISA FOLLOW-UP FORM
Date: Visit #:

Patient Label:

Date of birth: Age:
Gender:

ORBITOPATHY
Symptoms:

Progress:

Therapy:

THYROID
Symptoms:

Status:

Therapy:

GENERAL
Smoking:

Meds:

QOL: ☹ - - - - - - - - - - ☺

SUBJECTIVE	OBJECTIVE	OD	OS	
VISION				**Refractions**
				Wearing ______ + ______ X ______
Vision: n / abn	Central vision: sc / cc / ph	20/___	20/___	______ + ______ X ______
	with manifest	20/___	20/___	Manifest ______ + ______ X ______
				______ + ______ X ______
Color vis: n / abn	Color vision plates (HRR) / 14			
	Pupils (afferent defect)	y / n	y / n	
	Optic nerve: Edema	y / n	y / n	
	Pallor	y / n	y / n	
Progress: s / b / w	Macular/ lens pathology	y / n	y / n	
INFLAMM^N/ CONGESTION				**Inflammatory Index (worst eye/eyelid)**
	Caruncular edema (0-1)			Caruncular edema (0-1):
Retrobulbar ache	Chemosis (0-2)			Chemosis (0-2):
At rest (0-1)	Conjunctival redness (0-1)			Conj redness (0-1):
With gaze (0-1)	Lid redness (0-1)			Lid redness (0-1):
Lid swelling: y / n	Lid edema Upper (0-2)			Lid edema (0-2):
Diurnal variation: (0-1)	Lower (0-2)			Retrobulbar ache (0-2):
				Diurnal Variation (0-1):
Progress: s / b / w				**Total**: (10):
STRABISMUS/ MOTILITY				Prism Measure:
Diplopia:	Ductions (degrees):	+	+	↑
None (0)				
With gaze (1)				← →
Intermittent (2)				
Constant (3)	Restriction > 45°	0	0	
Head turn/ tilt: y / n	30-45°	1	1	↓
	15-30°	2	2	
Progress: s / b / w	< 15°	3	3	
APPEARANCE/EXPOSURE				Fat prolapse and eyelid position:
Lid stare y / n	Upper lid position: MRD	mm	mm	
	Scleral show (upper)	mm	mm	
	(lower)	mm	mm	
	Levator function	mm	mm	
Light sensitivity y / n	Lagophthalmos	mm	mm	
Bulging eyes y / n	Exophthalmometry (Base: mm)	mm	mm	
Tearing y / n	Corneal erosions	y / n	y / n	
Ocular irritation y / n	Corneal ulcers	y / n	y / n	
	IOP -straight	mmHg	mmHg	
Progress: s / b / w	-up	mmHg	mmHg	

DISEASE GRADE			Grade	Progress / Response	DISEASE ACTIVTY
V	(optic neuropathy)	y / n	/ 1	s / b / w	
I	(inflammation/congestion)	0-10	/ 10	s / b / w	Active
S	(diplopia)	0-3	/ 3	s / b / w	
	(restriction)	0-3	/ 3	s / b / w	Quiescent
A	(appearance/exposure):	normal - severe	/ 3	s / b / w	

MANAGEMENT **FOLLOW-UP INTERVAL:**

Downloadable from http://thyroideyedisease.org/downloads/

S: Strabismus/Motility Restriction

Three aspects are documented. Symptoms of diplopia are recorded using a modified Bahn-Gorman scale graded from 0 to 3. Ocular ductions are measured to the nearest 5° in four directions using the corneal light reflex technique; ocular restriction can be graded from 0 to 3 based on the range of ductions (0–15, 15–30, 30–45, >45°). Strabismus can be measured objectively by prism alternate cover testing in different gaze directions to plan surgical alignment.

A: Appearance/Exposure

This section records features relating to appearance and exposure. Photographs document appearance changes.

Risk Factors and Predictive Variables for Disease Severity

Because TED can present with a wide spectrum of orbital manifestations and activity levels, it would be useful to predict which patients are most likely to develop serious complications such as strabismus, corneal ulceration, or CON, so that these patients can be followed more closely and given preventive therapy as needed.

Risk factors for developing TED include smoking, life stressors, poorly controlled hypothyroidism following radioactive iodine, and a positive family history of orbitopathy [12, 13, 20]. Predictive variables for developing more serious consequences of TED include increasing age, male gender, smoking, and a rapid onset of orbitopathy [6]. Diabetics may have a higher risk of developing CON. Cigarette smoking correlates strongly with the development of TED and a progressively higher incidence of smoking is seen with more severe disease [32, 33].

Patients with TED are more likely to develop certain autoimmune diseases, including superior limbic keratitis (SLK), myasthenia gravis, diabetes mellitus, alopecia, and vitiligo [34].

Reactivation of disease is fairly uncommon, occurring in less than 5 % of individuals, and is sometimes associated with a major life stressor such as a family death, divorce, or loss of job [35].

The primary care physician or endocrinologist may be the first to make the diagnosis of TED, based primarily on clinical features and supported by imaging studies. In patients with a low-risk profile (non-smoking, younger females with slow onset of ocular changes), with milder clinical features, and with no history of recent progression, referral to an ophthalmologist is recommended on a non-urgent basis. Individuals undergoing radioactive iodine therapy for hyperthyroidism should be referred for ophthalmologic evaluation to help decide on prophylactic corticosteroid therapy. Individuals in a high-risk group (older, male, diabetic or smoker), with a recent history of progression, or with any moderate inflammatory changes, should be referred and seen by the ophthalmologist within a few weeks to consider therapy to avoid the onset of diplopia or CON. Patients with color or central visual loss, progressive diplopia, rapid deterioration in symptoms, or significant inflammatory scores should be seen within a few days. If corneal ulceration is suspected, patients should seen urgently by an ophthalmologist. In all cases, close communication between all involved physicians is essential.

References

1. Bahn RS. Graves' ophthalmopathy. N Engl J Med. 2010;362(8):726–38.
2. Dolman PJ. Evaluating graves orbitopathy. Best Pract Res Clin Endocrinol Metab. 2012;26(3):229–48.
3. Rootman J, Dolman PJ. Thyroid orbitopathy (Chapter 8). In: Diseases of the orbit. A multidisciplinary approach. Hagerstown: Lippincott Williams & Wilkins; 2003.
4. Rundle FF. Development and course of exophthalmos and ophthalmoplegia in Graves' disease with special reference to the effect of thyroidectomy. Clin Sci. 1945;5:177–94.
5. Rundle FF. Ocular changes in Graves' disease. QJM. 1960;29:113–26.
6. Dolman PJ, Rootman J. Predictors of disease severity in thyroid-related orbitopathy. (Chap 18) Orbital disease. Present status and future challenges. Boca Raton: Taylor and Francis; 2005
7. Cockerham KP, Mourits MP, McNab AA, et al. Does radiotherapy have a role in the management of thyroid orbitopathy? Debate. Br J Ophthalmol. 2002;86:102–4.

8. Kahaly G, Schrezenmeir J, Krause U, et al. Ciclosporin and prednisone vs prednisone in treatment of Graves' Ophthalmopathy: a controlled, randomized and prospective study. Eur J Clin Invest. 1986;16(5):415–22.
9. Gerding MN, Terwee CB, Dekker FW, et al. Quality of life in patients with Graves' Ophthalmopathy is markedly decreased: measurement by the medical outcomes study instrument. Thyroid. 1997;7(6):885–9.
10. Pritchard J, Horst N, Cruikshank W, et al. Igs from patients with Graves' disease induce the expression of T cell chemoattractants in their fibroblasts. J Immunol. 2002;168:942–50.
11. Pritchard J, Han R, Horst N, et al. Immunoglobulin activation of T cell chemoattractant expression in fibroblasts from patients with Graves' disease is mediated through the insulin-like growth factor 1 receptor pathway. J Immunol. 2003;170:6348–54.
12. Bartley GB. The epidemiologic characteristics and clinical course of ophthalmopathy associated with autoimmune thyroid disease in Olmsted County, Minnesota. Trans Am Ophthalmol Soc. 1994;92: 477–588.
13. Kendall-Taylor P, Perros P. Clinical presentation of thyroid associated orbitopathy. Thyroid. 1998;8: 427–8.
14. Perros P, Kendall-Taylor P. Natural history of thyroid eye disease. Thyroid. 1998;8:423–5.
15. Fatourechi V, Pajouhi M, Fransway AF. Dermopathy of Graves disease (pretibial myxedema). Review of 150 cases. Medicine (Baltimore). 1994;73(1):1–7.
16. Frueh BR, Musch DC, Garber FW. Lid retraction and levator aponeurosis defects in Graves' eye disease. Ophthalmic Surg. 1986;17:216–20.
17. Anderton LC, Neoh C, Walshaw D, Dickinson AJ. Reproducibility of clinical assessment in thyroid eye disease. In: Abstract of the European Society of Ophthalmic, Plastic and Reconstructive Surgery, Paris; 2000. p. 107.
18. Kendler DL, Lippa J, Rootman J. The initial clinical characteristics of Graves' orbitopathy vary with age and sex. Arch Ophthalmol. 1993;111:197–201.
19. Dolman PJ, Cahill K, Czyz CN, et al. Reliability of estimating ductions in thyroid eye disease: an International Thyroid Eye Disease Society Multicenter Study. Ophthalmology. 2012;119:382–9.
20. Regensburg NI, Wiersinga WM, Berendschot TT, et al. Densities of orbital fat and extraocular muscles in graves orbitopathy patients and controls. Ophthal Plast Reconstr Surg. 2011;27(4):236–40.
21. Polito E, Leccisotti A. MRI in Graves orbitopathy; recognition of enlarged muscles and prediction of steroid response. Ophthalmologica. 1995;209:182–6.
22. Kazim M, Trokel SL, Acaroglu G, Elliott A. Reversal of dysthyroid optic neuropathy following orbital fat decompression. Br J Ophthalmol. 2000;84(6):600–5.
23. McKeag D, Lane CM, Lazarus JH, et al. Clinical features of dysthyroid optic neuropathy: a European Group on Graves' Orbitopathy survey. Br J Ophthalmol. 2007;91:455–8.
24. Giaconi JA, Kazim M, Rho T, Pfaff C. CT scan evidence of dysthyroid optic neuropathy. Ophthal Plast Reconstr Surg. 2002;18(3):177–82.
25. Werner SC. Classification of the eye changes of Graves' disease. Am J Ophthalmol. 1969;68:646–8.
26. Boboridis K, Perros P. General management plan in Graves' orbitopathy: a multidisciplinary approach. Karger: Basel; 2007. p. 88–95.
27. Mourits MP, Prummel MF, Wiersinga WM, et al. Clinical activity score as a guide in the management of patients with Graves' Ophthalmopathy. Clin Endocrinol. 1997;47:9.
28. Martins JRM, Furlanetto RP, Oliveira LM, et al. Comparison of practical methods for urinary glycosaminoglycans and serum hyaluronan with clinical activity scores in patients with Graves' ophthalmopathy. Clin Endocrinol. 2004;60:726–33.
29. Gerding MN, van der Zant FM, et al. Octreotide-scintigraphy is a disease-activity parameter in Graves' ophthalmopathy. Clin Endocrinol. 1999;50:373–9.
30. Dolman PJ, Rootman J. VISA classification for Graves' orbitopathy. Ophthal Plast Reconstr Surg. 2006;22(5):319–24.
31. Fayers T, Dolman PJ. Validity and reliability of the TED-QOL: a new three-item questionnaire to assess quality of life in thyroid eye disease. Br J Ophthalmol. 2011;95:1670–4.
32. Prummel MF, Wiersinga WM. Smoking and risk of Graves' disease. JAMA. 1993;269:479–82.
33. Pfeilschifter J, Ziegler R. Smoking and endocrine ophthalmopathy: impact of smoking and current vs lifetime cigarette consumption. Clin Endocrinol (Oxf). 1996;45:477–81.
34. Cruz AA, Akaishi PM, Vargas MA, et al. Association between thyroid autoimmune dysfunction and non-thyroid autoimmune diseases. Ophthal Plast Reconstr Surg. 2007;23(2):104–8.
35. Selva D, Chen C, King G. Late reactivation of thyroid orbitopathy. Clin Exp Ophthalmol. 2004;32(1):46–50.

Emerging Role of Fibrocytes in the Pathogenesis of Thyroid Eye Disease

3

Terry J. Smith

Introduction

Graves' disease (GD) is among the most common autoimmune conditions affecting human beings with a prevalence of 1–3 % [1]. The cardinal features of GD include thyroid gland hypertrophy and hyperplasia. The underlying mechanism centers on generation of activating autoantibodies, known as thyroid stimulating immunoglobulins (TSI) that are directed against the thyrotropin (TSH) receptor (TSHR). This results in accelerated gland activity leading to thyroid hormone overproduction. This in turn leads to numerous metabolic consequences in peripheral tissues [1]. In addition to the pathological events confined to the thyroid, an autoimmunity-driven process, perhaps unrelated to derangements in thyroid function and known as thyroid-associated ophthalmopathy (thyroid eye disease, TED) manifests in orbital connectives tissues and those of the upper face [2]. Whether and how TSIs might play a direct role in the pathogenesis of TED remain topics of much investigation. Clinically important TED occurs in 25–50 % of individuals with GD. Periorbital edema, eyelid retraction, chemosis, and proptosis are among the signs found in TED. In extreme cases, vision may be threatened by compressive optic neuropathy or corneal ulceration, the latter constituting an ophthalmic emergency [2–4]. The disease profoundly affects quality of life by virtue of disfigurement and in the most severe cases loss of vision [5, 6]. TED may develop in individuals with no other signs of GD and without antecedent hyperthyroidism. Identity of factors underlying the variable presentation of GD and TED remain elusive. Typically, the disease runs a self-limited course with an active phase characterized by inflammation and tissue remodeling that lasts between 18 and 36 months [2]. This is followed by a stable phase where signs and symptoms remain static.

In this chapter recent findings are reviewed that link $CD34^+$ fibrocytes to the pathogenesis of GD. The potential role of fibrocytes in TED is emphasized. Fibrocytes are monocyte progenitor cells that derive from the bone marrow and participate in wound healing and tissue remodeling. We postulate that by virtue of their trafficking to the orbit, their expression of "thyroid-specific" proteins, production of cytokines, and their ability to present antigens, fibrocytes may direct the magnitude and quality of orbital immune reactivity in TED. Targeting these cells might prove an effective therapeutic strategy.

T.J. Smith, M.D. (✉)
Department of Ophthalmology and Visual Sciences, Kellogg Eye Center, University of Michigan, 1000 Wall St., Ann Arbor, MI 48105, USA

Internal Medicine, University of Michigan Medical School, Ann Arbor, MI, USA
e-mail: terrysmi@med.umich.edu

R.S. Douglas et al. (eds.), *Thyroid Eye Disease*,
DOI 10.1007/978-1-4939-1746-4_3, © Springer Science+Business Media New York 2015

Orbital Pathology Associated with TED

Since the first descriptions of GD nearly 200 years ago, the complex and dynamic relationship between thyroid centric GD and TED has puzzled physicians and scientists alike. Definitive elucidation of the relationship existing between thyroid and orbit remains unachieved. The histopathologic changes of TED include infiltration of connective tissues with mononuclear cells such as lymphocytes, macrophages, plasma cells, and rare mast cells [3]. In addition to cellular infiltrates, interstitial edema and accumulation of mucopolysaccharides, also known as glycosaminoglycans, such as hyaluronan in the extraocular muscles and orbital fat contributed to the expansion of tissues within the orbit [6]. This can culminate in tissue congestion and proptosis. The target antigen involved in the initial inflammatory response of TED remains uncertain. It has been postulated that this early response leads to fibroblast reactivity and provokes deposition of collagen, leaving fibrotic changes that limit the mechanical plasticity of the tissues involved.

The localized expression of thyroid antigens in the orbital space has been considered a potential explanation for the seemingly isolated involvement of the upper face and adjacent structure. Tao et al. first reported detection of thyroglobulin (Tg) in orbital tissues affected by TED [7]. Marino et al. more recently identified Tg within the orbit and in orbital fibroblasts from patients [8]. TSHR mRNA was initially detected in healthy and TED orbital tissues by Feliciello and colleagues [9]. Heufelder et al. [10] later detected TSHR mRNA in orbital fibroblasts, especially those from individuals with TED.

What Role Does TSHR Play in TED?

TSHR, a glycoprotein hormone receptor, is a member of the G protein-coupled receptor family [11]. It contains domains for ligand binding in the extracellular domain (ectodomain), one that spans the membrane bilayer (transmembrane), and an intracellular domain (endodomain). TSHR undergoes posttranslational intramolecular proteolytic cleavage, forming a two-subunit structure linked by a disulfide bond. This disulfide bond is prone to cleavage by matrix metalloprotease and protein disulfide isomerase, causing shedding of the A subunit, which exhibits immunoreactivity and is processed by antigen presenting cells. The generation of TSI results in activation of TSHR, unregulated thyroid hormone production, and development of goiter in GD.

Whether TSHR and TSI play a direct role in the development of TED remains uncertain, although strong circumstantial evidence supports their involvement [12]. After its initial cloning by Parmentier et al. [13], the receptor was characterized extensively and its pattern of expression was examined. Because of the close temporal relationship between the onset of thyroid dysfunction and development of TED, it was postulated that GD and TED might share a common autoantigen such as TSHR. TSHR is expressed widely in many tissues outside the thyroid, including the adrenal gland, skin, kidney, thymus, and several fat depots. Relevant to TED, TSHR can be detected in orbital fat/connective tissue, albeit at much lower levels than are found in thyroid epithelium [9]. Direct evidence that TSHR serves as intra-orbital autoantigen remains incomplete and no compelling demonstration of antigen-specific T cell infiltration in the orbit has been introduced.

Recent evidence has emerged suggesting that the IGF-1 receptor (IGF-1R) might play some role in TED [14]. IGF-1R is a tyrosine kinase receptor involved in proliferation and metabolic function of many cell types. It modulates apoptosis through the PI3K/AKT/FRAP/mTOR/p^{70s6k} pathway and is involved in thymic development and immune regulation through IGF-1R display on B and T cells. IGF-1R has been found to be overexpressed in several autoimmune diseases including Crohn's disease, pulmonary fibrosis, and multiple sclerosis [14].

Tramontano et al. first explored the individual and synergistic effects of IGF-1 and TSH on the growth of cloned rat thyroid follicular epithelium [15]. They demonstrated that IGF-1 and TSH each promoted DNA synthesis and cell proliferation. Further, IGF-1 seemed to enhance the effect of TSH on DNA synthesis with an effect the magnitude of which is greater than the sum of each. Substantial overlap between TSHR and IGF-1R downstream signaling was reported [16]. The receptors form a functional and physical complex and extensively utilize the Akt/FRAP/mTOR/P70^{s6k} pathway. Antibodies to either protein could pull down IGF-1Rβ and TSHR. Further, monoclonal antibodies used to block IGF-1R signaling also attenuated downstream signaling from TSHR [16, 17]. These studies suggest that IGF-1R transactivation could mediate at least some aspects of TSHR signaling.

Although TSHR is well established as the target autoantigen responsible for hyperthyroidism in GD, its role in TED remains uncertain. IGF-1R may also be involved. Weightman et al. demonstrated that IgG from patients with GD could displace ^{125}I-IGF-1 from the surface of human fibroblasts [18]. More recently IGF-1R has been shown to be expressed at a higher level by orbital fibroblasts in GD [19, 20]. Further, the frequency of IGF-1R^{+} orbital fibroblasts was three to four times higher in cultures from individuals with the disease. Both T and B cells from patients with GD also skewed towards the IGF-1R^{+} phenotype [21, 22] with CD8^{+}IGF-1R^{+} and CD4^{+}IGF-1R^{+} being extremely rare in the control population. The density of IGF-1R receptor on T cells, however, is similar in patients with GD and control lymphocytes. Similarly, the majority of T and B cells of unaffected monozygotic twins failed to exhibit a skewed IGF-1R^{+} phenotype [23]. Whether this cellular attribute represents an acquired characteristic is uncertain. Anti-IGF-1R antibodies were also detected in sera from patients with GD, whereas they were absent in controls [19, 20]. A subset of these antibodies appears to activate the IGF-1R pathway [19, 20, 24, 25] although the topic remains debated [26]. When treated with GD-IgG or IGF-1, TED orbital fibroblasts produced hyaluronan [27] and two powerful chemoattractants, IL-16 and RANTES, an induction which was mediated via the Akt/FRAP/mTOR/P70^{s6k} pathway [19]. Similar to fibroblasts, IGF-1R^{+} phenotype T cells have a growth advantage in vitro as display of IGF-1R may protect against Fas-mediated apoptosis [21].

Putative Importance of Fibroblast Heterogeneity in TED

When considering the underlying immunopathology associated with TED, one must first acknowledge the substantial limitations of our understanding. Much of what we don't know appears to be the consequence of the lack of robust animal models for the disease that recapitulate the ocular manifestations with high fidelity. Despite numerous attempts at replicating human TED in mouse models, important divergence between the phenotypes generated experimentally and human disease remains. Thus the vast majority of studies conducted to better understand the disease have been limited to those conducted in cultured orbital fibroblasts and immune-competent cells donated from individuals with GD and TED. Controls have traditionally come from healthy donors.

A striking characteristic of orbital fibroblasts, especially those from donors with TED, is the marked cellular heterogeneity in cultures [28, 29]. When orbital tissue explants are cultivated in plastic culture dishes, they exhibit multiple morphologies, including spindle-shaped cells and those with a fusiform appearance [30, 31]. Most are well arborized although the number of dendritic processes projecting from cell bodies varies. Others appear more angular. Among the first cell markers used to identify and distinguish between the various phenotypes was CD90 (also known as Thy-1). Earlier studies demonstrated that orbital fibroblasts, regardless of whether they derived from healthy tissues or those affected by TED are heterogeneous with regard to the surface display of Thy-1. When subjected to cytometric cell sorting, Thy-1^{+} and Thy-1^{-} cells respond differently to cytokines such as IL-1β and CD40 ligand. Levels of inflammation-related genes diverge in the two cell phenotypes.

Robust Responses of Orbital Fibroblasts to Specific Cytokines

Orbital fibroblasts express a distinctive set of proteins in response to pro-inflammatory cytokines. They display on their surfaces CD40, a member of the TNF-α receptor family [32]. Further, orbital fibroblasts from patients with TED displayed higher levels of CD40 than do those from healthy donors. CD40L induces the IL-6 gene. This cytokine in turn drives immunoglobulin synthesis and development of plasma cells. Hwang et al. reported a dramatic up-regulation of prostaglandin endoperoxide H synthase-2 (PGHS-2), the inflammatory cyclooxygenase, in orbital fibroblasts treated with CD40 ligand [33]. Leukoregulin and IL-1β also up-regulate PGHS-2 substantially in orbital fibroblasts [34, 35]. In each case, induction of PGHS-2 appears to be mediated by enhanced gene promoter activity and mRNA stability. It appears to be greater in orbital fibroblasts derived from those with TED than from healthy controls. The induction of the enzyme is coordinate with that of the microsomal PGE_2 synthase [32]. Further, the induction results in dramatically increased PGE_2 production. In addition to changing the morphology of orbital fibroblasts [31], PGE_2 influences B cell class-switching, T cell differentiation, and mast cell degranulation, all of which are intimately tied to the pathogenesis of TED.

Another cellular function greatly amplified by cytokines in orbital fibroblasts is the synthesis of high levels of hyaluronan and other abundant glycosaminoglycans. When exposed to leukoregulin, IFN-γ, CD40 ligand, or IL-1β, hyaluronan (HA) production is substantially up-regulated, a response mediated through the induction of UDP-glucose dehydrogenase and multiple members of the hyaluronan synthase family [36–38]. The rate of HA synthesis can be increased by approximately 15-fold over basal levels. Induction of these enzymes and HA synthesis can be attenuated substantially by glucocorticoids, actions which are mediated at the pre-translational level.

Details concerning the molecular basis for the divergent responses observed in orbital fibroblasts compared to those found in fibroblasts from other connective tissue depot have recently been brought to light. It would appear that the exaggerated responses in orbital fibroblasts may be due to differential profiles of IL-1 receptor antagonists (IL-1RA) [39]. These cytokines bind to IL-1 receptors and block the activities of IL-1α and IL-1β on the surface of target cells. Orbital fibroblasts, regardless of whether they derive from donors with TED, express extremely high levels of intracellular IL-1RA (icIL-1RA) but extremely low levels of secreted IL-1RA (sIL-1RA) when engaged by several inflammatory cytokines and TSH [39–41]. It is the latter form of the cytokine antagonist that appears to modulate the actions of IL-1α and IL-1β. This relative deficiency in sIL-1RA may underlie the exaggerated inductions in orbital fibroblasts such as the levels of PGHS-2.

Emergence of Fibrocytes as Potential Participants in TED

More recent studies have shed light on the potential involvement in TED of bone marrow-derived monocyte progenitor cells called fibrocytes. These cells resemble orbital fibroblasts under certain culture conditions (Fig. 3.1). They display the surface marker CD34 as well as the chemokine receptor CXCR4. These cells produce substantial levels of collagen 1. Fibrocytes were initially identified as important participants in wound healing and scar formation [42]. They exhibit a remarkable and characteristic repertoire of responses that result in terminal differentiation. For instance, when exposed to PPARγ activating ligands, fibrocytes differentiate into triglyceride bearing adipocytes. In contrast, when treated with TGF-β, they transition into a phenotype reminiscent of myofibroblasts. In that state, they express high levels of smooth muscle actin. The frequency of circulating $CD34^+$ fibrocytes is dramatically increased in a majority of patients with GD [43] (Fig. 3.2). The cells that they apparently differentiate into within the TED orbit, namely $CD34^+$ fibroblasts, can be identified in situ in orbital fat donated by patients with severe TED who are undergoing orbital decompression surgery. An interesting characteristic of fibrocytes, especially those coming from donors with GD is a

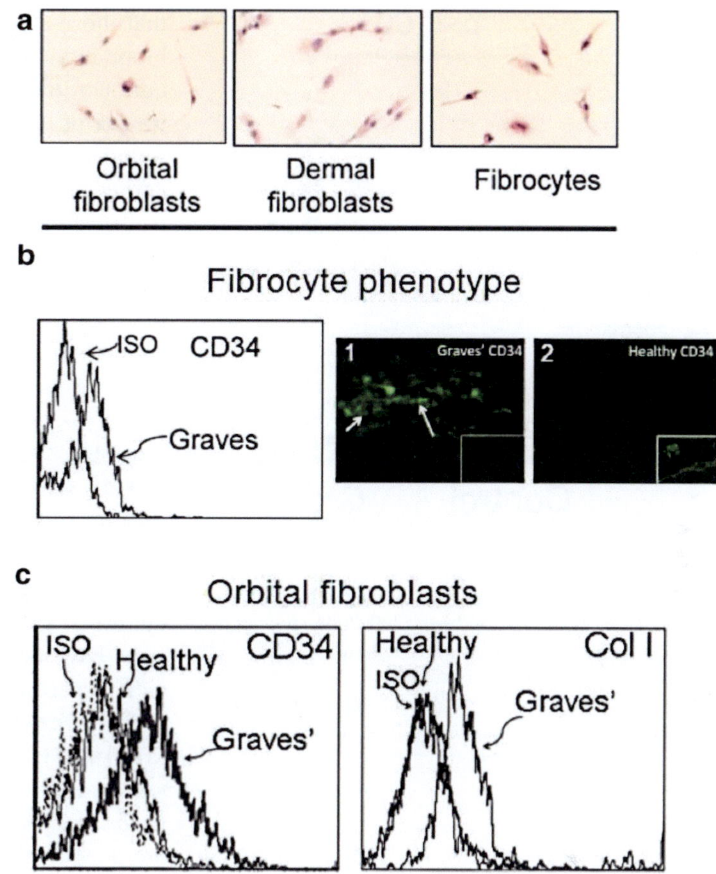

Fig. 3.1 (**a**) Similar spindle-shaped phenotypes among orbital fibroblasts, dermal fibroblasts, and fibrocytes (hematoxylin and eosin, ×20). (**b**) Fibrocytes from individuals with GD display cell surface receptor CD34. (1) Immunofloresence staining of CD34 in TAO-derived tissue (*inset* as negative control). (2) Absence of CD34 expression in healthy orbital tissue (*inset* as positive control). (**c**) Orbital fibroblasts from individuals with and without TAO display similar receptors as fibrocytes, as shown by flow cytometric analysis with anti-CD34 and anti-Col I antibodies. (Reprinted with permission; Douglas et al. Increased generation of fibrocytes in thyroid-associated ophthalmopathy, Copyright 2010. The Endocrine Society)

high level of TSHR expression. In fact, levels of TSHR on the surface of fibrocytes and the frequency of circulating TSHR$^+$ fibrocytes seem to be increased in GD [44]. The TSHR expressed by fibrocytes is functional in that when ligated either with TSH or TSI, the cells express extremely high levels of several proinflammatory cytokines, including IL-6, IL-8, TNFα, and IL-1β. Unlike orbital fibroblasts, fibrocytes exposed to TSH or TSI express relatively high levels of both sIL-1RA and icIL-1RA. Further, when CD34$^+$ orbital fibroblasts are segregated from CD34$^-$ cells, they express high levels of sIL-1RA.

The mechanism through which TSH and TSI up-regulate IL-6 production in fibrocytes has been at least partially solved recently. Raychaudhuri and colleagues [45] found that the induction of IL-6 is completely independent of adenylate cyclase activation or the generation of cAMP. In these cells, TSH activates PDK1, AKT/PKB and PKC pathways, and disruption of any of these pathways attenuates the induction of IL-6. Further, the isoenzyme, PKCβII is expressed and utilized in mediating the responses to TSH in fibrocytes. The study further compared the induction of IL-6 in fibrocytes with those occurring in orbital fibroblasts derived from patients with GD and TED. It would appear that as circulating fibrocytes transition to CD34$^+$ orbital fibroblasts, PKCβII expression and usage disappear and that PKCμ becomes expressed. Further, following the cellular transition, PKCμ signaling then becomes an indispensible component of the signaling to IL-6 expression. When TED-derived orbital fibroblasts which uniquely contain CD34$^+$ cells are isolated from their CD34$^-$ counterparts by flow cytometry-based cell sorting, expression of PKCμ is extinguished and PKCβII again becomes detectable and thus the profile of PKC isoenzymes reverts to that of the circulating fibrocyte.

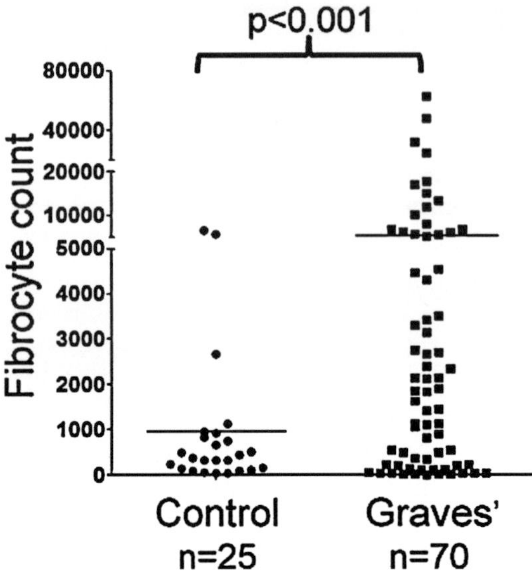

Fig. 3.2 Abundance of fibrocytes cultivated from PBMCs of individuals with GD (5,268 ± 1,260 fibrocytes per 10^6 PBMCs, $n=70$) and from healthy individuals (954 ± 329 fibrocytes per 10^6 PBMCs $n=25$) ($p<0.001$). (Reprinted with permission; Douglas et al. Increased generation of fibrocytes in thyroid-associated ophthalmopathy, Copyright 2010. The Endocrine Society)

IL-6 up-regulation following TSH treatment in fibrocytes and orbital fibroblasts results both from a coordinate activation of the IL-6 gene promoter and from enhanced IL-6 mRNA stability. Further, the transcriptional activity of the IL-6 gene can be traced to a CREB binding element extending from −213 to −208 nt, and to an NF-κB site extending from −78 to −62 nt. Thus TSHR signaling appears to involve a robust, cyclic AMP-independent set of pathways in non-thyroid epithelial cell types such as fibrocytes. Armed with these insights, it may be possible to interrogate multiple potentially attractive therapeutic targets for interrupting IL-6 expression in the context of GD and TED.

Fibrocytes Express Multiple "Thyroid-Specific Proteins"

Another interesting aspect of the CD34 fibrocyte is its expression of multiple "thyroid-specific" proteins. Fernando and colleagues [46] reported that those cultivated from circulating peripheral blood mononuclear cells express not only TSHR but also low levels of Tg mRNA. Levels of the transcript are considerably lower than those found in thyroid tissue. Tg resolved on polyacrylamide gel electrophoresis as a 305 kDa protein. Both ^{125}Iodine and ^{35}S methionine can be incorporated into Tg expressed by fibrocytes. siRNAs targeting Tg attenuated the synthesis of the protein. Tg gene promoter is active in fibrocytes. Compared with Tg levels found in fibrocytes, those in orbital fibroblasts from donors with GD were substantially lower. When GD-orbital fibroblasts were sorted into pure CD34$^+$ and CD34$^-$ populations, Tg mRNA expression segregated to CD34$^+$ fibroblasts. Tg expression is considerably greater in CD34$^+$ fibroblasts than in the mixed cell population found in parental cultures. Two additional thyroid-specific proteins have been detected in the protein expression repertoire of fibrocytes, namely sodium iodide symporter (NIS) and thyroid peroxidase (TPO) [47]. Levels of NIS and TPO mRNAs are substantially lower than those found in thyroid tissue and FRTL-5 cells in culture. However they are adequately abundant to result in translation into detectable protein. They are considerably higher than those detected in dermal fibroblasts or orbital fibroblasts from healthy individuals and those with TED. The expression of multiple autoantigens suggested that a specific transcription factor might be involved, namely the autoimmune regulator protein (AIRE) [44]. AIRE is a major determinant of intra-thymic education that allows the negative selection of autoreactive thymocytes. In fibrocytes, AIRE mRNA and protein are detectable but at extremely low levels compared to thymus. Interruption of AIRE expression using small interfering RNAs resulted in substantial reductions in the steady state mRNA levels of TSHR, Tg, TPO, and NIS (Fig. 3.3). Further, knocking down AIRE expression also reduced levels of PAX8 and TTF1, the two transcription factors closely associated with expression of these proteins in thyroid epithelium. To confirm the importance of AIRE in this specific context, fibrocytes cultivated from an individual with APS 1 syndrome were also

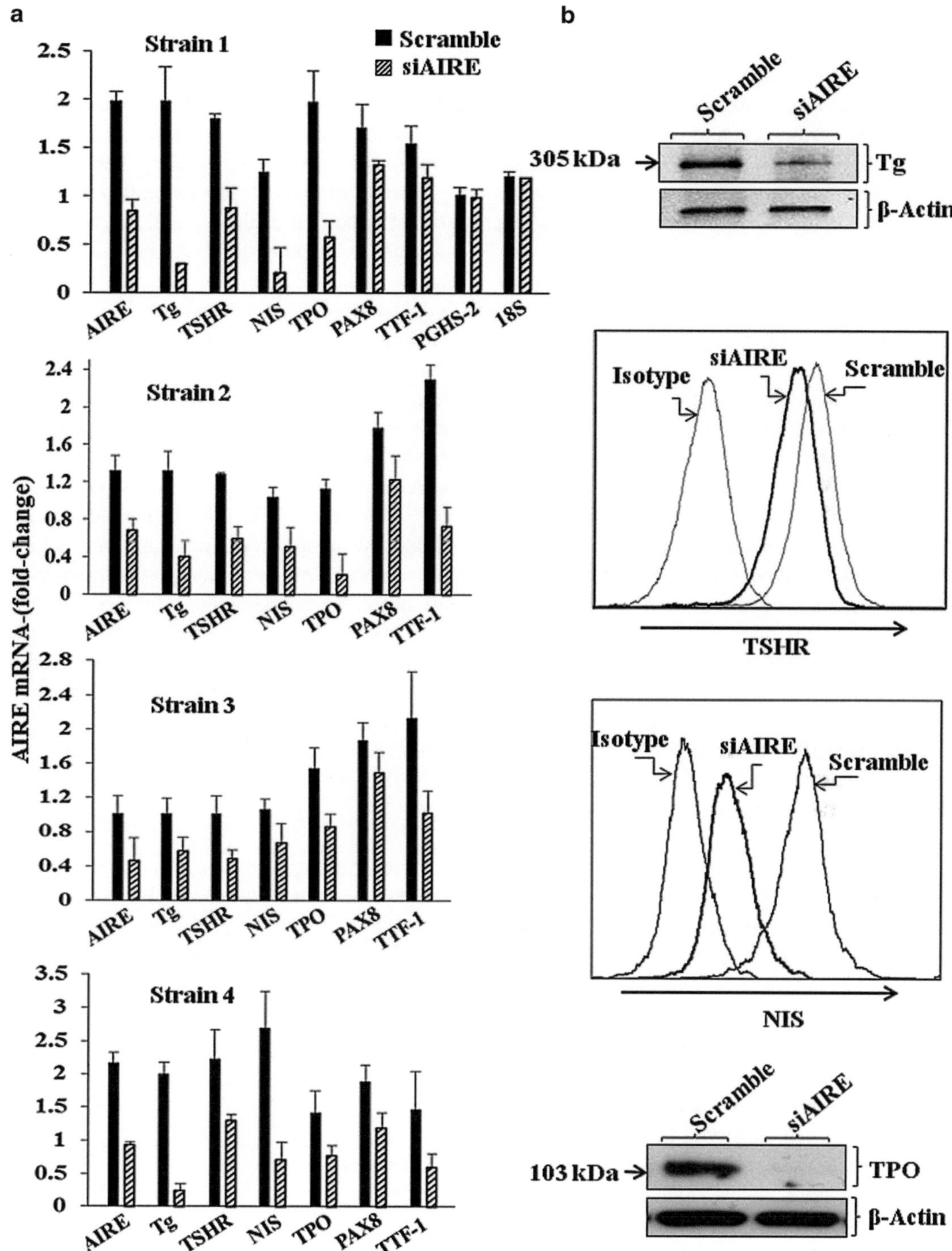

Fig. 3.3 Knocking down AIRE expression reduces Tg, TSHR, NIS, TPO, PAX8, and TTF-1 but not PGHS-2 or 18S RNA. (**a**) Fibrocytes from four different donors were treated with scrambled (control) siRNA or one targeting AIRE. Data are expressed as mean ± SD of three independent determinations. (**b**) Fibrocyte cultures were transfected with control siRNA or AIRE-targeting siRNA. Radiolabeled Tg, unlabeled TSHR, NIS, and TPO proteins were knocked-down by interrupting AIRE expression. (Reprinted with permission; Fernando et al. Copyright 2014. The Endocrine Society)

interrogated for levels of thyroid proteins and found to be significantly below those found in an unaffected first degree relative. AIRE expression in fibrocytes is the consequence of an active AIRE gene promoter and remarkably stable AIRE mRNA. The implications of these findings to the biology of fibrocytes and the tissues which they infiltrate include the suggestion that AIRE is an important component of extra thyroidal autoimmunity related to peripheral loss of tolerance to thyroid-associated proteins such as thyroglobulin, TPO, and TSHR. Further, they suggest that fibrocytes may be capable of synthesizing thyroid hormones or their derivatives. The array of self-antigens expressed by fibrocytes does not appear to be limited to those associated with autoimmune thyroid disease. Fernando et al. reported recently that IA-2 and ICA69 can also be detected in these cells, findings with implications for type 1 diabetes mellitus [48]. In addition to their expression of these proteins, fibrocytes express high levels of MHC Class II and can present antigens to T cells [49].

Could Identification of Fibrocytes as Participants in TED Disclose Additional Therapeutic Targets?

Despite substantial efforts to understand better the mechanisms responsible for the initiation of GD and the factors that overarch involvement of the orbit in TED, current knowledge remains mired in uncertainty. Much of this can be attributed to an absence of preclinical models that faithfully recapitulate the human disease. These deficits have resulted in substantial unmet need in how we treat this disease. Especially during the active phase when surgery is frequently discouraged, medical options are limited. Nonspecific anti-inflammatory agents, including corticosteroids, nonsteroidal agents (PGHS-2 inhibitors), and antimetabolites may lessen the symptoms directly caused by inflammation. But none of these agents is thought to alter the clinical course of TED. More recently, targeted strategies, many repurposed from other diseases, have been used on an ad hoc basis. Anti-CD20 monoclonal antibody (rituximab) is the currently best-studied among these and the results of two separate prospective trials are eagerly awaited. Other biologics, such as those that interrupt cytokine networks, have yet to be studied in a manner that could lead to conclusions about their efficacy. Their roles in the therapy of active TED remain to be established. Further, all of these candidate agents are associated with potentially serious side effects. Thus, we continue to rely on surgical intervention for ocular rehabilitation.

Recognition of the potential involvement of fibrocytes in GD and TED widens the horizons for future inquiry into disease mechanisms. It may be possible to directly target specific aspects of their behavior as potential mediators of the immune reactivity systemically as well as within the orbit space. To be certain, TED is a complex autoimmune condition with numerous molecular and cellular underpinnings. We are only now beginning to understand the underlying processes. Further insights into the potential roles fibrocytes play in the disease, especially the initial phases, should bring us closer to developing more effective treatments.

Acknowledgments The valuable assistance of Yao Wang in identifying reference material for this chapter is gratefully acknowledged as is the great help provided by Ms. Justyna Piernicka. This work was supported in part by National Institutes of Health grants EY008976, EY011708, DK063121, Core Center for Vision grant EY007003 from the National Eye Institute, an unrestricted grant from Research to Prevent Blindness, and the Bell Charitable Foundation.

References

1. Werner SC, Ingbar SH, Braverman LE, Utiger RD. Werner and Ingbar's the thyroid: a fundamental and clinical text. 7th ed. Philadelphia: Lippincott-Raven; 1996. p. 1124.
2. Bahn RS. Graves' ophthalmopathy. N Engl J Med. 2010;362:726–38.
3. Wang Y, Smith TJ. Current concepts in the molecular pathogenesis of thyroid-associated ophthalmopathy. Invest Ophthalmol Vis Sci. 2014;55:1735–48.
4. Douglas RS, Gupta S. The pathophysiology of thyroid eye disease: implications for immunotherapy. Curr Opin Ophthalmol. 2011;22:385–90.
5. Kazim M, Goldberg RA, Smith TJ. Insights into the pathogenesis of thyroid-associated orbitopathy:

evolving rationale for therapy. Arch Ophthalmol. 2002;120:380–6.
6. Prabhakar BS, Bahn RS, Smith TJ. Current perspective on the pathogenesis of Graves' disease and ophthalmopathy. Endocr Rev. 2003;24:802–35.
7. Tao TW, Cheng PJ, Pham H, et al. Monoclonal antithyroglobulin antibodies derived from immunizations of mice with human eye muscle and thyroid membranes. J Clin Endocrinol Metab. 1986;63:577–82.
8. Marinò M, Lisi S, Pinchera A, et al. Identification of thyroglobulin in orbital tissues of patients with thyroid-associated ophthalmopathy. Thyroid. 2001;11:177–85.
9. Feliciello A, Porcellini A, Ciullo I, et al. Expression of thyrotropin-receptor mRNA in healthy and Graves' disease retro-orbital tissue. Lancet. 1993;342:337–8.
10. Heufelder AE, Dutton CM, Sarkar G, et al. Detection of TSH receptor RNA in cultured fibroblasts from patients with Graves' ophthalmopathy and pretibial dermopathy. Thyroid. 1993;3:297–300.
11. Szkudlinski MW, Fremont V, Ronin C, et al. Thyroid-stimulating hormone and thyroid-stimulating hormone receptor structure-function relationships. Physiol Rev. 2002;82:473–502.
12. Wiersinga WM. Autoimmunity in Graves' ophthalmopathy: the result of an unfortunate marriage between TSH receptors and IGF-1 receptors? J Clin Endocrinol Metab. 2011;96:2386–94.
13. Parmentier M, Libert F, Maenhaut C, et al. Molecular cloning of the thyrotropin receptor. Science. 1989; 246:1620–2.
14. Smith TJ. Insulin-like growth factor-I regulation of immune function: a potential therapeutic target in autoimmune diseases? Pharmacol Rev. 2010;62:199–236.
15. Tramontano D, Cushing GW, Moses AC, et al. Insulin-like growth factor-I stimulates the growth of rat thyroid cells in culture and synergizes the stimulation of DNA synthesis induced by TSH and Graves'-IgG. Endocrinology. 1986;119:940–2.
16. Tsui S, Naik V, Hoa N, et al. Evidence for an association between thyroid-stimulating hormone and insulin-like growth factor 1 receptors: a tale of two antigens implicated in Graves' disease. J Immunol. 2008;181:4397–405.
17. Chen H, Mester T, Raychaudhuri N, et al. Teprotumumab, an IGF-1R blocking monoclonal antibody inhibits TSH and IGF-1 action in fibrocytes. J Clin Endocrinol Metab. 2014;99:E1635–40.
18. Weightman DR, Perros P, Sherif IH, et al. Autoantibodies to IGF-1 binding sites in thyroid associated ophthalmopathy. Autoimmunity. 1993;16:251–7.
19. Pritchard J, Horst N, Cruikshank W, Smith TJ. Igs from patients with Graves' disease induce the expression of T cell chemoattractants in their fibroblasts. J Immunol. 2002;168:942–50.
20. Pritchard J, Han R, Horst N, Cruikshank WW, Smith TJ. Immunoglobulin activation of T cell chemoattractant expression in fibroblasts from patients with Graves' disease is mediated through the insulin-like growth factor I receptor pathway. J Immunol. 2003; 170:6348–54.
21. Douglas RS, Gianoukakis AG, Kamat S, Smith TJ. Aberrant expression of the insulin-like growth factor-1 receptor by T cells from patients with Graves' disease may carry functional consequences for disease pathogenesis. J Immunol. 2007; 178:3281–7.
22. Douglas RS, Naik V, Hwang CJ, et al. B cells from patients with Graves' disease aberrantly express the IGF-1 receptor: implications for disease pathogenesis. J Immunol. 2008;181:5768–74.
23. Douglas RS, Brix TH, Hwang CJ, et al. Divergent frequencies of IGF-I receptor-expressing blood lymphocytes in monozygotic twin pairs discordant for Graves' disease: evidence for a phentotypic signature ascribable to nongenetic factors. J Clin Endocrinol Metab. 2009;95:1797–802.
24. Minich WB, Dehina N, Welsink T, et al. Autoantibodies to the IGF1 receptor in Graves' orbitopathy. J Clin Endocrinol Metab. 2013;98:752–60.
25. Varewijck AJ, Boelen A, Lamberts SW. Circulating IgGs may modulate IGF-I receptor stimulating activity in a subset of patients with Graves' ophthalmopathy. J Clin Endocrinol Metab. 2013;98: 769–76.
26. Smith TJ. Is IGF-I receptor a target for autoantibody generation in Graves' disease? J Clin Endocrinol Metab. 2013;98:515–8.
27. Smith TJ, Hoa N. Immunoglobulins from patients with Graves' disease induce hyaluronan synthesis in their orbital fibroblasts through the self-antigen, IGF-1 receptor. J Clin Endocrinol Metab. 2004;89: 5076–80.
28. Smith TJ, Sempowski GD, Wang HS, et al. Evidence for cellular heterogeneity in primary cultures of human orbital fibroblasts. J Clin Endocrinol Metab. 1995;80:2620–5.
29. Smith TJ, Koumas L, Gagnon A, et al. Orbital fibroblast heterogeneity may determine the clinical presentation of thyroid-associated ophthalmopathy. J Clin Endocrinol Metab. 2002;87:385–92.
30. Henrikson RC, Smith TJ. Ultrastructure of cultured human orbital fibroblasts. Cell Tissue Res. 1994;278: 629–31.
31. Smith TJ, Wang HS, Hogg MG, et al. Prostaglandin E2 elicits a morphological change in cultured orbital fibroblasts from patients with Graves ophthalmopathy. Proc Natl Acad Sci U S A. 1994; 91:5094–8.
32. Cao HJ, Wang HS, Zhang Y, et al. Activation of human orbital fibroblasts through CD40 engagement results in a dramatic induction of hyaluronan synthesis and prostaglandin endoperoxide H synthase-2 expression. Insights into potential pathogenic mechanisms of thyroid-associated ophthalmopathy. J Biol Chem. 1998;273:29615–25.
33. Hwang CJ, Afifiyan N, Sand D, et al. Orbital fibroblasts from patients with thyroid-associated ophthalmopathy overexpress CD40: CD154 hyperinduces IL-6, IL-8, and MCP-1. Invest Ophthalmol Vis Sci. 2009;50:2262–8.

34. Wang HS, Cao HJ, Winn VD, et al. Leukoregulin induction of prostaglandin-endoperoxide H synthase-2 in human orbital fibroblasts. An in vitro model for connective tissue inflammation. J Biol Chem. 1996; 271:22718–28.
35. Han R, Tsui S, Smith TJ. Up-regulation of prostaglandin E2 synthesis by interleukin-1beta in human orbital fibroblasts involves coordinate induction of prostaglandin-endoperoxide H synthase-2 and glutathione-dependent prostaglandin E2 synthase expression. J Biol Chem. 2002;277:16355–64.
36. Smith TJ, Wang HS, Evans CH. Leukoregulin is a potent inducer of hyaluronan synthesis in cultured human orbital fibroblasts. Am J Physiol. 1995;268:C382–8.
37. Kaback LA, Smith TJ. Expression of hyaluronan synthase messenger ribonucleic acids and their induction by interleukin-1beta in human orbital fibroblasts: potential insight into the molecular pathogenesis of thyroid-associated ophthalmopathy. J Clin Endocrinol Metab. 1999;84:4079–84.
38. Spicer AP, Kaback LA, Smith TJ, et al. Molecular cloning and characterization of the human and mouse UDP-glucose dehydrogenase genes. J Biol Chem. 1998;273:25117–24.
39. Li B, Smith TJ. Divergent expression of IL-1 receptor antagonists in CD34^{+} fibrocytes and orbital fibroblasts in thyroid-associated ophthalmopathy: contribution of fibrocytes to orbital inflammation. J Clin Endocrinol Metab. 2013;98:2783–90.
40. Li B, Smith TJ. Regulation of IL-1 receptor antagonist by TSH in fibrocytes and orbital fibroblasts. J Clin Endocrinol Metab. 2014;99:E625–33.
41. Li B, Smith TJ. PI3K/AKT pathway mediates induction of IL-1RA by TSH in fibrocytes: modulation by PTEN. J Clin Endocrinol Metab. 2014;99:3363–72.
42. Bucala R, Spiegel LA, Chesney J, et al. Circulating fibrocytes define a new leukocyte subpopulation that mediates tissue repair. Mol Med. 1994;1:71–81.
43. Douglas RS, Afifiyan NF, Hwang CJ, et al. Increased generation of fibrocytes in thyroid-associated ophthalmopathy. J Clin Endocrinol Metab. 2010;95:430–8.
44. Gillespie EF, Papageorgiou KI, Fernando R, et al. Increased expression of TSH receptor by fibrocytes in thyroid-associated ophthalmopathy leads to chemokine production. J Clin Endocrinol Metab. 2012;97:E740–6.
45. Raychaudhuri N, Fernando R, Smith TJ. Thyrotropin regulates IL-6 expression in CD34+ fibrocytes: clear delineation of its cAMP-independent actions. PLoS One. 2013;8:e75100.
46. Fernando R, Atkins S, Raychaudhuri N, et al. Human fibrocytes coexpress thyroglobulin and thyrotropin receptor. Proc Natl Acad Sci. 2012;109:7427–32.
47. Fernando R, Lu Y, Atkins SJ, et al. Expression of thyrotropin receptor, thyroglobulin, sodium-iodide symporter, and thyroperoxidase by fibrocytes depends on AIRE. J Clin Endocrinol Metab. 2014;155:E1236–44.
48. Fernando R, Vonberg A, Atkins SJ, et al. Human fibrocytes express multiple antigens associated with autoimmune endocrine disease. J Clin Endocrinol Metab. 2014;99:E796–803.
49. Chesney J, Bacher M, Bender A, et al. The peripheral blood fibrocyte is a potent antigen-presenting cell capable of priming naïve T cells in situ. Proc Natl Acad Sci U S A. 1997;94:6307–12.

4 Management of Hyperthyroidism in the Setting of Thyroid Eye Disease

Fatemeh Rajaii, Shivani Gupta, and Raymond S. Douglas

Introduction

Thyroid eye disease (TED) is a complex autoimmune disease with a poorly understood pathophysiology. It is often associated with Graves' disease and hyperthyroidism; however, the relationship between thyroid gland dysfunction and progression of TED is not well understood. Furthermore, the optimal treatment of hyperthyroidism in the context of TED is not well established.

The effects of treatment of hyperthyroidism on TED activity and progression are complex. Increased T3 levels are thought to be associated with a higher probability of developing or worsening TED, but the data have been inconsistent [1–3]. Furthermore, the development of hypothyroidism and increased TSH is associated with the onset or progression of TED, regardless of the thyroid treatment [2]. Consequently, the primary goal of thyroid treatment in TED patients is to achieve a euthyroid state with minimal endocrinologic exacerbations in an effort to reduce the likelihood of TED progression [4]. Available treatment modalities include anti-thyroid drugs (TDs), radioactive iodine (RAI), and surgical thyroidectomy. The ideal modality of hyperthyroid treatment that safely achieves a euthyroid state with minimal-to-no progression of TED is not well established and likely depends on the individual patient. This chapter will discuss the literature regarding the effects of each treatment modality on the development and progression of TED.

F. Rajaii, M.D., Ph.D. (✉) • S. Gupta, M.D., M.P.H.
R.S. Douglas
Division of Eye Plastic, Orbital, and Facial Cosmetic Surgery, Kellogg Eye Center, University of Michigan, 100 Wall St., Ann Arbor, MI 48105, USA
e-mail: frajaii@umich.edu

Endocrine Management and TED

Based on a survey of members of The Endocrine Society, American Thyroid Society, and American Association of Clinical Endocrinologists, anti-TDs are the preferred modality of management of uncomplicated GD (by 53.9 % of practitioners, with RAI being preferred by 45 %, and thyroidectomy preferred by 0.7 %) [5]. In patients with TED, practitioners increasingly prefer anti-TDs (62.9 %) and thyroidectomy (18.5 %). In this setting RAI is used less frequently (RAI without steroids by 1.9 %, RAI with steroids by 16.9 %) [5]. This change in preferred practice pattern reflects the concern about the effects of RAI on the onset or progression of TED.

Medical Therapy

The mainstay of medical therapy in the management of hyperthyroid patients is anti-TDs. Most anti-TDs belong to the thionamide class, which includes propylthiouracil (PTU), methimazole (MZ), and carbimazole. The latter is only available

R.S. Douglas et al. (eds.), *Thyroid Eye Disease*,
DOI 10.1007/978-1-4939-1746-4_4, © Springer Science+Business Media New York 2015

in Europe and Asia, while the former two are generally used in the United States. Chapter 1 discusses the relative merits of methimazole and recommends restricting the use of PTU to women in early pregnancy. These drugs reduce the production of thyroid hormone by inhibiting the coupling of iodothyronines [6]. In prescribing anti-TDs, two general strategies are used: the block-replace regimen and the titration regimen. In the block-replace regimen, thyroid hormone production is functionally "blocked" by a high dose of the anti-TD which completely suppresses hormone production and "replaced" by adding levothyroxine at a dose that achieves a euthyroid state. In contrast, the titration regimen consists of titrating down to the minimum dose of anti-TD needed to maintain a euthyroid state. A recent Cochrane review comparing anti-TD regimens demonstrated that the titration regimen is equally effective to the block-replace regimen for the management of hyperthyroidism with fewer adverse effects [7]. In most studies medical therapy for Graves' hyperthyroidism has not been associated with progression of orbitopathy [8]. In addition, there is a theoretical benefit to the use of anti-TDs because thyroid stimulating hormone receptor antibody (TSHR Ab) levels correlate with disease severity, and anti-TDs have been shown to cause a more rapid reduction in TSHR Ab levels than surgery or RAI [1, 9]. Further work is needed to determine whether there are significant differences in TED onset or progression in patients treated with anti-TDs with either the block-replace or titration regimen. Though often preferred, anti-TDs are not without side effects, which may include rash, fever, urticaria, and arthralgia in up to 5 % of patients [6]. Major side effects are rare but include agranulocytosis, hepatotoxicity, aplastic anemia, and vasculitis indicating that the use of anti-TDs should be closely monitored especially for long-term treatment.

Radioactive Iodine

RAI therapy uses the radioactive isotope ^{131}I to ablate thyroid follicular cells, which abrogates thyroid hormone production [6]. It is often first-line treatment for hyperthyroidism or in cases of recalcitrant hyperthyroidism following anti-TD treatment. The main contraindications to RAI are pregnancy and breastfeeding because the isotope crosses the placenta and is excreted in breast milk [10] (see Chap. 7). Achievement of a euthyroid state after RAI treatment may take several months, and sometimes a second treatment may be required.

RAI is the preferred modality for the treatment of uncomplicated GD among 45 % of practitioners in the United States [11, 12]. It effectively treats hyperthyroidism in nearly all patients but has a relapse rate of approximately 21–28 %. Relapse rates of up to 48 % have been reported in select patient groups and large goiter size is a risk factor for recurrent hyperthyroidism [5, 13]. Persistent hypothyroidism after RAI has been reported to worsen TED, so close monitoring of thyroid function and prompt replacement with levothyroxine is essential.

Several randomized trials have compared the effects of RAI and anti-TD on TED onset or progression. One randomized study with 4-year follow-up demonstrated that 39 % of patients treated with RAI experienced worsening or new onset TED, compared to 21 % of methimazole-treated patients [14]. In sub-group analysis, RAI was associated with an increased risk of development of new onset TED, but the rate of worsening of preexisting TED did not differ significantly between the two treatment groups [14]. Another randomized trial comparing RAI to anti-TD found that after 9 years, there was no difference in the percentage of patients with worsened or new onset TED, but that more patients treated with RAI had an improvement in TED compared to those treated with methimazole; euthyroid status after treatment correlated with improved TED in both treatment groups [15]. Similarly, a randomized trial from Hong Kong showed that at 2 years following treatment, the rates of developing new or worsened TED was not significantly different in patients treated with RAI alone or a 12-month course of methimazole, and the development of new or progression of TED was associated with hypothyroidism and increased TSH [2]. Therefore, randomized studies show that RAI may be associated with TED progression compared to anti-TDs, but this association may be secondary to increased rates of post-treatment hypothyroidism. Prevention of early hypothyroidism after treatment with RAI may prove beneficial in preventing the progression of TED.

RAI may also exacerbate TED secondary to increased antithyroid antibody levels. In a 5-year prospective randomized trial, patients treated with RAI had significantly higher TSHR Ab levels at all stages after treatment compared to patients treated with anti-TD or surgery [1, 9]. Given the correlation between TSI levels and TED severity and activity, this is a theoretical disadvantage to the use of RAI [16].

The use of prophylactic corticosteroids in conjunction with RAI can prevent progression of orbitopathy [3, 17–19]. A cohort study of TED patients treated with RAI demonstrated that prophylactic treatment with corticosteroids prevented worsening orbitopathy [19]. Other studies have shown that RAI treatment without corticosteroids was associated with the onset or progression of orbitopathy in 15 % of patients, but treatment with prednisone reduced the rate to 0 % [3]. In comparison, progressive or new orbitopathy was observed in 3 % of methimazole-treated patients [3]. No significant difference was seen in TED progression or incidence in patients treated with RAI and corticosteroids compared to those treated with methimazole; however, two-thirds of patients treated with RAI and corticosteroids had an improvement in the severity of TED, which was significantly higher than the proportion of patients treated with methimazole whose TED improved (2 %) [3]. Most of the changes in TED occurred within the first 6 months after treatment [3]. A systematic review of randomized controlled trials using RAI for hyperthyroidism showed a relative risk of 4.2 for the development or progression of TED when RAI was used compared to anti-TDs; the relative risk of severe TED was 4.3 for treatment with RAI compared to anti-TDs [18]. The use of prophylactic steroids with RAI, however, reduced the risk of progression of TED to 0 [18]. In summary, the data demonstrate that use of prophylactic glucocorticoids with RAI is effective in minimizing the risk for progression of orbitopathy, and furthermore may lead to improvement of TED.

The ideal protocol for steroid treatment is unknown. The European Group on Graves' Orbitopathy (EUGOGO) recommends starting prednisone 0.3–0.5 mg/kg/day orally 1–3 days after RAI and slowly tapering patients off over 3 months [6, 20]. A more recent retrospective study demonstrated that 0.2 mg/kg/day of prednisone, starting 1 day after RAI and tapered off over 6 weeks was as effective as a higher doses of 0.3–0.5 mg/kg/day [21]. More studies will be needed to establish the best glucocorticoid dosing regimen.

Thyroidectomy

Thyroid surgery is a rapid and effective method of treating hyperthyroidism in GD. Thyroidectomy may include either total or partial (subtotal) removal of the thyroid gland. The rate of recurrent hyperthyroidism after subtotal thyroidectomy has been reported to be as high as 9 %, which is significantly higher than after total thyroidectomy [22, 23]. Complications of thyroid surgery include recurrent laryngeal nerve palsy and hypoparathyroidism, which may be temporary or permanent. In a systematic review of both randomized and non-randomized studies, total thyroidectomy was associated with a higher rate of both temporary and permanent hypoparathyroidism than subtotal thyroidectomy [24]. The rate of permanent recurrent laryngeal nerve palsy was not significantly different between the two groups [24].

Three randomized controlled trials have compared the effects of total thyroidectomy and subtotal thyroidectomy on progression of TED and demonstrated that the majority of patients had improvement in TED after thyroidectomy (range 50–89 %) with no significant difference between the surgical groups [23, 25, 26]. A meta-analysis of randomized control trials comparing total thyroidectomy to subtotal thyroidectomy also showed that there is no significant difference in TED progression between the two groups. Recurrent hyperthyroidism was, however, observed more frequently in patients treated with subtotal thyroidectomy [22]. These findings were confirmed by a systematic review of both randomized and non-randomized studies [24]. Thus, the choice of subtotal or total thyroidectomy does not influence the progression of TED, in spite of differences in rates of postoperative recurrent hyperthyroidism and hypoparathyroidism.

Which Treatment Is Best for TED Patients?

One study compared the effects of methimazole, subtotal thyroidectomy, and RAI on progression of ophthalmopathy and found no significant difference in the rates of new or progressive ophthalmopathy in patients treated with methimazole (15 %) compared to surgery (11 %), but a significant increase in the onset or progression of TED was seen following RAI treatment [1]. Another systematic review has shown that the rate of recurrent hyperthyroidism is significantly higher with anti-TDs (53 %) compared to either RAI (15 %) or thyroidectomy (10 %), while the difference between RAI and thyroidectomy is not statistically significant [27].

Taken together, the decision about how best to treat hyperthyroidism in a given patient should be based upon three goals: (1) achieving rapid and stable euthyroidism, (2) minimizing complications, and (3) preventing the new development or worsening of TED. For patients with mild to moderate TED, anti-TDs are the first line of treatment because they may reduce hyperthyroidism and its effects without permanently altering the thyroid gland by surgery or radio-ablation. However, they are not without side effects. If patients are unable to be rendered euthyroid with anti-TDs in a timely fashion or if side effects are intolerable, then it is reasonable to proceed with thyroidectomy or RAI. Thyroidectomy has the theoretical advantage of reducing antithyroid antibody levels and any antigenic material within the explanted thyroid gland with up to 90 % of patients achieving undetectable THSR Ab levels by postoperative year 4 [9]. For patients who require definitive treatment of hyperthyroidism but who prefer medical therapy or have contraindications to surgery, RAI with prophylactic steroids is a safe alternative, provided that care is taken to prevent post-procedural hypothyroidism. RAI should be avoided in pregnant women in children, as discussed in Chap. 7).

Conclusions

When choosing an appropriate treatment plan for hyperthyroidism in GD, there are many factors to consider, including patient factors, risks and benefits of the various treatment options and the possibility of contributing to new onset or progressive TED. No single therapy can be viewed as a magic bullet to ideally manage hyperthyroidism and improve TED. Use of anti-TD, RAI with corticosteroids, or thyroidectomy does not increase the rates of developing new onset or worsening of TED, in contrast to RAI without corticosteroids. Thus, each modality may be considered for patients without TED, or with mild TED, depending on their endocrine status, potential contraindications, and preferences. For patients with severe TED, however, thyroidectomy may be preferable due to the rapid correction of hyperthyroidism, reduced burden of antithyroid antibodies, and the lower risk of progression of TED compared to RAI [6].

References

1. Tallstedt L, Lundell G, Tørring O, Wallin G, Ljunggren JG, Blomgren H, Taube A. Occurrence of ophthalmopathy after treatment for Graves' hyperthyroidism. The Thyroid Study Group. N Engl J Med. 1992;326(26):1733–8.
2. Kung AW, Yau CC, Cheng A. The incidence of ophthalmopathy after radioiodine therapy for Graves' disease: prognostic factors and the role of methimazole. J Clin Endocrinol Metab. 1994;79(2):542–6.
3. Bartalena L, Marcocci C, Bogazzi F, Manetti L, Tanda ML, Dell'Unto E, Bruno-Bossio G, Nardi M, Bartolomei MP, Lepri A, Rossi G, Martino E, Pinchera A. Relation between therapy for hyperthyroidism and the course of Graves' ophthalmopathy. N Engl J Med. 1998;338(2):73–8.
4. Prummel MF, Wiersinga WM, Mourits MP, Koornneef L, Berghout A, van der Gaag R. Effect of abnormal thyroid function on the severity of Graves' ophthalmopathy. Arch Intern Med. 1990;150(5):1098–101.

5. Törring O, Tallstedt L, Wallin G, Lundell G, Ljunggren JG, Taube A, Sääf M, Hamberger B. Graves' hyperthyroidism: treatment with antithyroid drugs, surgery, or radioiodine–a prospective, randomized study. Thyroid Study Group. J Clin Endocrinol Metab. 1996;81(8):2986–93.
6. Hegedüs L, Bonnema SJ, Smith TJ, Brix TH. Treating the thyroid in the presence of Graves' ophthalmopathy. Best Pract Res Clin Endocrinol Metab. 2012;26(3):313–24.
7. Abraham P, Avenell A, McGeoch SC, Clark LF, Bevan JS. Antithyroid drug regimen for treating Graves' hyperthyroidism. Cochrane Database Syst Rev. 2010;(1):CD003420.
8. Bartalena L. The dilemma of how to manage Graves' hyperthyroidism in patients with associated orbitopathy. J Clin Endocrinol Metab. 2011;96(3):592–9.
9. Laurberg P, Wallin G, Tallstedt L, Abraham-Nordling M, Lundell G, Tørring O. TSH-receptor autoimmunity in Graves' disease after therapy with anti-thyroid drugs, surgery, or radioiodine: a 5-year prospective randomized study. Eur J Endocrinol. 2008;158(1): 69–75.
10. Sankar R, Sripathy G. Radioactive iodine therapy in Graves' hyperthyroidism. Natl Med J India. 2000; 13(5):246–51.
11. Wartofsky L, Glinoer D, Solomon B, Nagataki S, Lagasse R, Nagayama Y, Izumi M. Differences and similarities in the diagnosis and treatment of Graves' disease in Europe, Japan, and the United States. Thyroid. 1991;1(2):129–35.
12. Burch HB, Burman KD, Cooper DS. A 2011 survey of clinical practice patterns in the management of Graves' disease. J Clin Endocrinol Metab. 2012; 97(12):4549–58.
13. Chen JY, Huang HS, Huang MJ, Lin JD, Juang JH, Huang BY, Wang PW, Liu RT. Outcome following radioactive iodine therapy in Graves' disease. Changgeng Yi Xue Za Zhi. 1990;13(4):258–67.
14. Träisk F, Tallstedt L, Abraham-Nordling M, Andersson T, Berg G, Calissendorff J, Hallengren B, Hedner P, Lantz M, Nyström E, Ponjavic V, Taube A, Törring O, Wallin G, Asman P, Lundell G, Thyroid Study Group of TT 96. Thyroid-associated ophthalmopathy after treatment for Graves' hyperthyroidism with antithyroid drugs or iodine-131. J Clin Endocrinol Metab. 2009;94(10):3700–7.
15. Chen DY, Schneider PF, Zhang XS, Luo XY, He ZM, Chen TH. Changes in graves' ophthalmopathy after radioiodine and anti-thyroid drug treatment of Graves' disease from 2 prospective, randomized, open-label, blinded end point studies. Exp Clin Endocrinol Diabetes. 2014;122(1):1–6.
16. Ponto KA, Kanitz M, Olivo PD, Pitz S, Pfeiffer N, Kahaly GJ. Clinical relevance of thyroid-stimulating immunoglobulins in graves' ophthalmopathy. Ophthalmology. 2011;118(11):2279–85.
17. Bartalena L, Marcocci C, Bogazzi F, Panicucci M, Lepri A, Pinchera A. Use of corticosteroids to prevent progression of Graves' ophthalmopathy after radioiodine therapy for hyperthyroidism. N Engl J Med. 1989; 321(20):1349–52.
18. Acharya SH, Avenell A, Philip S, Burr J, Bevan JS, Abraham P. Radioiodine therapy (RAI) for Graves' disease (GD) and the effect on ophthalmopathy: a systematic review. Clin Endocrinol (Oxf). 2008;69(6): 943–50.
19. Stan MN, Durski JM, Brito JP, Bhagra S, Thapa P, Bahn RS. Cohort study on radioactive iodine-induced hypothyroidism: implications for Graves' ophthalmopathy and optimal timing for thyroid hormone assessment. Thyroid. 2013;23(5):620–5.
20. Bartalena L, Baldeschi L, Dickinson AJ, Eckstein A, Kendall-Taylor P, Marcocci C, Mourits MP, Perros P, Boboridis K, Boschi A, Currò N, Daumerie C, Kahaly GJ, Krassas G, Lane CM, Lazarus JH, Marinò M, Nardi M, Neoh C, Orgiazzi J, Pearce S, Pinchera A, Pitz S, Salvi M, Sivelli P, Stahl M, von Arx G, Wiersinga WM. Consensus statement of the European group on Graves' orbitopathy (EUGOGO) on management of Graves' orbitopathy. Thyroid. 2008;18(3):333–46.
21. Lai A, Sassi L, Compri E, Marino F, Sivelli P, Piantanida E, Tanda ML, Bartalena L. Lower dose prednisone prevents radioiodine-associated exacerbation of initially mild or absent graves' orbitopathy: a retrospective cohort study. J Clin Endocrinol Metab. 2010;95(3):1333–7.
22. Guo Z, Yu P, Liu Z, Si Y, Jin M. Total thyroidectomy vs bilateral subtotal thyroidectomy in patients with Graves' diseases: a meta-analysis of randomized clinical trials. Clin Endocrinol (Oxf). 2013;79(5): 739–46.
23. Barczyński M, Konturek A, Hubalewska-Dydejczyk A, Gołkowski F, Nowak W. Randomized clinical trial of bilateral subtotal thyroidectomy versus total thyroidectomy for Graves' disease with a 5-year follow-up. Br J Surg. 2012;99(4):515–22.
24. Feroci F, Rettori M, Borrelli A, Coppola A, Castagnoli A, Perigli G, Cianchi F, Scatizzi M. A systematic review and meta-analysis of total thyroidectomy versus bilateral subtotal thyroidectomy for Graves' disease. Surgery. 2014;155(3):529–40.
25. Järhult J, Rudberg C, Larsson E, Selvander H, Sjövall K, Winsa B, Rastad J, Karlsson FA, TEO Study Group. Graves' disease with moderate-severe endocrine ophthalmopathy-long term results of a prospective, randomized study of total or subtotal thyroid resection. Thyroid. 2005;15(10):1157–64.
26. Witte J, Goretzki PE, Dotzenrath C, Simon D, Felis P, Neubauer M, Röher HD. Surgery for Graves' disease: total versus subtotal thyroidectomy-results of a prospective randomized trial. World J Surg. 2000;24(11): 1303–11.
27. Sundaresh V, Brito JP, Wang Z, Prokop LJ, Stan MN, Murad MH, et al. Comparative effectiveness of therapies for Graves' hyperthyroidism: a systematic review and network meta-analysis. J Clin Endocrinol Metab. 2013;98:3671–7.

5 Smoking and Prevention of Thyroid Eye Disease

Wilmar M. Wiersinga

Introduction

Thyroid eye disease (TED, also called Graves' Ophthalmopathy, Graves' Orbitopathy, or Thyroid Associated Ophthalmopathy,) is one of the phenotypes of Graves' disease. In about 90 % of TED patients, the ophthalmopathy occurs in conjunction with Graves' hyperthyroidism, the most prevalent phenotype of Graves' disease in which TSH receptor stimulating antibodies (TSHR-Ab) induce excessive thyroid hormone production. However, about 7 % of TED patients are euthyroid and 3 % are hypothyroid when the ophthalmopathy becomes clinically manifest [1, 2]. Remarkably, TSHR-Ab are present in the vast majority of these eu- or hypothyroid patients [3]. Experimental animal studies have shown that genetic immunization with the TSH receptor induces TSHR-Ab, hyperthyroidism and eye changes resembling TED [4]. The data provide fair evidence to consider TED and Graves' hyperthyroidism as phenotypic appearances of one and the same disease entity, namely Graves' disease.

Graves' disease is a complex multifactorial autoimmune disease in which the immune reaction against the TSH receptor develops in genetically susceptible subjects provoked by environmental factors. TED is present in about 25–35 % of patients diagnosed with Graves' hyperthyroidism [5, 6], although imaging studies have demonstrated subclinical TED in the majority of patients with Graves' hyperthyroidism without manifest TED [7]. The question thus arises why TED does not become clinically manifest in all patients. It could be related to differences in the prevalence of susceptibility genes between Graves' patients with and without TED. Available studies, however, have failed to find consistent differences in the genetic make-up between Graves' patients with and without TED [8]. Exposure to environmental factors including iodine intake, stress and smoking has each been linked to Graves' hyperthyroidism. Anecdotal reports mention great stress prior to development of TED, but formal studies comparing stress levels in patients with or without TED are lacking [9]. In contrast, there is good evidence that the prevalence of smoking among patients with Graves' hyperthyroidism is higher in the presence of TED than in the absence of TED [10]. Consequently it appears that smoking behaviour is one of the main determinants whether or not TED will become clinically manifest (Fig. 5.1).

We will review the association between smoking and TED, the biologic mechanism behind this association and whether the association indicates a causal relationship. We also discuss if cessation of smoking could prevent TED, and explore smoking cessation strategies.

W.M. Wiersinga, M.D., Ph.D. (✉)
Department of Endocrinology & Metabolism,
Academic Medical Center, University of Amsterdam,
Meibergdreef 9, Amsterdam 1105AZ,
The Netherlands
e-mail: w.m.wiersinga@amc.uva.nl

R.S. Douglas et al. (eds.), *Thyroid Eye Disease*,
DOI 10.1007/978-1-4939-1746-4_5, © Springer Science+Business Media New York 2015

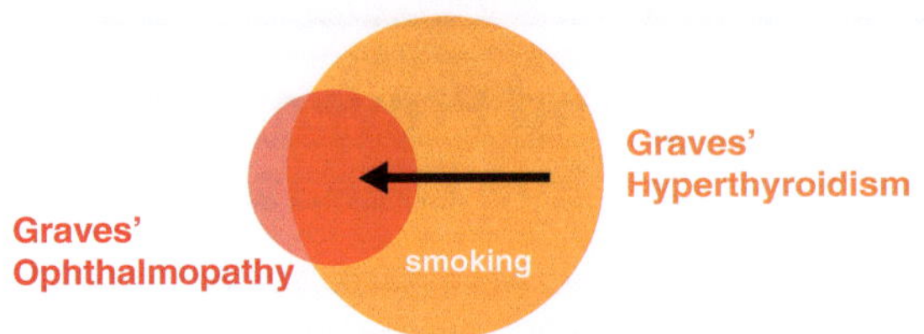

Fig. 5.1 Graves' ophthalmopathy or thyroid eye disease (TED) (*red circle*) occurs in 90 % of patients in conjunction with Graves' hyperthyroidism, but 10 % is euthyroid or hypothyroid. Patients with Graves' hyperthyroidism (*yellow circle*) have clinically manifest TED in about 25–35 %, and subclinical TED in the majority of the remaining 65–75 %. Smoking is a main determinant of the transition from subclinical to overt TED

Association Between Smoking and TED

A meta-analysis published in 2002 concluded that smoking increases the risk of TED beyond the risk associated with Graves' hyperthyroidism alone [10]. Comparison of smoking behaviour between patients with Graves' disease (Graves' hyperthyroidism, with cases of TED included in 5 of the 8 studies) and controls revealed current smoking as a risk factor for Graves' disease with an odds ratio of 3.30; there was no increased risk among former smokers (Table 5.1). When comparing TED patients with controls, the risk for ever smokers was significantly higher with an odds ratio of 4.40. Restricting the analysis to patients with Graves' hyperthyroidism with or without TED, current smoking significantly increases the risk of TED with an odds ratio of 2.18. Essentially similar results have been obtained in a systematic review published in 2008 [11]. The observed association between smoking and Graves' disease is somewhat stronger in women than in men [10], and found in diverse ethnic groups [5, 10, 12–14]. In view of the undisputed association between smoking and TED, the question emerges whether smoking has a causal relationship with TED.

Table 5.1 Meta-analyses of studies on the risk of Graves' disease associated with smoking

	Odds ratio (95 % confidence interval)
Graves' disease patients vs. controls	
Current smokers vs. never smokers	3.30 (2.09–5.22)
Ever smokers vs. never smokers	1.90 (1.42–2.55)
Ex-smokers vs. never smokers	1.41 (0.77–2.58)
Graves' ophthalmopathy vs. controls	
Ever smokers vs. never smokers	4.40 (2.88–6.73)
Graves' ophthalmopathy vs. Graves' disease	
Current smokers vs. never smokers	2.18 (1.51–3.14)
Ever smokers vs. never smokers	2.53 (1.70–3.77)

Data from [10]. Graves' disease patients refer to patients with Graves' hyperthyroidism, although in some studies these patients also had Graves' ophthalmopathy

Several features of the association suggest causality [15]:

1. *Strength*. There is some heterogeneity in the analysed studies, which differ in sample size, age and sex distribution, and definition of current smoking. Also, some studies do not discriminate between Graves' hyperthyroidism and TED, labelling all patients as Graves' disease. Most studies are cross-sectional with just a few being prospective. Despite these deficiencies, strong associations (high odds ratio) are found.
2. *Consistency*. The likelihood of a causal relationship increases if the association is observed in different populations. This certainly is true for TED: studies from various countries in Europe, Asia and the USA all identified smoking as a risk factor [10].
3. *Dose–response relationship*. A Japanese study describes an increased risk of Graves' hyperthyroidism with an increasing number of cigarettes smoked per day (odds ratio 3.7 for 1–10 cig./day and 5.1 for 21–40 cig./day, $p<0.01$ for trend) [13]. In a UK study among patients with Graves' hyperthyroidism, the proportion of patients with TED increased as cigarette

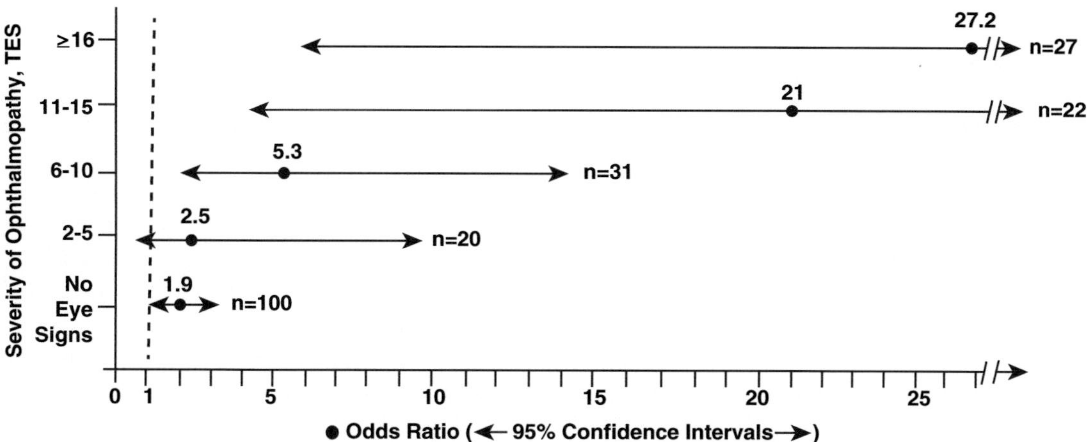

Fig. 5.2 The increase in the prevalence of smokers (represented by the odds ratio with 95 % confidence intervals) in relation to the severity of TED (assessed by the total eye score TES) in patients with Graves' hyperthyroidism. From Prummel MF, Wiersinga WM. Smoking and risk of Graves' disease. JAMA 1993; 269: 479–482. Reprinted with permission from American Medical Association

consumption increased ($p=0.008$) [12]. Many studies describe a dose–response relationship between current smoking and the severity of TED [10, 12]. In a retrospective survey the frequency of current smokers with moderate, severe and malignant TED was 64 %, 71 % and 87 %, respectively [16]. In another study smokers had more severe eye disease than nonsmokers as assessed by the total eye score (12.2 ± 6.9 vs. 8.6 ± 6.2; $p=0.03$), and patients with more severe forms of TED were more often smokers than those with no or less severe TED resulting in a significant increase in the odds ratio ($p<0.001$ by trend test) (Fig. 5.2) [17]. In a prospective study there was a significant increase in the relative risk for proptosis with increased smoking; the relative risk for diplopia was 1.8 for patients currently smoking 1–10 cigarettes daily, 3.8 for those smoking 11–20 cigarettes and 7.0 for patients smoking >20 cig./day [18]. In this study lifetime tobacco use was not an independent risk factor for the development of TED symptoms. A study from Korea reports that smoking status was a predictive risk factor for a severe course of TED and the development of optic neuropathy (odds ratios 6.57 and 10.0, respectively) [14]. The data support a quantitative relationship between current smoking and the severity of TED: the higher the number of daily cigarettes, the greater the severity of TED.

4. *Temporality*. To stop smoking apparently decreases the risk for Graves' disease, as the odds ratio is lower in ever smokers than in current smokers (but still significant) while it is no longer significant in former smokers (Table 5.1). In the prospective study by Pfeilschifter et al. [18], the incidence of TED among current smokers, former smokers and never smokers was 68.2 %, 64.0 % and 51.7 %, respectively; the incidence of proptosis in these groups was 49.0 %, 16.0 % and 18.6 %, and that of diplopia 27.9 %, 16.0 % and 8.9 %, respectively. The risk for TED was not increased in former smokers compared to never smokers (TED incidence RR 1.45, 95 % CI 0.90–2.33; proptosis incidence RR 0.90, 95 % CI 0.24–2.33; diplopia incidence RR 1.88, 95 % CI 0.46–7.73). When current smokers were subdivided in those smoking 1–10 cig./day, 11–20 cig./day and >20 cig./day, the incidence of proptosis in these three groups was 36.7 %, 59.5 % and 62.5 %, respectively; the incidence of diplopia in these groups was 16.3 %, 34.0 % and

62.5 %, respectively. Cessation of smoking may lead to a lower incidence of TED and to less severe TED.

5. *Specificity*. Is the risk of smoking specific for hyperthyroidism when it is caused by Graves' disease? Apparently so, because ever smoking was not associated with hyperthyroidism due to toxic nodular goitre (odds ratio 1.22, 95 % CI 0.96–1.55) [10]. Is the risk of smoking specific for Graves' disease and not for other autoimmune thyroid diseases? It appears so because recent epidemiological studies have demonstrated that smoking is associated with a lower occurrence of TPO- and Tg-antibodies and the development of overt autoimmune hypothyroidism (Hashimoto's disease) [19, 20]; cessation of smoking transiently increases the risk of developing overt hypothyroidism [21]. The contrasting effects of smoking on the risk of Graves' and Hashimoto's disease resemble the divergent effects of smoking on inflammatory bowel disease: smoking is a risk factor for Crohn's disease (odds ratio 1.61, 95 % CI 1.27–2.03), but has a protective effect for colitis ulcerosa (odds ratio 0.41, 95 % CI 0.34–0.48) [22]. Smoking is also a known risk factor for other autoimmune diseases like rheumatoid arthritis and systemic lupus erythematosus. Smoking is thus a disease modifier of many autoimmune conditions, but its consequences appear to be rather disease specific.
6. *Biological plausibility*. The studies reporting the association between smoking and Graves' disease might have been affected by confounding factors like iodine intake, stress exposure and alcohol intake. While possible, this seems unlikely for several reasons. First, the association has been observed in areas with iodine deficiency as well as in areas with sufficient iodine intake. Second, smoking behaviour might be related to stress, but smoking was still an independent risk factor for Graves' disease after adjustment for stressful life events [13]. Third, smoking behaviour might be connected with alcohol intake, but alcohol consumption has a protective effect on both Graves' hyperthyroidism and Hashimoto's hypothyroidism and its effects are independent of smoking [23, 24]. Confounding factors can never be excluded completely, but the association between smoking and TED apparently is with exposure to cigarette smoke itself and not with a factor connected with smoking behaviour. Although the pathogenesis of TED is still incompletely understood, a number of in vivo and in vitro studies report how smoking might favour the development of TED. This is discussed in the next section.

Taken together, the strong and consistent association between smoking and TED, the presence of a dose–response relationship, the temporality of the risk (which decreases after cessation of smoking), the specificity of the risk for Graves' disease and not for Hashimoto's disease and the biological plausibility of the association, all support the existence of a causal relationship between smoking and TED.

Biological Mechanisms Relating Smoking to TED

1. *Immunopathogenesis of TED*: *A synopsis* [25, 26]. The hallmark of TED is swelling of extraocular muscles and orbital fat. It is caused mostly by excessive secretion of glycosaminoglycans (very hydrophilic compounds which attract a lot of water) by activated orbital fibroblasts, and differentiation of a subset of orbital fibroblasts into mature adipocytes. Orbital fibroblasts have been recognized as the target cells of the orbital autoimmune attack in Graves' disease; they express low levels of TSH receptors, which however markedly increase upon differentiation into mature fat cells. Homing of immunocompetent cells to the orbit is facilitated by cytokine-induced expression of HLA and adhesion molecules on vascular endothelium. Graves' immunoglobulins induce orbital fibroblasts to secrete T cell chemoattractants. The numerous macrophages but also the few B cells in the orbit may act as antigen-presenting cells that in the setting of MHC class II molecules present linear TSHR peptides to T cells. Activated T cells release a

variety of inflammatory cytokines, chemokines and prostaglandins, causing inflammatory edema and proliferation of fibroblasts. The cytokine profile in the early stages of TED is predominantly derived from Th1-cells, inducing orbital fibroblasts to secrete cytokines and excessive amounts of glycosaminoglycans, which cause swelling of orbital tissues, in particular of extraocular muscles. A subset of fibroblasts differentiates into adipocytes under the influence of particular cytokines. In late stages of TED, the cytokine profile is mostly Th2-cell derived and the effect of Graves' IgG becomes more prominent in the process of adipogenesis. TSHR antibodies bind to TSHR on orbital fibroblasts, resulting in upregulation of hyaluronan synthase and excessive production of hyaluronan, one of the prevalent glycosaminoglycans in the orbit.

2. *Effect of smoking on immune responses in general.* The immunological effects of cigarette smoking have been studied extensively. However, it remains difficult to relate changes in the number of immunocompetent cells and the concentration of their products in the blood to functional alterations in other immunological compartments, and then to link these alterations to specific diseases. Adding to the complexity are the many components of cigarette smoke; some of these over 4,800 compounds are endotoxin (acting via Toll-like receptor 4), nicotine (acting via nicotinic acetylcholine receptor), reactive oxygen species/free radicals (acting via NOD-like receptor family, pyrin domain containing 3) and polycyclic aromatic hydrocarbons (acting via aryl hydrocarbon receptors) [27]. It has become clear that smoking affects both the innate and adaptive immune systems [28]. Cigarette smoke activates innate immune cells (like macrophages, dendritic cells, neutrophils and epithelial cells) via oxidative stress and by triggering pattern recognition receptors (PPR, such as Toll-like receptors, NOD-like receptors and purinergic receptors). The activation of PPR may occur directly by cigarette components or indirectly via the release of damage-associated molecular patterns (DAMP) by dying—autophagic death, apoptotic or necrotic—cells [27]. DAMPs can be released from injured cells due to exposure to tobacco smoke, oxidative stress, infections or tissue hypoxia. DAMPs released from stressed or dying cells include uric acid, heat shock proteins, β-defensins and interleukin-1α, among many others, and DAMPs released from the breakdown of extracellular matrix encompass glycosaminoglycans like hyaluronan, heparin sulphate, versican and biglycan (acting via Toll-like receptors) and fibronectin (acting via Toll-like receptor-4 and integrins). Following stimulation by PPR, the innate immune cells release pro-inflammatory cytokines and chemokines, reactive oxygen species (ROS) and proteolytic enzymes, such as neutrophil elastase and matrix metalloproteinases. Activated dendritic cells induce adaptive immune responses involving T helper (Th1 and Th17) CD4+ T cells, CD8+ cytotoxicity and B-cell responses. Cigarette smoke increases the production of many pro-inflammatory cytokines, such as TNF-α, Il-1, IL-6, IL-8, and decreases the production of anti-inflammatory cytokines such as IL-10 [28]. Smoking also induces oxidative stress, enhances the generation of free radicals, and decreases the level of antioxidants not only in the blood but also in aqueous humour and ocular tissue [29, 30].

3. *Effect of smoking on immune responses in TED: in vitro studies.* Cultures of human orbital fibroblasts have been used to explore how smoking might affect the immune response in TED. In the absence of a validated animal model of TED, the rationale of using orbital fibroblasts as a surrogate experimental model is that orbital fibroblasts on the one hand are the target cells of the orbital autoimmune attack and on the other hand also effector cells by their production and secretion of excessive amounts of glycosaminoglycans. Smoking reduces tissue oxygen tension by causing vasoconstriction and the formation of carboxyhemoglobin. Extraocular muscle fibroblasts when cultured under hypoxic conditions (5 % CO_2: 95 % N_2 vs. 5 % CO_2: 95 % air in normal conditions, resulting in PO_2 of

13 and 18.6 kPa, respectively), display a significant increase in glycosaminoglycan, protein and DNA synthesis, under both basal and cytokine-treated conditions [31]. Incubation of orbital fibroblasts with H_2O_2 increases the expression of heat shock protein-72 (HSP-72) [32]. Cultured orbital fibroblasts obtained from patients undergoing orbital decompression for severe TED did not express HLA-DR when treated with nicotine or tar; HLA-DR expression increased about threefold upon exposure to nicotine or tar in combination with interferon-γ [33]. Cigarette smoke contains large quantities of superoxide radicals and other ROS. Exposure of orbital fibroblasts to superoxide radicals, induced by adding xanthine oxidase and hypoxanthine to the culture medium, caused a dose-dependent proliferation of fibroblasts derived from TED patients but not from control fibroblasts; proliferation was inhibited by the xanthine-oxidase inhibitor allopurinol, the antioxidant nicotinamide and by methimazole [34]. In another experiment cultured orbital fibroblasts were exposed to cigarette smoke extract (CSE) [35]. Fibroblasts from TED patients and controls showed similar results. CSE did not affect ICAM1 (intercellular adhesion molecule-1) expression. CSE did stimulate hyaluronic acid production in a dose-dependent manner, with 5 % CSE causing an increase of 44 % ($p=0.001$); 5 % CSE compares to 40 cigarettes daily. CSE also increased adipogenesis in a dose-dependent manner, as did interleukin-1; the effect of 5 % CSE is approximately half that seen with 0.1 ng/mL IL-1. The effects of CSE and IL-1 on adipogenesis were synergistic: the degree of adipogenesis in the well containing 5 % CSE and 0.1 ng/mL IL-1 was double the magnitude of the sum of the values obtained from either stimulus alone, and reduced by 82 % by addition of an anti-IL-1 antibody. Lastly, CSE and H_2O_2 (used as a control) dose-dependently stimulated intracellular ROS production and adipogenesis in orbital fibroblasts from TED patients and control subjects [36]. The effects of 2 % CSE and 10 μM H_2O_2 were similar. Addition of quercetin, a flavonoid phytoestrogen with antifibrotic properties, inhibited adipogenesis by reducing ROS generation in vitro. Quercetin thus holds promise as a therapeutic option in TED patients [37, 38].

Taken together, the results with cultured orbital fibroblasts strongly support the notion that exposure to cigarette smoke is causally connected with TED. Oxidative stress plays a major role in TED as several studies have indicated greater oxidative DNA damage, lipid peroxidation and ROS production in cultured orbital fibroblasts from TED patients relative to normal orbital fibroblasts [39–41]. Cigarette smoking greatly increases oxidative stress. It induces expression of HLA-DR and HSP-72 on orbital fibroblasts, which is involved in antigen recognition and T cell recruitment. It causes orbital fibroblasts to proliferate, to produce excessive amounts of glycosaminoglycans and to differentiate into adipocytes. Many of these effects of smoking are dose dependent, and may occur or are potentiated in a particular cytokine environment. Smoking-induced hypoxia may further aggravate these events.

4. *Effect of smoking on immune responses in TED: in vivo studies*. Several studies have investigated whether smokers differ from nonsmokers with respect to serum concentrations of adhesion molecules, cytokines and TSHR antibodies. TED patients had higher levels of the adhesion molecules sICAM-1, sVCAM-1 and sELAM-1 than Graves' disease patients without TED or healthy controls; only sICAM-1 correlated with the severity of TED. Smoking was independently associated with higher levels of sICAM-1 and lower levels of sVCAM-1 in both TED patients and controls; it did not affect sELAM-1 [42]. Serum concentrations of IL-1α, IL-1β and TNFα were not influenced by smoking or the presence of TED [43–45]. Soluble interleukin-1 receptor antagonist (sIL-1RA) levels, however, were lower in smokers than in nonsmokers with TED; baseline sIL-1RA and its increase during immunosuppressive treatment were lower in nonresponders than in responders to therapy [43]. It was suggested that measurement of sIL-1RA might predict the therapeutic response.

However, subsequent studies could not confirm these findings since they reported similar sIL-1RA concentrations between smokers and nonsmokers and between responders and nonresponders to immunosuppression in TED patients [44–47]. Serum sIL-2R, IL-6, IL-6R, TNFαRI, TNFαRII and sCD30 concentrations were all higher in TED patients than in healthy controls, but levels did not differ between smokers and nonsmokers [47]. Serum IL-6 and IL-6R are higher in active than in inactive TED [44].

Serum concentrations of IL-1β, s IL-1RA, TNFα, IL-6 and sIL-6R were not different in Graves' disease patients with or without TSHR antibodies [44]. Although the serum concentration of TSHR antibodies is higher in TED than in Graves' patients without TED, the levels are not different between smokers and nonsmokers [16, 48]. No correlation was found between smoking (as assessed by urinary levels of cotinine, the major metabolite of nicotine) and the level of TSHR antibodies in TED [49]. Another study in TED patients likewise found no difference in TSHR antibodies between smokers and nonsmokers [50]. Serum concentrations of TSHR antibodies are higher in patients with a severe course of TED compared with patients with a mild course of TED, but this relationship of TSHR antibodies to TED severity was independent from smoking [51].

An early report distinguished TED patients without restrictive myopathy (type I) and with restrictive myopathy (type II); 63 % of type I and 83 % of type II were smokers [52]. The data suggest smoking affects enlargement of extraocular muscles to a greater extent than enlargement of the orbital fat/connective tissue compartment. A subsequent volumetric study, however, observed a direct relationship between orbital connective tissue volume and current smoking, whereas extraocular muscle volume was not influenced by smoking [53]. In contrast, a recent study in consecutive-untreated TED patients found that smoking did not influence orbital fat volume, but that smokers had significantly larger extraocular muscle volumes than nonsmokers [54].

Taken together, the higher serum concentrations of some adhesion molecules and cytokines in smokers as well as the differential effect of smoking on orbital fat and muscle enlargement provides some evidence regarding the mechanism by which smoking is causally related to TED.

Smoking and Prevention of TED

The concept of prevention is illustrated in Fig. 5.3. Primary prevention aims at keeping the disease from occurring at all by removing risk factors. Secondary prevention is directed at early detection when the disease is still asymptomatic and when early treatment can stop the disease from progressing. Tertiary prevention refers to those clinical activities that prevent further deterioration or reduce complications after the disease has declared itself [55].

1. *Primary prevention.* The biological plausibility of a causal relationship between smoking and TED suggests that to refrain from smoking may diminish the chance to develop both Graves' disease and TED. This notion is strongly supported by the significant odds for current smokers to contract Graves' disease, whereas the odds are lower in ever smokers and not significant in former smokers [10]. Indeed current, but not lifetime, tobacco consumption constitutes a risk for the incidence of proptosis and diplopia in Graves' patients [18].

   Indirect evidence for the efficacy of smoking cessation as primary prevention of TED comes from questionnaire studies. A European survey in 1996 revealed that 43 % of physician respondents thought TED was decreasing in frequency, and 12 % thought it to be increasing [56]. The supposed decrease most likely was attributed to a secular trend towards a lower prevalence of smoking in most European countries. It is remarkable that all respondents from Hungary and Poland (where the proportion of smokers in the general population had increased since the fall of the Berlin Wall) indicated an increased incidence of TED.

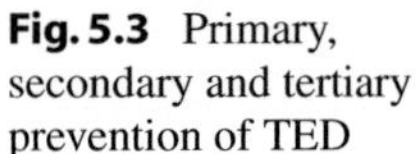

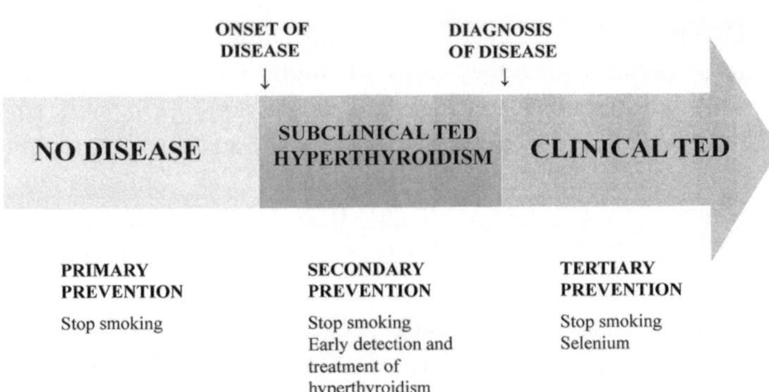

Fig. 5.3 Primary, secondary and tertiary prevention of TED

Table 5.2 Frequency of childhood TED in pediatric Graves' hyperthyroidism as a function of smoking prevalence among teenagers in their country of origin

Smoking prevalence (%)	Graves' hyperthyroidism	Thyroid eye disease	Thyroid eye disease among children	
			≤10 year (%)	11–18 years (%)
≥25	644 (100 %)	236 (36.6 %)	52	48
20–25	818 (100 %)	223 (27.3 %)	15	85
<20	452 (100 %)	117 (25.9 %)	24	76

Data from [57]

Another European questionnaire survey collected data on pediatric Graves' disease [57]. The prevalence of TED among children with Graves' hyperthyroidism was 30 %. When grouped according to smoking prevalence among teenagers in the country of origin, it became evident that TED frequency was the highest in countries in which teenagers smoked most (Table 5.2). Divided by age, the highest proportion of children with TED 10 years of age or younger was found in countries where the smoking prevalence was highest. As it is unlikely that children ≤10 year smoke, the results are best explained by passive smoking as a result of living in an environment in which 25 % or more of their peers smoke.

2. *Secondary prevention.* In patients with newly diagnosed Graves' hyperthyroidism without clinically manifest TED, the majority will have some enlargement of extraocular muscles as evident from orbital imaging [7]. What can be done at this stage of subclinical TED in terms of preventing progression to clinically manifest TED? A study in the UK noted a substantial decline in the prevalence of TED among newly diagnosed patients with Graves' hyperthyroidism: it was 57 % in 1960 and 35 % in 1990. The proportion of patients with severe TED (diplopia or optic nerve compression) also fell in this period from 30.4 to 20.7 % [58]. It is highly likely that the introduction of more reliable tests of thyroid function (the sensitive TSH assay became widely available in the 1980s, greatly facilitating diagnosis of thyrotoxicosis in family practices) leading to earlier diagnosis and treatment of thyrotoxicosis is responsible for this trend to fewer and less severe TED. Diagnosis of hyperthyroidism rather early in the natural history of the disease is likely associated with less severe hyperthyroidism, and recovery of the euthyroid state may be relatively fast. This likely limits the vicious cycle of hyperthyroidism worsening the autoimmunity and autoimmunity worsening the hyperthyroidism [59]. Circumstantial evidence indicates that cessation of smoking at this stage most likely will decrease the risk of progression to overt TED. When antithyroid drugs are chosen for treating hyperthyroidism, smokers display a

much slower reduction in TSHR antibodies than nonsmokers [48]. Smokers also have a higher recurrence rate after discontinuation of antithyroid drugs than nonsmokers [60–62]. The recurrence risk in patients with negative TSHR antibodies at discontinuation of antithyroid drugs was 57 % in smokers and 18 % in nonsmokers; if TSHR antibodies were positive, recurrences occurred in 100 % of smokers and in 86 % of nonsmokers [59]. When ^{131}I therapy is chosen to treat Graves' hyperthyroidism, there is approximately a 15 % chance of developing or worsening TED; this risk can be diminished by a preventive course of steroids [63, 64]. Smoking increases this risk fourfold (from 6 % in nonsmokers to 23 % in smokers, relative risk 3.94, 95 % CI 1.41–11.02), and improvement of eye changes with steroids is four times less likely in smokers (from 64 % in nonsmokers to 15 % in smokers, relative risk 0.23, 95 % CI 0.14–0.40).

3. *Tertiary prevention*. When the disease has become clinically manifest, circumstantial evidence indicates it is likely still worthwhile to stop smoking in order to improve the outcome of TED. In a series of patients treated with steroids followed by retrobulbar irradiation, baseline characteristics of TED were not different between smokers and nonsmokers [50]. However, improvement of the clinical activity score and eye muscle motility occurred significantly faster and to a greater extent in nonsmokers than smokers. There was also a dose–response relationship in that improvements were inversely correlated to the erythrocyte content of the hemoglobin adduct *N*-2-hydroxyethylvaline, a parameter of long-term smoking. Two other studies also describe better outcomes of orbital irradiation in nonsmokers than in smokers [65, 66]. Finally, strabismus surgery was required more often in active smokers than in nonsmokers at presentation with TED (26 % vs. 14 %, hazard ratio 2.19) [67]. The data suggest that smoking cessation early in the disease improves outcomes.

   Selenium administration has proven to prevent progression of mild TED to more severe TED, and therefore can be labelled as tertiary prevention. In a placebo-controlled randomized clinical trial in patients with mild TED, sodium selenite (100 μg orally twice daily for 6 months) improved quality-of-life, clinical activity score, eyelid aperture and soft tissue signs compared to placebo; the improvement was maintained at 1 year [68]. TED improved in 61 % in the selenium group vs. 36 % in the placebo group, and worsened in 7 % in the selenium group vs. 26 % in the placebo group ($p=0.01$). Smoking status had no apparent influence on the effect of different treatments. As increased generation of oxygen-free radicals plays a pathogenic role in TED [32, 34, 39], the efficacy of selenium might be explained from its antioxidant action [69]. The study was conducted in several European countries, in which ambient selenium intake is low. Whether the same positive results will be obtained in countries with sufficient selenium intake like the USA is not known. One might hypothesize that selenium would also be effective in early stages of thyroid autoimmunity or in moderate-to-severe stages of TED; evidence to support that hypothesis is currently lacking.

Cessation of Smoking

Attempts to quit smoking are notorious for their failures. Efficacy of methods to stop smoking are as follows: written self-help leaflets 1 %, proactive telephone counselling 2 %, brief opportunistic advice from a doctor 2 %, intensive behavioural support from a specialist 7 %, bupropion 9 %, nicotine replacement therapy (NRT) 5–12 %, intensive behavioural support + buproprion + NRT 13–19 %. The low success rates are sobering, but can we do any better in TED patients? One is inclined to think so for a number of reasons. First, most TED patients are women and are concerned about the effect of the ophthalmopathy on their appearance. Second, one can provide rather accurate information on the risk of smoking for their specific disease, in contrast to general remarks on the increased risk of smoking for the development of cancer and cardiovascular disease.

Smokers will have a greater chance for recurrent Graves' hyperthyroidism after a course of antithyroid drugs, a four times higher chance for worsening of eye changes after ^{131}I therapy and a fourfold lower chance that this post-radioiodine worsening can be prevented by steroids. Outcomes of treatment with glucocorticoids or retrobulbar irradiation are also less favourable in smokers than in nonsmokers. Nevertheless, standard advice against smoking does not seem to be very effective in TED patients [70]. Even showing unpleasant photos of patients with advanced stages of TED was unlikely to make smokers quit [71]. Interventional programs specifically designed for TED patients might be very helpful. So far, however, formal studies on the success rate of quitting smoking have not been done in TED patients, nor has it been formally proven that the outcome of the ophthalmopathy will indeed be better after cessation of smoking.

Every effort should be made to help TED smokers to stop smoking, and it might well be that the mere presence of TED provides a golden opportunity to get a higher success rate of quitting smoking than usual. The patient should receive specific counseling from the treating physician, and referral to smoking clinics should be considered. Two recent papers detail strategies to help a smoker who is struggling to quit [72, 73]. Table 5.3 provides evidence for the efficacy (i.e. prolonged abstinence at least 6 months from the start of treatment) of various approaches [72, 74].

Table 5.3 Meta-analyses of studies on the efficacy of methods for smoking cessation

	Odds ratio (95 % confidence interval)
Nonpharmacological methods	
Brief advice vs. no advice or usual care	1.66 (1.42–1.94)
Brief counselling vs. no advice or usual care	1.84 (1.60–2.13)
Pharmacological methods	
Nicotine replacement therapy vs. placebo	1.84 (1.71–1.99)
Buproprion vs. placebo	1.82 (1.60–2.06)
Varenicline	2.88 (2.40–3.47)

Data from the Cochrane Database of systematic reviews [72, 74]

Smokers who are using NRT, buproprion or varenicline when trying to quit, double their odds of success. NRT and bupropion show equal efficacy; varenicline is superior to single forms of NRT and to bupropion. The most effective way to use NRT is to combine the long-acting nicotine patch with a shorter-acting product (lozenge, gum, inhaler or nasal spray) and extend treatment beyond 12 weeks [72]. The new drug cytosine (a nicotine receptor partial agonist) seems also to be effective with a risk ratio of 3.98 (2.01–7.87). On current evidence, none of the treatments appear to have an incidence of adverse events that would mitigate their use [74, 75].

A new player in the field is the electronic cigarette. An Internet survey in 2010 reveals the reasons why people use e-cigarettes: perception that it was less toxic than tobacco (84 %), to deal with craving for tobacco (79 %) and withdrawal symptoms (67 %), to quit smoking or avoid relapsing (77 %) [76]. Participants in a longitudinal internet survey from 2011 to 2013 were mostly former smokers (72 %), and 76 % were using e-cigarettes daily; it was concluded that e-cigarettes may contribute to relapse prevention in former smokers and smoking cessation in current smokers [77]. A randomized controlled trial for smoking cessation reported a verified abstinence at 6 months of 7.3 % with nicotine e-cigarettes, 5.8 % with nicotine patches and 4.1 % with placebo e-cigarettes [78]. The power of the study was insufficient to demonstrate superiority of e-cigarettes.

References

1. Eckstein A, Loesch C, Glowacka D, et al. Euthyroid and primarily hypothyroid patients develop milder and significantly more asymmetric Graves' ophthalmopathy. Br J Ophthalmol. 2009;93:1052–6.
2. Kashkouli MB, Pakdel F, Kiavash V, Heidari I, Heirati A, Jam S. Hyperthyroid vs hypothyroid eye disease: the same severity and activity. Eye. 2011;25:1442–6.
3. Khoo DH, Eng PH, Ho SC, et al. Graves' ophthalmopathy in the absence of elevated free thyroxine and triiodothyronine levels: prevalence, natural history and thyrotropin receptor antibody levels. Thyroid. 2000;10:1093–100.
4. Moskhelgosha S, So PW, Deasy N, Diaz-Cano S, Banga P. Cutting edge: retrobulbar inflammation, adipogenesis, and acute orbital congestion in a preclinical

female mouse model of Graves' orbitopathy induced by thyrotropin receptor plasmid-in vivo electroporation. Endocrinology. 2012;154:3008–15.
5. Lim SL, Lim AK, Mumtaz M, et al. Prevalence, risk factors, and clinical features of thyroid-associated ophthalmopathy in multiethnic Malaysian patients with Graves' disease. Thyroid. 2008;18:1297–301.
6. Tanda ML, Piantanida E, Liparulo L, et al. Prevalence and natural history of Graves' orbitopathy in a large series of patients with newly diagnosed Graves' hyperthyroidism at a single center. J Clin Endocrinol Metab. 2012;98:1443–9.
7. Werner SC, Coleman DJ, Franzen LA. Ultrasonographic evidence of a consistent orbital involvement in Graves' disease. N Engl J Med. 1974; 290:1447–50.
8. Bednarczuk T, Gopinath B, Ploski R, Wall JR. Susceptibility genes in Graves' ophthalmopathy: searching for a needle in a haystack? Clin Endocrinol. 2007;67:3–19.
9. Falgarone G, Heshmati HM, Cohen R, Reach G. Role of emotional stress in the pathophysiology of Graves' disease. Eur J Endocrinol. 2013;168:R13–8.
10. Vestergaard P. Smoking and thyroid disorders—a meta-analysis. Eur J Endocrinol. 2002;146:153–61.
11. Thornton J, Kelly SP, Harrison RA, Edwards R. Cigarette smoking and thyroid eye disease: a systematic review. Eye. 2007;21:1135.
12. Tellez M, Cooper J, Edmonds C. Graves' ophthalmopathy in relation to cigarette smoking and ethnic origin. Clin Endocrinol. 1992;36:291–4.
13. Yoshiuchi K, Kumano H, Nomura S, et al. Stressful life events and smoking were associated with Graves'disease in women, but not in men. Psychosom Med. 1998;60:182–5.
14. Lee JH, Lee SY, Yoon JS. Risk factors associated with the severity of thyroid-associated orbitopathy in Korean patients. Korean J Ophthalmol. 2010;24: 267–73.
15. Hegedus L, Brix TH, Vestergaard P. Relationship between cigarette smoking and Graves' ophthalmopathy. J Endocrinol Invest. 2004;27:265–71.
16. Winsa B, Mandahl A, Karlsson FA. Graves' disease, endocrine ophthalmopathy and smoking. Acta Endocrinol. 1993;128:156–60.
17. Prummel MF, Wiersinga WM. Smoking and risk of Graves' disease. JAMA. 1993;269:479–82.
18. Pfeilschifter J, Ziegler R. Smoking and endocrine ophthalmopathy: impact of smoking severity and current vs lifetime cigarette consumption. Clin Endocrinol. 1996;45:477–81.
19. Effraimidis G, Tijssen JGP, Wiersinga WM. Discontinuation of smoking increases the risk of developing thyroid peroxidase antibodies and/or thyroglobulin antibodies: a prospective study. J Clin Endocrinol Metab. 2009;94:1324–8.
20. Effraimidis G, Strieder TGA, Tijssen JGP, et al. Natural history of the transition from euthyroidism to overt autoimmune hypo- or hyperthyroidism: a prospective study. Eur J Endocrinol. 2011;164:107–13.
21. Carle A, Bulow-Pedersen I, Knudsen N, et al. Smoking cessation is followed by a sharp but transient rise in the incidence of overt autoimmune hypothyroidism—a population-based, case–control study. Clin Endocrinol. 2012;77:764–72.
22. Arnson Y, Shoenfeld Y, Amital H. Effects of tobacco smoke on immunity, inflammation and autoimmunity. J Autoimmunity. 2010;34:1258–65.
23. Carle A, Bulow-Pedersen I, Knudsen N, et al. Moderate alcohol consumption may protect against overt autoimmune hypothyroidism: a population-based case-control study. Eur J Endocrinol. 2012;167:483–90.
24. Carle A, Bulow-Pedersen I, Knudsen N, et al. Graves' hyperthyroidism and moderate alcohol consumption: evidence for disease prevention. Clin Endocrinol. 2013;79:111–9.
25. Wiersinga WM. Autoimmunity in Graves' ophthalmopathy: the result of an unfortunate marriage between TSH receptors and IGF-1 receptors? J Clin Endocrinol Metab. 2011;96:2386–94.
26. Smith TJ, Hegedus L, Douglas RS. Role of insulin-like growth factor-1 (IGF-1) pathway in the pathogenesis of Graves' orbitopathy. Best Pract Res Clin Endocrinol Metab. 2012;26:291–302.
27. Brusselle GG, Joos GF, Bracke KR. New insights into the immunology of chronic obstructive pulmonary disease. Lancet. 2011;378:1015–26.
28. Arnson Y, Shoenfeld Y, Amital H. Effects of tobacco smoke on immunity, inflammation and autoimmunity. J Autoimmun. 2010;34:J258–65.
29. Cheng AC, Pang CP, Leung AT, Chua JK, Fan DS, Lam DS. The association between cigarette smoking and ocular diseases. Hong Kong Med J. 2000;6: 195–202.
30. Edirisinghe I, Rahman I. Cigarette smoke-mediated oxidative stress, shear stress, and endothelial dysfunction: role of VEGFR2. Ann N Y Acad Sci. 2010;1203: 66–72.
31. Metcalfe RA, Weetman AP. Stimulation of extraocular muscle fibroblasts by cytokines and hypoxia: possible role in thyroid-associated ophthalmopathy. Clin Endocrinol. 1994;40:67–72.
32. Heufelder AE, Wenzel BE, Bahn RS. Methimazole and propylthiouracil inhibit the oxygen free radical-induced expression of a 72 kilodalton heat shock protein in Graves' retroocular fibroblasts. J Clin Endocrinol Metab. 1992;74:737–42.
33. Mack WP, Stasior GO, Cao HJ, Stasior OG, Smith TJ. The effects of cigarette smoke constituents on the expression of HLA-DR in orbital fibroblasts derived from patients with Graves' ophthalmopathy. Ophthal Plast Reconstr Surg. 1999;15:260–71.
34. Burch HB, Lahiri S, Bahn RS, Barnes S. Superoxide radical production stimulates retroocular fibroblast proliferation in Graves' ophthalmopathy. Exp Eye Res. 1997;65:311–6.
35. Cawood TJ, Moriarty P, O'Farrelly C, O'Shea D. Smoking and thyroid-associated ophthalmopathy: a novel explanation of the biological link. J Clin Endocrinol Metab. 2007;92:59–64.

36. Yoon JS, Lee HJ, Chae MK, Lee SY, Lee EJ. Cigarette smoke extract-induced adipogenesis in Graves' orbital fibroblasts is inhibited by quercetin via reduction in oxidative stress. J Endocrinol. 2013;216:145–56.
37. Lisi S, Botta R, Lemmi M, et al. Quercetin decreases proliferation of orbital fibroblasts and their release of hyaluronic acid. J Endocrinol Invest. 2011;34:521–7.
38. Yoon JS, Chae MK, Lee SY, Lee EJ. Anti-inflammatory effect of quercetin in a whole orbital tissue culture of Graves' orbitopathy. Br J Ophthalmol. 2012;96:1117–21.
39. Lu R, Wang P, Wartofsky L, et al. Oxygen free radicals in interleukin-1β-induced glycosaminoglycan production by retro-ocular fibroblasts from normal subjects and Graves' ophthalmopathy patients. Thyroid. 1999; 9:297–303.
40. Bartalena L, Tanda ML, Piantanida E, Lai A. Oxidative stress and Graves' ophthalmopathy: in vitro studies and therapeutic implications. Biofactors. 2003;19:155–63.
41. Tsai CC, Wu SB, Cheng CY, et al. Increased oxidative DNA damage, lipid peroxidation, and reactive oxygen species in cultured orbital fibroblasts from patients with Graves' ophthalmopathy: evidence that oxidative stress has a role in this disorder. Eye. 2010;24:1520–5.
42. Wakelkamp IM, Gerding MN, van der Meer JW, Prummel MF, Wiersinga WM. Smoking and disease severity are independent determinants of serum adhesion molecules in Graves' ophthalmopathy. Clin Exp Immunol. 2002;127:316–20.
43. Hofbauer LC, Muhlberg T, Konig A, Heufelder G, Schworm HD, Heufelder AE. Soluble interleukin-1 receptor antagonist serum levels in smokers and nonsmokers with Graves' ophthalmopathy undergoing orbital radiotherapy. J Clin Endocrinol Metab. 1997;82: 2244–7.
44. Salvi M, Pedrazzoni M, Girasole G, et al. Serum concentrations of proinflammatory cytokines in Graves' disease: effect of treatment, thyroid function, ophthalmopathy and cigarette smoking. Eur J Endocrinol. 2000;143:197–202.
45. Liu G, Wu Z, Yang H, et al. Study on IL-1alpha, IL-1beta and sIL-1ra in sera of patients with Graves' ophthalmopathy. Yan Ke Xue Bao. 2002;18:151–5.
46. Bartalena L, Manetti L, Tanda ML, et al. Soluble interleukin-1 receptor antagonist concentration in patients with Graves' ophthalmopathy is neither related to cigarette smoking nor predictive of subsequent response to glucocorticoids. Clin Endocrinol. 2000;52:647–51.
47. Wakelkamp IM, Gerding MN, van der Meer JW, Prummel MF, Wiersinga WM. Both Th1- and Th2-derived cytokines in serum are elevated in Graves' ophthalmopathy. Clin Exp Immunol. 2000;121:453–7.
48. Nyirenda MJ, Taylor PN, Stoddart M, et al. Thyroid-stimulating hormone-receptor antibody and thyroid hormone concentrations in smokers vs nonsmokers with Graves' disease treated with carbimazole. JAMA. 2009;301:162–4.
49. Czarnywoitek A, Zgorzalewicz-Stachowiak M, Florek E, et al. The level of cotinine—marker of tobacco smoking—in patients with hyperthyroidism. Endokrynol Pol. 2006;57:612–8.
50. Eckstein A, Quadbeck B, Mueller G, et al. Impact of smoking on the response to treatment of thyroid associated ophthalmopathy. Br J Ophthalmol. 2003;87: 773–6.
51. Eckstein AK, Plicht M, Lax H, et al. Thyrotropin receptor autoantibodies are independent risk factors for Graves' ophthalmopathy and help to predict severity and outcome of the disease. J Clin Endocrinol Metab. 2006;91:3464–70.
52. Nunery WR, Martin RT, Heinz GW, Gavin TJ. The association of cigarette smoking with clinical subtypes of ophthalmic Graves' disease. Ophthal Plast Reconstr Surg. 1993;9:77–82.
53. Szucs-Farkas Z, Toth J, Kollar J, et al. Volume changes in intra- and extraorbital compartments in patients with Graves' ophthalmopathy: effect of smoking. Thyroid. 2005;15:146–51.
54. Regensburg NI, Wiersinga WM, Berendschot TT, Saeed P, Mourits MP. Effect of smoking on orbital fat and muscle volume in Graves' orbitopathy. Thyroid. 2011;21:177–81.
55. Wiersinga WM, Bartalena L. Epidemiology and prevention of Graves' ophthalmopathy. Thyroid. 2002;12: 855–60.
56. Weetman AP, Wiersinga WM. Current management of thyroid-associated ophthalmopathy in Europe. Results of an international survey. Clin Endocrinol. 1998;49:21–8.
57. Krassas GE, Segni M, Wiersinga WM. Childhood Graves' ophthalmopathy: results of a European questionnaire study. Eur J Endocrinol. 2005;153: 515–21.
58. Perros P, Kendall-Taylor P. Natural history of thyroid eye disease. Thyroid. 1998;8:423–5.
59. Laurberg P. Remission of Graves' disease during antithyroid drug therapy. Time to reconsider the mechanism? Eur J Endocrinol. 2006;155:783–6.
60. Glinoer D, de Nayer P, Bex M, et al. Effect of L-thyroxine administration, TSH-receptor antibodies and smoking on the risk of recurrence in Graves' hyperthyroidism treated with antithyroid drugs: a double-blind prospective randomized study. Eur J Endocrinol. 2001;144:475–83.
61. Nedrebo BG, Holm PL, Uhlving S, et al. Predictors of outcome and comparison of different drug regimens for the prevention of relapse in patients with Graves' disease. Eur J Endocrinol. 2002;147:583–9.
62. Hoermann R, Quadbeck B, Roggenbuck U, et al. Relapse of Graves' disease after successful outcome of antithyroid drug therapy: results of a prospective study on the use of levothyroxine. Thyroid. 2002;12: 1119–28.
63. Bartalena L, Marcocci C, Bogazzi F, et al. Relation between therapy for Graves' hyperthyroidism and the course of Graves' ophthalmopathy. N Engl J Med. 1998;338:73–8.
64. Traisk F, Tallstedt L, Abraham-Nordling M, et al. Thyroid-associated ophthalmopathy after treatment

for Graves' hyperthyroidism with antithyroid drugs of iodine-131. J Clin Endocrinol Metab. 2009;94: 3700–7.
65. Abboud M, Arabi A, Salti I, Geara F. Outcome of thyroid associated ophthalmopathy treated by radiation therapy. Radiat Oncol. 2011;6:46.
66. Prabhu RS, Liebman L, Wojno T, Hayek B, Hall WA, Crocker I. Clinical outcomes of radiotherapy as initial local therapy for Graves' ophthalmopathy and predictors of the need for post-radiotherapy decompressive surgery. Radiat Oncol. 2012;7:95.
67. Rajendram R, Bunce C, Adams GG, Dayan CM, Rose GE. Smoking and strabismus surgery in patients with thyroid eye disease. Ophthalmology. 2011;118: 2493–7.
68. Marcocci C, Kahaly GJ, Krassas GE, et al. Selenium and the course of mild Graves' orbitopathy. N Engl J Med. 2011;364:1920–31.
69. Rayman MP. Selenium and human health. Lancet. 2012;379:1256–68.
70. Karadimas P, Bouzas EA, Mastorakos G. Advice against smoking is not effective in patients with Graves' ophthalmopathy. Acta Med Austriaca. 2003; 30:59–60.
71. Christensen HD. Can repulsive photos make smokers quit?http://sciencenordic.com/can-repulsive-photos-make-smokers-quit
72. Rigotti NA. Strategies to help a smoker who is struggling to quit. JAMA. 2012;308:1573–80.
73. Fiore MC, Baker TB. Treating smokers in the health care setting. N Engl J Med. 2011;365:1222–31.
74. Cahill K, Stevens S, Perera R, Lancaster T. Pharmacological interventions for smoking cessation: an overview and network meta-analysis. Cochrane Database Syst Rev. 2013;(5):Art No. CD009329. doi: 10.1002/14651858.CD009329.pub2
75. Mills EJ, Thorlund K, Eapen S, Wu P, Prochaska JJ. Cardiovascular events associated with smoking cessation pharmacotherapies: a network meta-analysis. Circulation. 2014;129:28–41.
76. Elter JF, Bullen C. Electronic cigarette: users profile, utilization, satisfaction and perceived efficacy. Addiction. 2011;106:2017–28.
77. Elter JF, Bullen C. A longitudinal study of electronic cigarettes. Addict Behav. 2014;39:491–4.
78. Bullen C, Howe C, Laugesen M, et al. Electronic cigarettes for smoking cessation: a randomised controlled trial. Lancet. 2013;382:1629–37.

6 Nutrition and Supplements in Thyroid Eye Disease

Claudio Marcocci and Francesca Menconi

Thyroid eye disease (TED) occurs in approximately 50 % of Graves' disease (GD) patients [1]. The minority of patients (about 5 %) present with moderate-to-severe and active eye disease, which is commonly treated with intravenous (iv) glucocorticoids in the active phase [2, 3]. The majority of TED patient present with mild ocular involvement and usually do not receive any intervention apart from supportive measures (artificial tears, ointments, sunglasses). However, a substantial proportion of patients with mild TED suffer from a significant decrease in their quality of life (QoL). Furthermore, studies on the natural history of mild TED have reported a spontaneous improvement in about 50 % of the patients, stability in 34 %, and worsening in 16 % [4]. Hence, an intervention would be justified in patients with mild TED in order to improve quality of life, reduce ocular signs and symptoms, and, above all, prevent disease progression. Treatment should be well tolerated, safe, and widely available. Supplements have been shown to be beneficial in several conditions and could meet the above-mentioned treatment requirements. Based on the complex pathogenetic mechanisms at play in TED, which include humoral and cell-mediated immunity, cytokine production, and oxidative stress, the trace element selenium, which is known to have both antioxidant and immunomodulating properties, could represent a therapeutic option for patients with mild TED.

C. Marcocci (✉) • F. Menconi
Department of Clinical and Experimental Medicine, University of Pisa, Via Paradisa 2, Pisa 56124, Italy
e-mail: claudio.marcocci@med.unipi.it

Selenium

Selenium is a trace mineral discovered in 1817 by the Swedish chemist Berzelius. Selenium is incorporated as selenocysteine in selenoproteins. The most important selenoproteins, glutathione peroxidase (GPXs), thioredoxin reductases (TRs) and deiodinases (D1, D2, or D3), are highly expressed in the thyroid and contribute to maintenance of cell reduction–oxidation balance [5].

The main selenium dietary sources are meat, fish, shellfish, offal, eggs, and cereals. The bioavailability of selenium in each food is different (e.g., lower in fish and higher in cereals). Reasons for this variability relate to the selenium content of the soil where crops and fodder are grown and on other factors including the presence of ions that can complex with selenium, soil pH, and selenium speciation [6]. The mean value of daily selenium intake in Europe is 40 μg, while in the United States is 93 μg in women and 134 μg in men. The daily-recommended selenium intake is 53 μg in women and 60 μg in men [6].

Selenium intake is widely variable in different parts of the word. For instance, selenium intake

R.S. Douglas et al. (eds.), *Thyroid Eye Disease*,
DOI 10.1007/978-1-4939-1746-4_6, © Springer Science+Business Media New York 2015

is very high in North America but low in most European countries, particularly in Eastern Europe [7]. It is therefore important to test selenium plasma concentration in order to avoid selenium supplementation in subjects whose plasma selenium concentration is greater than 122 μg/L [7]. Indeed, it has been reported that excessive supplementation may increase risk of type 2 diabetes and certain malignancies [6, 8]. Selenium status can be assessed by measuring total selenium concentration or the concentration of circulating selenoproteins. Two soluble selenoproteins, glutathione peroxidase-3 and selenoprotein P, account for blood selenium content [7].

Selenium-containing supplements generally contain either selenomethionine or sodium selenite as the active ingredient. Both selenomethionine and selenite compounds can be used for biosynthesis of selenoproteins. However, once selenoproteins are saturated, only selenomethionine causes an additional increase in serum selenium concentration through its unregulated incorporation into proteins, while selenite is excreted. Thus, selenomethionine-containing supplements have the potential to cause selenium excess, whereas those containing selenite do not.

As mentioned before, selenium is incorporated into selenoproteins, mostly enzymes, in which selenium acts as a reduction–oxidation center and functions as an antioxidant. Selenium also has an immunomodulary effect and may be beneficial in patients with autoimmune thyroid diseases [9, 10].

Role of Oxidative Stress in the Pathogenesis of TED

TED is the most common extra thyroidal manifestation of GD. Although its pathogenesis is still controversial, TED is believed to be due to an autoimmune reaction against antigen(s) shared by the orbital tissue and the thyroid. The activation of orbital T lymphocytes initiates a cascade of events leading to increased production of cytokines, growth factors, and reactive oxygen species (ROS) [11]. The inflammatory process leads to an increased proliferation of adipocytes and orbital fibroblasts and overproduction of hydrophilic glycosaminoglycans (GAG). As a consequence the volume of orbital structures (fibroadipose tissue and extraocular muscles) increases and leads to impaired ocular motility, diplopia, and proptosis [12].

Several in vitro and in vivo studies have reported a potential role of ROS in the pathogenesis of TED [13]. Furthermore, cigarette smoking, the most important environmental factor involved in the development and progression of TED, has been shown in vitro to enhance the generation of ROS and cripple the antioxidant defense [13] (see Chap. 5).

In vitro studies have also been performed using cultured orbital fibroblasts obtained from patients with TED undergoing orbital decompression. In 1992, Heufelder et al. reported an increased expression of heat shock protein 72 (HSP 72) under stressful conditions in cultured TED patients fibroblasts compared with control fibroblasts, indicating that the increased capacity to induce HSP 72 may play a role in the inflammatory process affecting the orbital tissue in TED [14]. The same authors also reported that simultaneous treatment or pretreatment of TED fibroblast cultures with anti-oxidative agents or antithyroid drugs reduced the HSP 72 expression enhanced by H_2O_2 or heat stress [15]. A few years later Burch et al. showed a greater superoxide-induced proliferation of orbital fibroblasts from TED patients compared with control fibroblasts, suggesting that ROS may contribute to the abundant orbital fibroblast proliferation in TED [16]. Similarly, oxygen free radicals were shown to increase the IL-1β-induced GAG accumulation in retro-ocular fibroblasts from normal subjects and TED patients [17]. More recent studies confirmed a role of oxidative stress in the pathogenesis of TED, showing increased oxidative DNA damage, lipid peroxidation, and higher intracellular ROS in orbital fibroblasts from TED patients compared with controls [18–20].

Significant support for a pathogenic role of oxidative stress in TED has been found in human studies. Bednarek et al. studied 47 patients with recently diagnosed GD with and without active TED. Plasma concentrations of superoxide dismutases (SOD) and catalase, but not of GPXs and glutathione reductase, were increased in GD patients compared with healthy controls. Restoration of euthyroidism with methimazole led to normalization of all the above markers only in patients without TED, suggesting that orbital inflammation is related to the increased circulating markers of the oxidative status [21]. Similarly, urinary concentrations of 8-hydroxy-2′-deoxyguanosine (8-OHdG), a marker of oxidative DNA damage, were shown to be higher in patients with active TED compared to healthy controls. Furthermore, a significant decrease in 8-OHdG was observed during and after oral glucocorticoids administration and 8-OHdG urinary levels paralleled TED clinical activity and ophthalmopathy index scores. Interestingly, two patients in the study group experienced a relapse of TED (during or after glucocorticoid treatment), which was associated with an increase in urinary 8-OHdG [22]. The same authors examined the relationship between oxidative DNA damage, as evaluated by 8-OHdG urinary levels, and TED activity in an extended cohort of patients and found that the Clinical Activity Score (CAS) was significantly correlated with 8-OHdG levels. Smokers had higher levels of urinary 8-OHdG compared to nonsmoker TED patients.

Akarsu et al. recently investigated the relationship between oxidative stress and glucocorticoid treatment in patients with TED. They measured serum levels of malondialdehyde (MDA), another marker of the oxidative status, in a series of TED patients who underwent treatment with either iv or oral glucocorticoids, in GD patients without TED, and in healthy controls. MDA was significantly higher in TED patients compared to GD patients (without TED) and healthy controls. Moreover the MDA concentration correlated with the CAS and was significantly lower in TED patients treated with iv glucocorticoids compared with those untreated [23].

Taken together, these data support the notion that oxidative stress plays an important role in orbital inflammatory process in TED patients. Furthermore, human studies suggest that parameters of oxidative status might be used in clinical practice for evaluation of TED activity and as predictor of response to treatment and recurrence of the orbital disease.

Selenium in the Management of TED

The rationale for the use of selenium in the management of TED is based upon its antioxidant and immunomodulatory effects.

In 2000, a small pilot study reported encouraging results on the use of antioxidant treatment in patients with mild or moderately severe TED [24]. In this study, patients with newly diagnosed ophthalmopathy were treated for 3 months with oral allopurinol (300 mg/day) and nicotinamide (300 mg/day) or placebo. Improvement of TED was observed in 9 of 11 (82 %) patients treated with the antioxidant mixture and only in 3 of 11 (27 %) patients treated with placebo. Soft tissue involvement was the feature that improved the most in the active treatment group and no side effects of the antioxidant treatment were reported [24].

Recently, the European Group on Graves' Orbitopathy (EUGOGO; http://www.eugogo.eu) reported the results of a randomized, double-blind, placebo-controlled trial on the effect of selenium supplementation in patients with mild TED [25].

The study included 159 patients with recent onset TED (less than 18 months). Other inclusion criteria were as follows: (a) at least one sign of mild TED (e.g., NO SPECS class 2 soft tissue swelling [26]), according to the Color Atlas edited by EUGOGO (http://www.eugogo.eu); (b) euthyroidism (whether due to methimazole treatment, disease remission, or status post RAI or thyroidectomy); (c) no previous treatment for TED, except for supportive measures. Patients were assigned to one of the following treatments: selenium (sodium selenite 100 μg twice daily, for a total of 91.3 μg daily), pentoxifylline (600 mg twice daily), or placebo (twice daily). Treatment was given for 6 months, followed by a 6-month monitoring period.

Patients were evaluated at baseline and after 3, 6, and 12 months. The treating physicians were unaware of the treatment received by the patient. Quality of life (QoL) was evaluated at each visit using a disease-specific questionnaire (GO-QoL), available on http://www.eugogo.eu [27, 28]. Thyroid function and antithyroid antibodies were checked at each visit. Side effects from medication received were recorded at each visit.

Ophthalmologic assessment included eyelid aperture (measured in mm); soft tissue involvement (according to the Color Atlas, available on http://www.eugogo.eu); proptosis (measured in mm using the same exophthalmometer); extraocular muscle involvement (evaluated by the extent of ductions in degrees); and visual acuity (in decimals using the Snellen chart). In addition, the CAS and the Gorman's diplopia score were recorded. The CAS is calculated giving 1 point to each of the following symptoms and/or signs: spontaneous retro-ocular pain, pain on attempted eye movement, redness of the conjunctiva, redness of the eyelids, chemosis, swelling of the caruncle, and swelling of the eyelids [29]. The Gorman's score is a subjective diplopia assessment that consists of four categories: (a) no diplopia (absent); (b) diplopia when tired or when first awakening (intermittent); (c) diplopia at extremes of gaze (inconstant); (d) continuous diplopia in primary or reading position (constant) [30].

The primary end points of the study were changes in the eye findings at 6 months, performed by a blinded ophthalmologist; and changes in quality of life, assessed with GO-QoL questionnaires filled out by the patient at each visit. The evaluation criteria are reported in Table 6.1. Secondary outcomes of the study were variations in the CAS and diplopia (according to the Gorman Score).

Table 6.1 Evaluation of primary outcomes in patients with mild thyroid eye disease (TED) treated with selenium or placebo

Overall ophthalmic outcome
1. *Improvement* in one eye of at least one of the following measures, without worsening in any of these measures in either eye
(a) Eyelid aperture reduction by at least 2 mm
(b) Improvement by at least one grade in the NOSPECS classification for Class 2 signs [26]
(c) Exophthalmos reduction by at least 2 mm
(d) Ocular motility improvement by at least 8° in any duction
2. Worsening, if any of the following occurred
(a) Worsening by at least one grade in any of the NOSPECS classes [26]
(b) Appearance of a new NOSPECS class [26]
(c) Any sign of optic nerve involvement: decrease in visual acuity by at least one line on the Snellen chart, impaired color vision, presence of a relative afferent pupillary defect, or other concern for optic nerve compression
TED-specific Quality of Life (GO-QoL) questionnaire
1. *Improvement*, when an increase of six or more points on either one (or both) the GO-QoL scales (functioning and appearance) occurred[a]
2. Worsening, when a decrease of six points on any one of the two scales occurred[b]

[a]GO-QoL questionnaire measures health-related quality of life of patients with Graves' orbitopathy [30]. It quantifies limitations in visual functioning as a consequence of decreased visual acuity and/or diplopia (eight questions), and limitations in psychosocial functioning as a consequence of a changed appearance (eight questions)

[b]A change of at least six points on one or both GO-QoL subscales was considered as an important change in daily functioning for TED patients [27]. This cut-off value was derived from a previous study in which the minimal clinically important difference (MCID), defined as the smallest difference in score on the domain of interest which patients perceive as benefit and which would mandate, in the absence of troublesome side effects and costs, a change in the patient's management in either GO-QoL subscales appeared to be six points

The overall ophthalmologic outcome at the end of the treatment (6 months) was significantly better in the selenium group compared to the placebo group ($P=0.01$) (Fig. 6.1). TED improved in 61 % of patients in the selenium group and in 36 % of patients in the placebo group and worsened in 7 % of the former and in 26 % of the latter group. The ophthalmologic outcome was similar when patients were evaluated 6 months after treatment withdrawal, indicating the persistence of the beneficial effect of selenium beyond the active treatment period (Fig. 6.1). Soft tissue involvement and eyelid aperture were the major determinants of the more favorable outcome in the selenium group (Fig. 6.2). Proptosis and ocular motility did not change; however very few patients had motility impairment at start of study (data not shown).

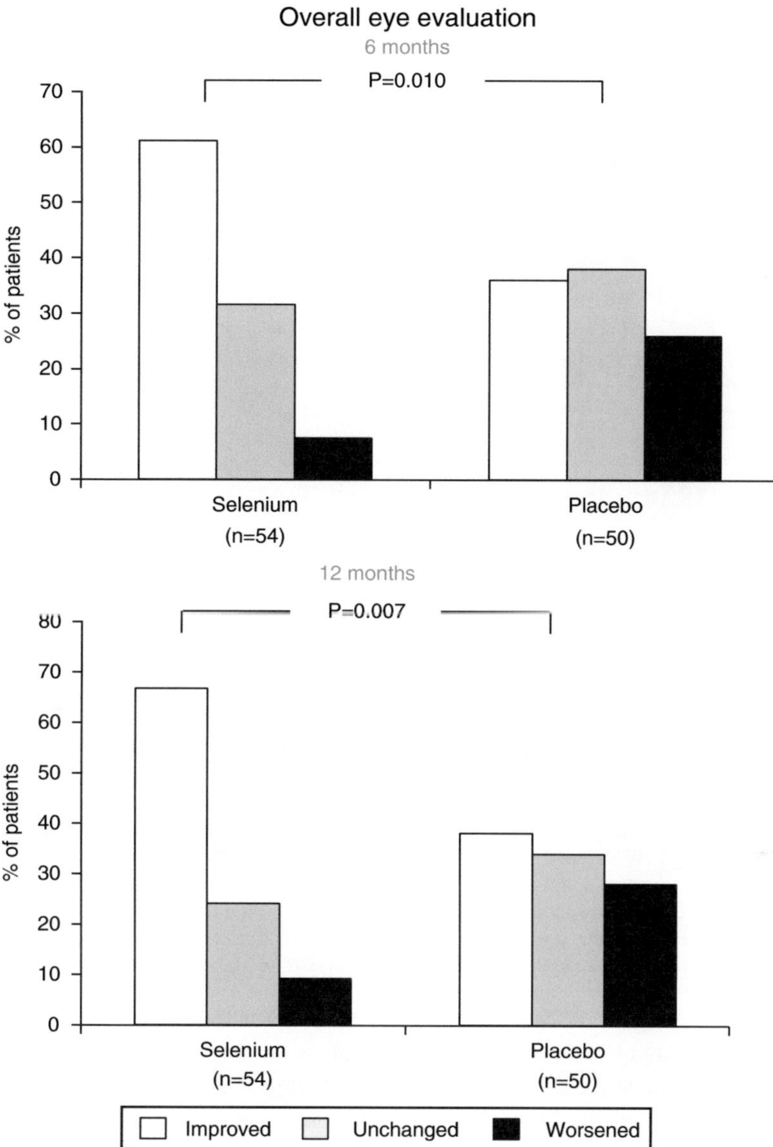

Fig. 6.1 Overall eye evaluation at 6 and 12 months in patients with mild TED treated with selenium (100 μg twice daily) or placebo (twice daily). Ophthalmologic outcomes were scored as improved, unchanged, or worsened according to the criteria reported in Table 6.1 (derived from data of Marcocci et al. [25]). *P* values were calculated using the X^2 test

The GO-QoL includes a "visual functioning" score and an "appearance" score. Baseline GO-QoL showed a mild to moderate impairment in quality of life with no differences between the two groups of patients. After 6 months of treatment, a greater proportion of patients receiving selenium showed an improvement of visual functioning (33/53, 62 %) and appearance (40/53, 75 %) scores compared with those treated with placebo. This better outcome in patients treated with selenium was confirmed by the overall GO-QoL evaluation, which includes changes in both subscales (Fig. 6.3).

The CAS improved after 6 and 12 months in all patients (Fig. 6.4). However, the reduction of CAS in selenium supplemented patients was

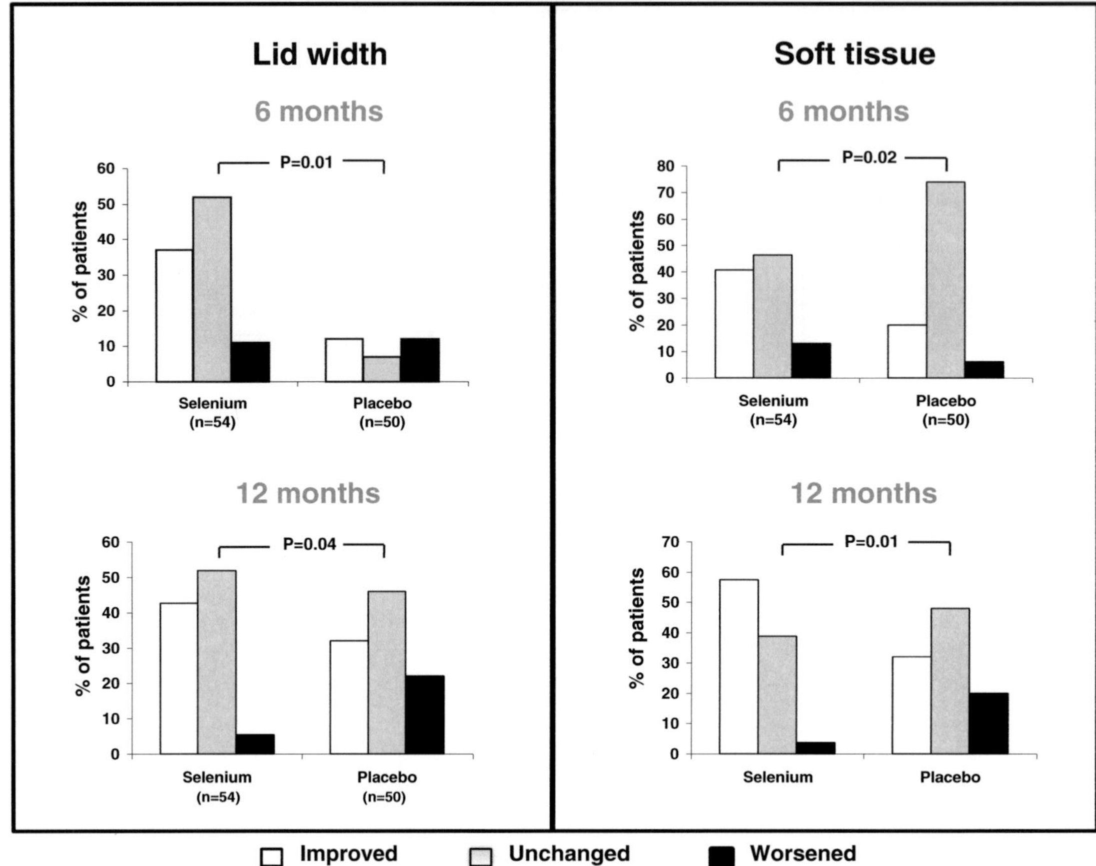

Fig. 6.2 Changes in lid aperture and soft tissue at 6- and 12-month evaluation, in TED patients treated with selenium and placebo. Changes were scored according to criteria reported in Table 6.1, as improved, unchanged, or worsened. X^2 test was used to calculate P values (derived from data of Marcocci et al. [25])

significantly greater compared to the placebo group ($p<0.001$). Diplopia score did not change significantly in any group during the study (data not shown).

No drug-related adverse effects were recorded.

In summary, this study reported a beneficial effect of selenium treatment in patients with mild TED both in terms of quality of life and ocular involvement. It supports the hypothesis that an intervention aimed at restoring the balance of the antioxidant/oxidant status could help patients with mild TED [25].

Two potential limitations of this study were the lack of information regarding the changes of serum selenium concentration after selenium selenite treatment and, secondly, the inclusion of patients coming from areas of marginal selenium deficiency. Therefore, further studies should be performed in selenium-sufficient areas in order to prove a beneficial effect of selenium supplementation in non-selenium-deplete patients.

Despite these limitations, selenium supplementation appears to reduce the severity of TED signs and symptoms in a selenium-deficient population. Whether this effect may also be seen with additional antioxidant supplements remains to be seen.

Some concerns on the safety of selenium supplementation have been raised particularly for patients living in selenium-sufficient areas. The Nutritional Prevention of Cancer trial, performed in the United States, reported a potential risk of

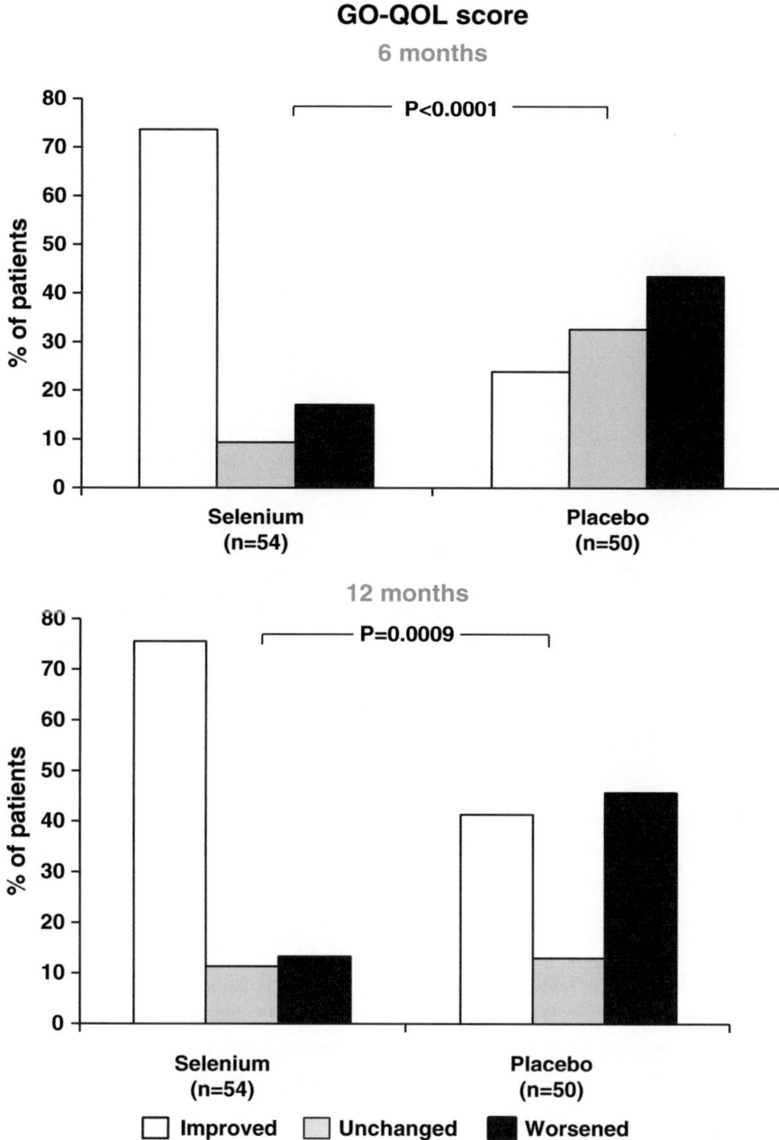

Fig. 6.3 Changes of GO-QoL at 6 and 12 months in patients with mild TED randomly assigned to treatment with selenium or placebo. Changes of QoL were scored as improved, unchanged, or worsened according to predefined criteria (Table 6.1). *P* values were calculated with the X^2 test (derived from data of Marcocci et al. [25])

developing type 2 diabetes in patients supplemented with 200 μg selenium daily for up to 12 years [8]. Assessment of diabetes was the secondary end point of the study and diabetes occurrence was self-reported. The study showed an increased incidence of diabetes in patients supplemented with selenium compared with those given placebo; the development of diabetes correlated with higher serum selenium concentration [8].

Population studies on serum selenium levels and diabetes have provided conflicting results. A National Health and Nutrition Examination Survey, designed to evaluate the association of serum selenium concentration and type 2 diabetes in US population, found a higher prevalence of diabetes in patients with high serum selenium levels [31]. On the other hand, a study performed in the elderly French population found

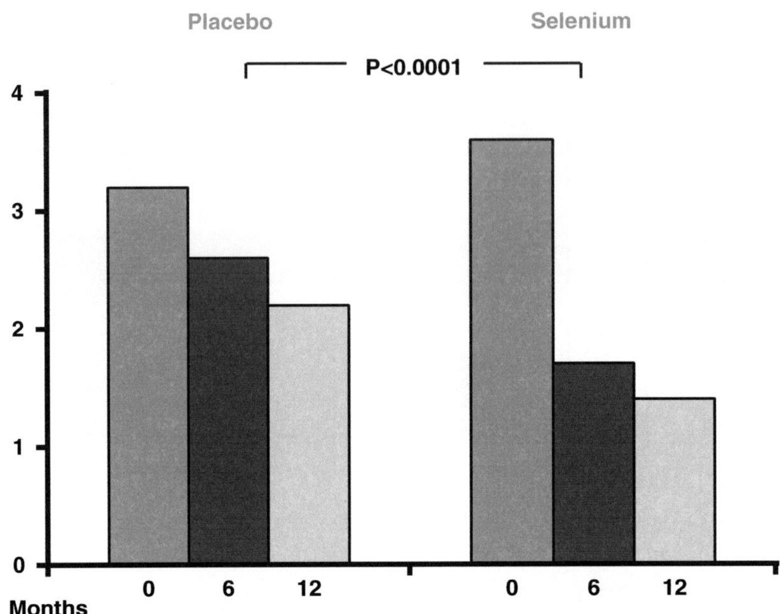

Fig. 6.4 Clinical Activity Score (CAS) evaluation at 6- and 12-month in patients supplemented with selenium or placebo. The Mann–Whitney test was used to calculate the *P* value (derived from data of Marcocci et al. [25])

a sex-specific (male) protective effect of higher selenium levels on the occurrence of dysglycemia [32]. An association of selenium supplementation with glaucoma has also been reported [33].

Patients included in our study originated from moderately selenium-deficient areas and were supplemented with a relatively low dose of sodium selenite (equivalent to 91.3 μg of selenium) for 6 months. Blood sugar was not routinely measured, but no significant changes of glycemia were observed in a subgroup of patients enrolled in Greece over the 6-month treatment. No cases of glaucoma were found in the selenium-treated cohort. Thus, it is reasonable to conclude that a 6-month selenium supplementation in selenium-deficient areas is a safe and beneficial treatment option in patients with mild TED [25].

Concluding Remarks

Due to the lack of safe and well-tolerated treatments, patients with mild TED represent a challenge for the endocrinologist and ophthalmologist caring for them. Recent studies on the use of antioxidant supplements, such as selenium, have opened the possibility of a new therapeutic tool in TED. A 6-month course of selenium supplementation has been shown to result in improvement of quality of life, amelioration of eye signs and symptoms, and prevention of worsening TED. Thus, we believe that a 6-month course of selenium supplementation should be offered to all patients with mild TED together with supportive measures. Further studies are needed to evaluate the benefit of selenium treatment in patients with more severe TED, and of antioxidants the potential role of antioxidants in preventing the new onset or worsening of TED in high-risk patients.

References

1. Bartalena L, Pinchera A, Marcocci C. Management of Graves' ophthalmopathy: reality and perspectives. Endocr Rev. 2000;21(2):168–99.
2. Bartalena L, Baldeschi L, Dickinson A, Eckstein A, et al.; European Group on Graves' Orbitopathy (EUGOGO). Consensus statement of the European Group on Graves' orbitopathy (EUGOGO) on

management of GO. Eur J Endocrinol. 2008;158(3): 273–85.
3. Marcocci C, Marinò M. Treatment of mild, moderate-to-severe and very severe Graves' orbitopathy. Best Pract Res Clin Endocrinol Metab. 2012;26(3):325–37.
4. Menconi F, Profilo MA, Leo M, Sisti E, et al. Spontaneous improvement of untreated mild Graves' ophthalmopathy: the rundle curve revisited. Thyroid. 2014;24(1):60–6.
5. Drutel A, Archambeaud F, Caron P. Selenium and the thyroid gland. Clin Endocrinol (Oxf). 2013;78:155–64.
6. Rayman MP. Selenium and human health. Lancet. 2012;379:1256–68.
7. Duntas LH. Selenium and the thyroid: a close-knit connection. J Clin Endocrinol Metab. 2010;95(12):5180–8.
8. Stranges S, Marshall JR, Natarjan R, et al. Effects of long term supplementation on the incidence of type 2 diabetes: a randomized trial. Ann Intern Med. 2007; 147:217–23.
9. Rayman MP. The importance of selenium to human health. Lancet. 2000;356:233–41.
10. Hoffmann PR, Berry MJ. The influence of selenium on immune responses. Mol Nutr Food Res. 2008;52: 1273–80.
11. Marcocci C, Leo M, Altea MA. Oxidative stress in Graves' disease. Eur Thyroid J. 2012;2:80–7.
12. Bahn RS. Graves' ophthalmopathy. N Engl J Med. 2010;362:726–38.
13. Bartalena L, Tanda ML, Piantanida E, Lai A. Oxidative stress and Graves' ophthalmopathy: in vitro studies and therapeutic implications. Biofactors. 2003;19:155–63.
14. Heufelder AE, Wenzel BE, Bahn RS. Enhanced induction of a 72 kDa heat shock protein in cultured retroocular fibroblasts. Invest Ophthalmol Vis Sci. 1992;33(2):466–70.
15. Heufelder AE, Wenzel BE, Bahn RS. Methimazole and propylthiouracil inhibit the oxygen free radical-induced expression of a 72 kilodalton heat shock protein in Graves' retroocular fibroblasts. J Clin Endocrinol Metab. 1992;74(4):737–42.
16. Burch HB, Lahiri S, Bahn RS, Barnes S. Superoxide radical production stimulates retroocular fibroblast proliferation in Graves' ophthalmopathy. Exp Eye Res. 1997;65:311–6.
17. Lu R, Wang P, Wartofsky L, Sutton BD, Zweier JL, Bahn RS, Garrity J, Burman KD. Oxygen free radicals in interleukin-1beta-induced glycosaminoglycan production by retro-ocular fibroblasts from normal subjects and Graves' ophthalmopathy patients. Thyroid. 1999;9(3):297–303.
18. Hondur A, Konuk O, Dincel AS, Bilgihan A, Unal M, Hasanreisoglu B. Oxidative stress and antioxidant activity in orbital fibroadipose tissue in Graves' ophthalmopathy. Curr Eye Res. 2008;33:421–7.
19. Tsai CC, Wu SB, Cheng CY, Kao SC, Kau HC, Chiou SH, Hsu WM, Wei YH. Increased oxidative DNA damage, lipid peroxidation, and reactive oxygen species in cultured orbital fibroblasts from patients with Graves' ophthalmopathy: evidence that oxidative stress has a role in this disorder. Eye (Lond). 2010;24:1520–5.
20. Tsai CC, Wu SB, Cheng CY, Kao SC, Kau HC, Lee SM, Wei YH. Increased response to oxidative stress challenge in Graves' ophthalmopathy orbital fibroblasts. Mol Vis. 2011;17:2782–8.
21. Bednarek J, Wysocki H, Sowiński J. Oxidative stress peripheral parameters in Graves' disease: the effect of methimazole treatment in patients with and without infiltrative ophthalmopathy. Clin Biochem. 2005;38(1):13–8.
22. Tsai CC, Kao SC, Cheng CY, Kau HC, Hsu WM, Lee CF, Wei YH. Oxidative stress change by systemic corticosteroid treatment among patients having active graves ophthalmopathy. Arch Ophthalmol. 2007;125(12):1652–6.
23. Akarsu E, Buyukhatipoglu H, Aktaran S, Kurtul N. Effects of pulse methylprednisolone and oral methylprednisolone treatments on serum levels of oxidative stress markers in Graves' ophthalmopathy. Clin Endocrinol (Oxf). 2011;74(1):118–24.
24. Bouzas EA, Karadimas P, Mastorakos G, Koutras DA. Antioxidant agents in the treatment of Graves' ophthalmopathy. Am J Ophthalmol. 2000;129:618–22.
25. Marcocci C, Kahaly GJ, Krassas GE, Bartalena L, et al.; European Group on Graves' Orbitopathy. Selenium and the course of mild Graves' orbitopathy. N Engl J Med. 2011;364:1920–31.
26. Werner SC. Modification of the classification of the eye changes of Graves' disease: recommendation of the Ad Hoc Committee of the American Thyroid Association. J Clin Endocrinol Metab. 1977;44: 203–4.
27. Terwee CB, Gerding MN, Dekker FW, Prummel MF, Wiersinga WM. Development of a disease specific quality of life questionnaire for patients with Graves' ophthalmopathy: the GO-QOL. Br J Ophthalmol. 1998;82:773–9.
28. Terwee CB, Dekker FW, Mourits MP. Interpretation and validity of changes in scores on the Graves' ophthalmopathy quality of life questionnaire (GO-QOL) after different treatments. Clin Endocrinol (Oxf). 2001;54:391–8.
29. Mourits MP, Prummel MF, Wiersinga WM, Koornneef L. Clinical activity score as a guide in the management of patients with Graves' ophthalmopathy. Clin Endocrinol (Oxf). 1997;47:9–14.
30. Bahn RS, Gorman CA. Choice of therapy and criteria for assessing treatment outcome in thyroid-associated ophthalmopathy. Endocrinol Metab Clin North Am. 1987;16:391–407.
31. Bleys J, Navas-Acien A, Guallar E. Serum selenium and diabetes in U.S. adults. Diabetes Care. 2007;30: 829–34.
32. Akbaraly TN, Arnaud J, Rayman MP, Hininger-Favier I, Roussel AM, Berr C, Fontbonne A. Plasma selenium and risk of dysglycemia in an elderly French population: results from the prospective Epidemiology of Vascular Ageing Study. Nutr Metab (Lond). 2010;7:21.
33. Sheck L, Davies J, Wilson G. Selenium and ocular health in New Zealand. N Z Med J. 2010;123:85–94.

7 Pregnancy and Childhood Thyroid Eye Disease

Andrew G. Gianoukakis, Teeranun Jirajariyavej, Rebecca A. Hicks, and Jennifer K. Yee

Thyroid eye disease (TED) occurs infrequently during pregnancy and childhood. However, pregnancy and childhood are periods of tolerance formation and immune system development. During this time, the host immune system may uniquely alter the disease presentation and course of autoimmune diseases such as Graves' disease (GD) and TED.

Pregnancy and Thyroid Eye Disease

Autoimmune Disease and Pregnancy

T and B cells recognize self or foreign antigens presented on the cell surface of antigen presenting cells by a major histocompatibility complex (MHC) molecule called human leukocyte antigen (HLA). Autoimmune diseases involve an immune reaction to self-antigens possibly due to defects in T and/or B cell selection or regulation. This phenomenon may be selective to certain organs or specific tissues [1].

During pregnancy, the maternal immune system skews toward an immune tolerant state in order to host the fetus [1, 2]. Multiple adaptive mechanisms are invoked to achieve peripheral tolerance, including clearance of fetal reactive cells and inhibition of immunoreactive pathways (inflammatory cytokine and chemokine pathways as well as the complement system) [1]. Amelioration of autoimmune disease such as GD and rheumatoid arthritis (RA) is often observed during pregnancy [1, 3]; other autoimmune diseases such as systemic lupus erythematosus (SLE) can exhibit an unpredictable course, with disease remaining stable or deteriorating during pregnancy [1]. In the postpartum period, the maternal immune system "reverts" to normal. As relative maternal immune tolerance subsides, postpartum exacerbation or the de novo appearance of autoimmune disease is commonly noted [2].

One proposed pathogenic mechanism for autoimmune disease in pregnancy is fetal–maternal microchimerism. This is a phenomenon by which cells from the fetus traverse the placenta, enter the maternal circulation, and establish cell lineages within the mother [4]. Microchimerism refers to the harboring of small numbers of cells

A.G. Gianoukakis, M.D. (✉)
Department of Medicine, Division of Endocrinology and Metabolism, Harbor-UCLA Medical Center, 1124 West Carson St., RB-1, Torrance, CA 90502, USA
e-mail: agianouk@ucla.edu

T. Jirajariyavej, M.D.
Department of Medicine, Division of Endocrinology and Metabolism, Harbor-UCLA Medical Center, 1000 W. Carson St., Box 446, Torrance, CA 90508-0446, USA

R.A. Hicks, M.D. • J.K. Yee, M.D.
Department of Pediatrics, Division of Endocrinology and Metabolism, Harbor-UCLA Medical Center, 1124 West Carson St., RB-1, Box 446, Torrance, CA 90502, USA

R.S. Douglas et al. (eds.), *Thyroid Eye Disease*,
DOI 10.1007/978-1-4939-1746-4_7, © Springer Science+Business Media New York 2015

that originate from a genetically different individual, in this case, the fetus. Male fetal–maternal microchimerism is evident when cells harboring a Y chromosome are detected in women with a previous male pregnancy. Methods used to detect fetal cells in the maternal circulation include quantitative PCR or fluorescence in situ hybridization (FISH) [1, 4]. Fetal–maternal microchimerism was found to occur commonly in pregnancy, with the number of fetal microchimeric cells increasing as pregnancy progresses, peaking at time of delivery and decreasing in the postpartum period [4, 5]. The association of fetal microchimerism with autoimmunity is suggested by the accumulation of fetal cells at maternal sites often involved in autoimmunity such as the thyroid, skin, and pancreas [6]. Microchimeric cells can persist in the maternal blood and tissues for decades. Whether such cells of fetal origin can represent the target of an immune response in the mother as immune tolerance subsides in the postpartum period remains a topic of interest and investigation [7].

Several studies have linked fetal microchimerism to autoimmune thyroid disease (ATD). In ATD, fetal microchimeric cells of male fetal origin have been detected with greater frequency in the thyroid gland of women with Hashimoto's thyroiditis (HT) and GD compared to those without ATD [4]. In particular, Klintschar et al. showed that microchimerism was detected in 8 of 17 cases (47 %) of HT but only 1 of 25 cases (4 %) of nodular goiter [8]. Further investigation using quantitative real-time PCR detected microchimeric cells in 8 of 21 cases (38 %) of HT (ranging from 15 to 4,900/100,000 cells), versus in 1 of 18 cases (5.5 %) of nodular goiters and none of 17 healthy thyroid glands (Fig. 7.1) [9]. These differences in prevalence of microchimerism among patients with ATD compared to nodular goiter or healthy controls reached statistical significance ($p<0.01$, Fisher's exact test). Another study analyzing immunohistology of paraffin-embedded thyroid specimens taken at surgery (from 25 HT, 15 GD, and 9 nodular goiter patients), detected Y-chromosome-specific staining more frequently in HT (60 %) and GD (40 %) compared to follicular adenoma (22.2 %) [10]. Differences between groups in the latter study did not reach statistical significance. Furthermore, a large community-based study found no association between parity and the presence of thyroid autoantibodies and suggested a lesser role of fetal microchimerism in autoimmunity [11].

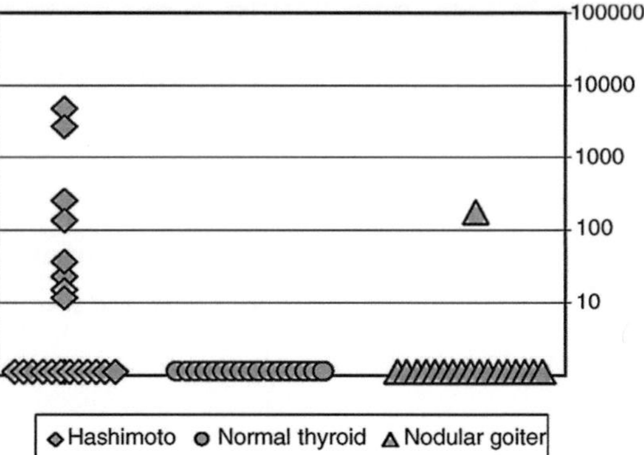

Fig. 7.1 Number of male genomes detected per 100,000 female genomes in the thyroid of women with Hashimoto's thyroiditis, nodular goiter, and normal thyroid [9]. Reprinted with permission from Bioscientifica Ltd.

Maternal autoimmune responses may also target the fetus when autoantibodies cross the placenta, as evidenced by transplacental transfer of maternal thyroid autoantibodies to the TSH receptor (TRAbs) in some infants born to mothers with GD (see section "Neonatal Thyrotoxicosis ("Neonatal Graves' Disease")"). Typically, neonatal thyrotoxicosis occurs in the first few days of life and can last up to 4 months, by which time the maternal antibodies are cleared from the infant's circulation [12].

Graves' Disease in Pregnancy and Postpartum

Hyperthyroidism occurs in 0.1–0.4 % of pregnancies [13]. Autoimmune thyroid dysfunction represents the most common cause of hyperthyroidism in pregnancy [14, 15]. While GD accounts for 80 % of these cases and the majority were present prior to pregnancy, GD can rarely develop de novo during pregnancy [16, 17]. The hyperthyroidism of GD is caused by thyroid stimulating immunoglobulins (TSI) binding and activating the TSH receptor, and inducing excess synthesis and secretion of thyroid hormone [17, 18].

The clinical presentation of GD in pregnancy and postpartum is similar to the general adult population. Classic clinical manifestations include diffuse goiter, anxiety, palpitations, tremor, heat intolerance, and thyroid associated manifestations such as ophthalmopathy and dermopathy. Multiple thyroid autoantibodies target the thyroid epithelial cell TSH receptor. Patients with GD can produce activating (TSI), blocking (TBIIs), and neutral thyroid receptor autoantibodies (TRAbs). The interplay of these autoantibodies during the immune tolerance of pregnancy is complex.

During pregnancy, the differential diagnosis of hyperthyroidism in the majority of cases involves distinguishing between GD and gestational hyperthyroidism, which is limited to the first half of pregnancy. Both entities are characterized by elevated free T4 (FT4) and suppressed serum TSH levels. The presence of serum markers of thyroid autoimmunity (TSI, thyroid autoantibodies) can help distinguish between these two diagnoses.

In the postpartum period, new onset GD should be distinguished from postpartum and subacute thyroiditis. New onset postpartum GD occurs 20-fold less commonly than postpartum thyroiditis [19]. The majority of cases of postpartum GD (95 %) exhibit serum positivity for TRAbs [20]. The presence of ophthalmopathy can also help to distinguish postpartum GD from postpartum thyroiditis.

Although exacerbations of GD early in pregnancy are sometimes observed, the disease most often abates after the first trimester. TRAbs are present in over 95 % of patients with active GD and high titers may remain following radioiodine treatment [21]. Pregnancy is associated with a decrease in thyroid autoantibody titers [14, 22] with TRAbs appearing to reach their lowest levels during the third trimester (Fig. 7.2) [23, 24]. A number of studies have examined changes in TRAbs [23–25] and other antithyroid antibodies [26] during pregnancy. Kamijo studied changes in TRAb levels during pregnancy, using four different methods of detection [24]. The author was able to demonstrate a significant decrease in TRAb titers as pregnancy progressed [24]. Similarly, Gonzalez-Jimenez et al. reported that TRAb levels decreased significantly ($p < 0.01$) during pregnancy in active GD patients [23]. However Tamaki et al. demonstrated that TRAb levels do not always decline during pregnancy in active GD [25]. The immune tolerance of pregnancy is believed to play a role in the decrease of thyroid autoantibody titers, including anti-peroxidase antibodies (anti-TPOAb), thyroglobulin autoantibodies (Anti-TgAb), and TRAbs. The decline of autoantibody levels is

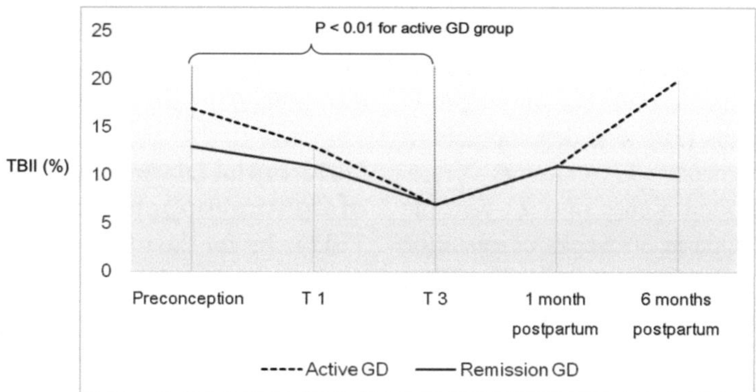

Fig. 7.2 TBII levels nadir in the third trimester of pregnancy. Preconception, first trimester (T1), third trimester (T3), early (1 month) and late (6 months) postpartum levels in pregnant women with active-GD and remission-GD are shown. There was a statistically significant decrease in mean levels from preconception (17 %) to third trimester (7 %) in the active GD group ($p < 0.01$). Adapted from [23]

anticipated to begin by approximately 20 weeks of gestation. Persistence of maternal TRAbs is important as they have the potential to impact the fetal and neonatal thyroidal status. As noted above, maternal antithyroid antibodies may cross the placenta, particularly when they remain at high levels after week 25. The transfer of stimulatory or inhibitory TRAbs to the fetus may lead to a transient fetal and neonatal hyper- or hypothyroidism.

The American Thyroid Association recommends a determination of serum TRAbs by 24–28 weeks gestation in the following cases:

- Pregnant women with active hyperthyroidism
- Previous history of radioiodine treatment
- Previous history of delivering an infant with hyperthyroidism
- Total thyroidectomy treatment of hyperthyroidism in pregnancy

This recommendation intends to identify pregnancies at risk of maternal–fetal transfer of antithyroid autoantibodies. A TRAb value over three times the upper limit of normal is an indication for close monitoring of the fetus. High TRAb titers between 22 and 26 weeks of gestation represent a risk factor for fetal or neonatal hyperthyroidism [21].

Thyroid Eye Disease in Pregnancy

TED is responsible for approximately 50 % of orbital disorders in the general population [27], and is characterized by inflammation, edema, secondary fibrosis, and extra-ocular muscle involvement. This classic presentation is seen in 70 % of TED patients [28]. The development of TED during pregnancy is extremely rare. Germain et al. reported a case of a 23-year-old euthyroid primigravida at 30 weeks of gestation who developed severe sight-threatening TED. Functionally active TRAbs were demonstrated using a cyclic adenosine monophosphate (cAMP) biological assay [29].

The rare occurrence of worsening TED and the rare development of new onset TED in pregnancy is attributed to the immune tolerant state and decreasing TRAb levels [2].

Studies of TED During Pregnancy and Postpartum

TED progression in pregnancy is rare and to our knowledge, there are no published studies of TED during pregnancy and the postpartum period. Only a very limited number of cases have been reported [29–32]. The severity of TED in the adult ranges from mild to severe, with only 5 % considered severe [33]. Data on prevalence or severity of TED in pregnancy are not available. The peak female age distribution of TED is from 40s to 60s, representing the post-reproductive age [34]. One case report of severe TED in pregnancy described a 22-year-old primigravida, who presented at 30 weeks of gestation with progressive worsening of vision and swollen eyes over a period of 2 months. The patient had been diagnosed with GD 3 years prior and had been treated with radioiodine and rendered euthyroid after the treatment. Physical examination revealed marked bilateral periorbital edema, exophthalmos, limitation of left abduction, decreased visual acuity, and dyschromatopsia bilaterally. Her thyroid function tests were within normal range and TSI = 434 % (normal < 130 %) were detected. On brain CT, bilateral optic nerve compression was suspected. The patient was treated with high-dose steroids, methylprednisolone 300 mg twice daily, without significant improvement. The concern for permanent nerve damage secondary to optic nerve compression prompted surgical orbital wall decompression within 3 days of admission. Steroid therapy was continued and tapered postoperatively. In follow-up, the patient demonstrated improvement of visual acuity, proptosis, lid lag, as well as color discrimination [30].

Differential Diagnosis of Ophthalmopathy in Pregnancy

TED is by far the most common cause of extra-ocular muscle enlargement in adults [27]. As in any adult, other causes of ophthalmopathy should be considered and excluded before diagnosing TED in pregnancy (Table 7.1). The differential diagnosis of TED in pregnancy includes myasthenia gravis (MG), retro-ocular tumors, carotid-cavernous fistula, and other inflammatory ophthalmopathies.

Table 7.1 Differential diagnosis of TED in pregnancy

Diagnosis	Clinical manifestations
TED	Usually bilateral and associated with hyperthyroidism MRI: Orbital fat and extraocular muscle involvement with tendon sparing
Ocular Myasthenia Gravis	Weakness usually involves one or more ocular muscles without overt pupillary abnormality. Ptosis which shifts from one eye to the other is virtually pathognomonic of Myasthenia Gravis
Orbital inflammation of muscle (orbital myositis or orbital pseudotumor)	Clinical diagnosis is made by exclusion of other conditions. Unilateral disease is very common but bilateral presentations are not uncommon, especially in children. Symptoms usually acute in onset with proptosis and inflammatory sign such as pain, swelling, and erythema CT scan: Moderately enhanced focal or diffuse mass frequently accompanied by infiltration of orbital fat MRI: Proptosis, optic nerve thickening, uveal-scleral thickening, lacrimal gland infiltration, and extraocular muscle involvement with muscle tendon and sheath enlargement can differentiate this diagnosis from TED
Carotid-cavernous fistula	History: Preceding trauma and surgical manipulations, recent childbirth or pregnancy. The onset is rapid with pulsating exophthalmos, ocular bruit, diplopia, headache, conjunctival chemosis, increased intraocular pressure, and a reduction in vision CT scan: Enlargement of the superior ophthalmic vein and to a lesser extent, enlargement of extraocular muscles
Orbital lymphoid tumor	Orbit, lacrimal glands, eyelids, or conjunctiva can be affected. Most often presents as a (1) nontender, firm, subcutaneous mass in the anterior orbit; (2) conjunctival salmon-patch infiltrate; or (3) eyelid infiltration
Orbital cellulitis	Should be suspected in any pregnant patient with a preceding history of upper respiratory tract infection, trauma, dental infection, or dental procedure. Commonly presents with fever, malaise, and pain with eye movement. CT scan: preseptal cellulitis appears as an area of hyper-attenuation with swelling of anterior orbital tissues and obliteration of adjacent fat planes. MRI: hypointense on T1-weighted, hyperintense on T2-weighted images

MG is important to consider in the differential because of the overlapping patient demographics and clinical findings with TED. Women are affected by MG nearly three times more often than men before age 40, but the incidence is higher in males after age 50, and roughly equal in men and women during puberty [35]. MG usually affects women in their third decade of life. Pregnancy is considered a precipitating factor for MG. Although the disease course is variable, pregnant patients face risk of exacerbation, respiratory failure, adverse drug response, crisis, and death. A study by Batocchi et al. reported that MG worsened in 10 (19 %) of 54 patients followed during pregnancy. Approximately 60 % of exacerbations occurred during the first trimester, and approximately 28 % of patients deteriorated immediately after delivery [36]. Thyroid disorders also represent an exacerbating factor for MG. The clinical presentation of MG associated with ATD is frequently limited to double vision [37]. Diplopia, intermittent ptosis, and incomplete eyelid closure are the most common presenting symptoms occurring in approximately 85 % of patients with MG [38]. The symptoms are a result of the involvement of extraocular muscles, levator, and orbicularis oculi in MG. Symptoms can fluctuate in severity, worsening with exertion, and improving with rest. Fatigue upon exertion is essential to making the diagnosis and differentiating MG from TED. Gaze-evoked nystagmus and Cogan's lid twitch represent clinical signs characteristic of MG. Ptosis and/or exotropia are rarely seen in TED. If ptosis, exotropia, or weakness of the orbicularis oculi muscle develops in a patient with TED, coincidence of MG should be considered.

Due to the trophic factors elaborated in pregnancy, orbital tumors such as lymphoid tumors, cavernous hemangiomas, and meningiomas can proliferate and become manifest during pregnancy. Any of these can present like TED.

Carotid-cavernous fistula is an abnormal communication between the internal and external carotid arteries in the cavernous sinus and represents a rare cause of exophthalmos in the adult, which can also manifest in pregnancy. Pertinent histories include recent trauma, surgical manipulations as well as pregnancy or recent childbirth. Patients could present with increasing proptosis, conjunctival chemosis, ocular pulsation, and progressive vision loss [27].

Orbital cellulitis can also masquerade as TED during pregnancy. Patients may present with proptosis, double vision, fever, malaise, and pain with eye movement. Orbital cellulitis should be suspected in any pregnant patient with a preceding history of upper respiratory tract infection, trauma, dental infection, or dental procedure. A thorough history and physical examination are crucial in establishing the diagnosis [27].

Therapeutic Options for TED During Pregnancy

The majority of GD patients exhibit mild and nonprogressive ocular involvement that tends to improve spontaneously [39]. Therefore, most TED pregnant patients would be expected to require only local measures for symptomatic relief.

For the rare case of severe TED that does not improve during pregnancy, more aggressive medical, and possibly surgical, therapy may be indicated. As noted elsewhere, the severity and activity of TED are not synonymous, but both are important in the assessment of TED patients including those who are pregnant. Similar to the nonpregnant adult, patients with active eye disease during pregnancy are expected to respond to medical treatment, whereas surgical treatment is indicated for the rare case of unresponsive, sight-threatening TED.

It is necessary to identify patients with sight-threatening TED, including compressive optic neuropathy (CON), corneal breakdown, or occasionally, globe subluxation [40, 41]. This group of patients must be treated urgently and aggressively [34, 42], and treatment should not be delayed on account of pregnancy. The optimal initial treatment for CON is high-dose systemic steroids (see medical management below). Suboptimal response to steroids is an indication for surgical decompression.

The Therapeutic Interventions for TED During Pregnancy Include

Local Measures

Eye shades/sunglasses help alleviate photophobia and shield the eyes from dust and wind. Saline artificial tears can alleviate foreign body sensation, dry eyes, and the gritty sensation. Raising the head of the bed at night may be of some help to reduce periorbital edema in addition to diuretics. Elimination of controllable risk factors for TED progression such as smoking is critical, not only for the benefit of TED but also for the pregnancy. Nocturnal taping of the eyes can be helpful when lagophthalmos is present and prisms can be used to improve cases of mild diplopia. Understanding the natural history of the disease and providing reassurance is one of the most important therapeutic measures since the chance of progression of TED to more severe forms is very low [40]. All the above supportive measures can be safely implemented during pregnancy. Diuretic use to decrease swelling is debatable for routine treatment of TED.

Medical Therapy

Both hyper- and hypothyroidism can influence the course of TED. Patients with uncontrolled thyroid hormone levels are more likely to exhibit severe TED than euthyroid patients. Anti-thyroid drugs (anti-TDs) do not appear to have a negative influence on the course of TED. Medical treatment is usually followed by a fall in serum antibody concentrations, suggesting a waning of autoimmunity [43]. Since obstetrical and medical complications are directly related to thyroid status during pregnancy, patients should be euthyroid before conceiving. Anti-TDs are the mainstay of treatment during pregnancy. The American Thyroid Association recommends propylthiouracil (PTU) for the first trimester, due to the risk of methimazole (MMI) embryopathy [44]. Following the first trimester, patients on PTU should be switched to MMI in order to decrease the incidence of hepatotoxicity related to PTU. Thyroid function tests should be monitored monthly during pregnancy [15, 21].

Glucocorticoid therapy has been shown to reduce interferon gamma-induced HLA-DR expression in vitro [43–46]. Current recommendations for the treatment of acute and moderate-to-severe TED in adults is a course of 0.5 g of methylprednisone IV once weekly for 6 weeks, followed by 0.25 g/week for 6 weeks. If the patient fails to respond, treatment may be stopped after 6 weeks of 0.5 g/week dosing [47]. Currently there are no specific dosing recommendations for pregnancy. Glucocorticoids, however, have been widely used during pregnancy for the treatment of a variety of medical conditions. They are categorized as a class C pregnancy risk and should be given only if the potential benefits justify the potential risk to the fetus. Various animal studies showed that high doses of glucocorticoid can lead to an increased incidence of cleft palate in exposed offspring [48, 49]. However, several subsequent reports in which pregnant women were treated with glucocorticoids throughout the first trimester for various medical conditions did not reveal a consistent pattern of embryopathy [50]. Glucocorticoids do not appear to have major teratogenic potential [51]. Glucocorticoids during pregnancy, however, may increase the risk of premature rupture of the membranes and intrauterine growth restriction [52, 53]. Antenatal exposure to a relatively large dose of synthetic glucocorticoids is associated with suppression of the hypothalamic-pituitary-adrenal axis [54]. Other maternal adverse effects include pregnancy-induced hypertension, gestational diabetes, osteoporosis, and infection [51]. Therefore, when systemic glucocorticoids are needed in pregnancy, it is generally recommended to use the lowest effective dose for the shortest duration of time, avoiding high doses during the first trimester [55]. Glucocorticoids are metabolized in the placenta by a crucial enzyme, 11-beta-hydroxysteroid dehydrogenase-2. Prednisolone-related drugs (methylprednisone, prednisolone, and prednisone) are mostly metabolized to inactive forms by this enzyme and thus only approximately 10 % of the total dose compared to 33 % of betamethasone and 50 % of dexamethasone will enter the fetal circulation [56].

Prednisone and prednisolone have been measured in breast milk. Levels of prednisolone, the active form of prednisone measured in the milk, are typically less than 0.1 % of the total prednisone dose, even for a dose up to 80 mg. This corresponds to less than 10 % of an infant's endogenous cortisol production [57] and therefore does not pose a clinically significant risk to a nursing infant. Nonetheless, exposure may be minimized if nursing is performed 3–4 h after a dose [57]. The American Academy of Pediatrics considers steroid therapy compatible with breastfeeding [57]. Guidelines from the National Heart, Lung and Blood Institute for the management of asthma also note that maternal use of systemic glucocorticoids is not a contraindication to breastfeeding [58].

Other Alternative Medical Treatments

In nonpregnant women, some studies have found that selenium may lower anti-TPOAb titers. The European Group on Graves' Orbitopathy (EUGOGO) consortium conducted a trial to compare selenium use with placebo or pentoxifylline. Several ocular parameters (eye involvement ($P=0.01$), progression of TED ($P=0.01$) as well as quality of life outcome measures ($P<0.001$)) improved in the selenium-treated group compared to placebo without significant side effects (see Chap. 6 for a full discussion) [59]. The selenium levels of the study population were marginally low and this may have biased in favor of a positive selenium treatment response [59]. Although selenium levels can be low in full-term pregnant women compared with nonpregnant women, the risk to benefit comparison does not support routine selenium supplementation during pregnancy [21]. Currently, there is an ongoing study on selenium supplementation in pregnancy where secondary outcomes will examine maternal and fetal risks.

Somatostatin Analogs

Four large double-blind, placebo-controlled studies of somatostatin analogs have shown no significant effects on TED compared with placebo [60–63]. Somatostatin analogs are listed as a category B pregnancy drug. Since somatostatin analogs cross the placenta, potential adverse fetal outcomes must be considered. Several papers reported the safe and effective use of these analogs in pregnancy for various therapeutic indications [64–66].

Rituximab: Rituximab has been assigned a pregnancy category C by the FDA. Because human IgG is known to traverse the placenta, rituximab may potentially cause fetal B-cell depletion. Post-marketing data indicate that B-cell lymphocytopenia generally lasts less than 6 months in infants exposed to the medication in utero. It is only recommended for use in pregnant women when the drug is clearly necessary. Rituximab use during breastfeeding is also not recommended since the drug is excreted in breast milk.

Azathioprine: Azathioprine is a pregnancy category D drug. Azathioprine should not be given during pregnancy and breastfeeding.

In summary, rituximab and azathioprine are contraindicated in pregnancy for the treatment of TED.

Orbital Radiotherapy

Orbital irradiation has been shown to be moderately useful as monotherapy [40]. The main benefit is an improvement in motility [34]. Nonetheless, orbital radiotherapy is contraindicated in pregnancy.

Surgical Therapy

Orbital decompression can be safely performed during pregnancy for severe CON unresponsive to a short course of systemic glucocorticoids or if sight is threatened by corneal exposure. If ophthalmopathy is severe but inactive, orbital decompression may also be performed. Reducing proptosis and decompressing the optic nerve can be achieved by a variety of decompression techniques (see Chaps. 11 and 12). One of the most feared complications of orbital decompression is postoperative diplopia. Extraocular muscle or eyelid surgery is often needed for full rehabilitation but can be delayed until after delivery.

Although orbital decompression is sometimes performed as first-line treatment for CON, most patients will still require glucocorticoid therapy; whereas less than half of patients treated with glucocorticoids initially will require orbital decompression [67]. Although it is preferable to operate on a pregnant patient during the second trimester [68, 69], emergencies require intervention regardless of gestational age.

Thyroidectomy

Whether or not thyroidectomy affects the course of TED remains unsettled. In many studies [41, 70, 71], different thyroid surgeries (subtotal versus total thyroidectomy) seem to carry very low risk for progression of TED [40]. Thyroidectomy is not recommended as first-line therapy for hyperthyroid GD, regardless of pregnancy status, but it should be considered in the event of contraindications to anti-TD therapy [21]. If thyroidectomy is indicated during pregnancy, the optimal time to perform surgery is in the second trimester [21].

With regard to the need for oculoplastic referral, it is the authors' opinion that because of the rare occurrence of TED during pregnancy and the limited therapeutic options, there should be a very low threshold for referral to oculoplastic specialists.

Summary

TED during pregnancy is a relatively uncommon occurrence in clinical practice. The prevalence of moderate-to-severe TED during pregnancy should decrease with treatment of preexisting TED prior to conception. Studies are needed to better understand the natural course of TED during pregnancy as well as the short- and long-term consequences of the differing therapeutic options. An endocrinologist, ophthalmologist, and obstetrician should be members of a multidisciplinary patient care team.

Pediatric Thyroid Eye Disease

Neonatal Thyrotoxicosis ("Neonatal Graves' Disease")

Neonatal thyrotoxicosis (referred to as "neonatal Graves' disease" in the pediatric literature) is uncommon, comprising no more than 1 % of childhood cases of hyperthyroidism, and presenting in less than 2 % of infants born to mothers with a

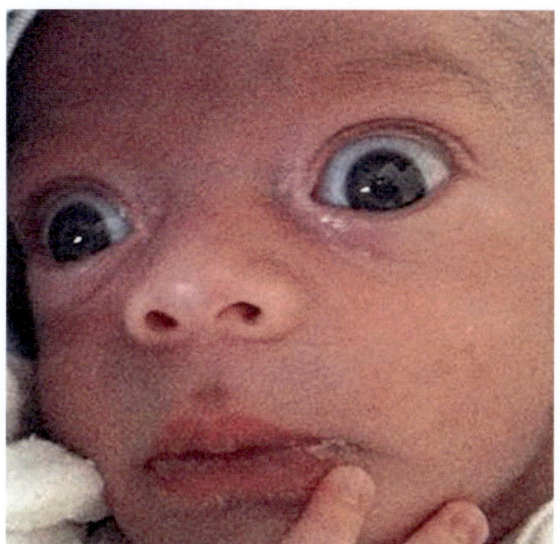

Fig. 7.3 Characteristic stare of an infant with neonatal thyrotoxicosis. The infant was born to a mother with a history of Graves' disease, treated with radioactive iodine a decade earlier. Tachypnea, tachycardia, poor feeding, and the ocular appearance of the infant prompted evaluation for neonatal thyrotoxicosis (Figure courtesy of Moran Gotesman, MD)

history of GD [72]. Most cases of neonatal thyrotoxicosis result from transplacental passage of maternal thyroid-stimulating immunoglobulins in utero. Even more rarely, there have been case reports of neonatal thyrotoxicosis due to activating mutations of the TSH receptor (TSHR) [73]. According to Wiersinga et al., true clinically significant TED has never been observed in neonatal thyrotoxicosis [74]. However, a prominent stare may be present (Fig. 7.3), providing a clinical clue to neonatal thyrotoxicosis. A maternal history of GD is often not elicited if the mother is being treated for hypothyroidism after radioactive iodine (RAI) ablation. The characteristic stare may prompt the clinician to inquire further into the maternal history, observe the infant for additional clinical signs such as tachycardia and poor feeding, and perform a laboratory evaluation.

Pediatric Graves' Disease

In children, the signs and symptoms of GD may develop gradually, often leading to a delayed diagnosis. Nonspecific clinical features such as difficulty concentrating and faltering academic achievement may be attributed to other conditions such as attention deficit hyperactivity disorder (ADHD). In children, long-term treatment with anti-TDs represents first-line therapy. Most children who are treated appropriately do not suffer long-term sequelae. However, delayed diagnosis has been associated with abnormal neurodevelopment (hyperactivity, psychomotor delay, and mental retardation) and altered skeletal maturation, including craniosynostosis and advanced bone age in younger children [75, 76].

Epidemiology of Pediatric Graves' Disease

The frequency of thyrotoxicosis ranges from 0.1 in 100,000 in young children (i.e., prior to adolescence) to 3.0 in 100,000 in adolescents [7]. Although GD represents the most common cause of thyrotoxicosis, it only affects 0.02 % of all children [78]. GD comprises 10–15 % of thyroid disorders in patients under 18 years of age, is rare under the age of 5, has a peak incidence at 10–15 years of age, and more commonly affects female pediatric patients [75]. Mild signs and symptoms of TED, including lid retraction and lid lag, are common (25–60 %) in pediatric thyrotoxicosis [78]. However, severe TED is rarely seen in pediatric patients. Bartley et al. studied subjects in Olmsted County, Minnesota, and found that only 6/120 cases of TED occurred in patients under the age of 20 years [79]. The reported incidence rate of TED in male children is 0 per 100,000 for ages 5–9 and 15–19 years, and 1.7 per 100,000 for ages 10–14 years. The reported incidence rate of TED in female children is 3.5 per 100,000 for ages 5–9 years, 1.8 per 100,000 for ages 10–14 years, and 3.3 per 100,000 for ages 15–19 years [74, 79].

Clinical Features of Pediatric Graves' Disease

Pediatric GD may present with many of the same signs and symptoms as in adults, including heat intolerance (61 %), tremor (49 %), and ophthalmopathy (43 %) [80]. Additionally, children with GD may often present with decreased academic performance (50 %) [80]. Favorable predictors of long-term remission include age less than 12 years old, free thyroxine (FT4) level <35–50 pmol/L at diagnosis, initial response to therapy, TSH receptor antibody levels ≤4 times the upper limit of normal, Caucasian ethnicity, and having other autoimmune condition(s) [81, 82].

Thyrotoxicosis has deleterious physiologic effects on children, including low bone mineral density and increased bone turnover, advancement of bone age leading to a lower than predicted final height, diminished left ventricular reserve, thyrotoxic ophthalmologic signs, and cognitive/neuropsychiatric deficits (hyperactivity, irritability, anxiety, and impaired school attention). Correction of the thyrotoxicosis in a timely manner usually reverses the adverse physiologic effects of thyrotoxicosis. Thus, in most children there do not seem to be long-term sequelae as long as the hyperthyroidism is corrected without delay [83].

Treatment of Pediatric Graves' Disease

In adult GD, the standard of care is a 12–18-month trial of anti-TDs followed by definitive therapy (i.e., RAI or thyroidectomy) if remission is not achieved. In contrast, pediatric GD is commonly treated for years with anti-TDs - typically methimazole - as long as the patient tolerates the therapy and euthyroidism can be achieved. Propylthiouracil (PTU) is avoided in the treatment of hyperthyroidism in children due to reports of PTU-induced liver failure (also discussed in chapter 1) [54]. The preference for medical management arises from the theoretical fear of radioiodine-induced thyroid malignancy, as well as the fear of potential morbidity and mortality associated with thyroidectomy [75, 80, 84]. After discontinuation of anti-TD therapy, over 50 % of pediatric patients will remain in remission for at least 2 years; however, relapse rates remain high and on the order of 36–47 % [75, 85–88]. Sustained disease remission for over 2 years post anti-TD therapy is less common in children (15–30 %) compared to adults (40–60 %), and may take up to 10 years to achieve [75, 83, 84, 88]. Gruniero-Papendieck et al. reported that in children who did not receive definitive treatment, the rate of persistent GD at 10 years was 31 % [77]. Up to 28 % of pediatric patients on anti-TD therapy experience adverse effects, and severe complications such as agranulocytosis, aplastic anemia, hepatotoxicity, and mortality have been reported, for PTU in particular [83].

Thyroidectomy and radioiodine represent definitive treatment options. Sherman et al. retrospectively investigated 78 patients under 18 years of age who underwent thyroidectomy for GD. The surgical indication for more than half the patients was failed medical therapy (60 %). Other indications included intolerance to anti-TDs (9 %), severe thyrotoxicosis, severe TED (concern for worsening with RAI), significant thyromegaly (gland >30 g), suspicious/malignant thyroid nodule, and unwillingness to receive RAI. Postoperative morbidity was transient and consisted of hypocalcemia (96 %) and unilateral recurrent laryngeal nerve palsy (1 %). It should be noted that the surgery was performed by experienced thyroid surgeons in a high-volume center [80]. Additional indications leading to thyroidectomy over RAI included age less than 10 years (due to theoretical higher risk of thyroid malignancy with RAI in this age group) and consideration of pregnancy in late adolescent females (TRAb levels can transiently increase and persist for at least 5 years after ablation, thus increasing risk of fetal/neonatal GD in the offspring) [75, 89–91].

Although radiation-induced thyroid malignancy as evidenced by the Chernobyl nuclear accident is a concern, retrospective studies suggest a very low risk of malignancy associated with RAI therapy. Patients with GD who are over 10 years old can be treated with RAI with the consultation of a pediatric ophthalmologist prior to ablation [75, 91]. Published retrospective studies with up to 36 years of follow-up have not supported the concerns of increased thyroid malignancy post RAI in the pediatric population [90–92]. In a retrospective review of the medical records of 78 pediatric patients who underwent thyroidectomy at Mayo Clinic, 4 patients (5 %) were incidentally found to have thyroid malignancies on histologic examination [80]. Thus, pediatric patients may harbor occult thyroid malignancy irrespective of RAI therapy.

TED in Children

Definition of TED

The definition of TED with respect to adults has been reviewed elsewhere in this textbook. In children, Antoniazzi et al. defined TED as clinical signs of ocular involvement in patients with GD (lid retraction, lid lag, or stare), who also have exophthalmos or signs of enlarged extraocular muscles on orbital MRI [93].

Epidemiology, Risk Factors, and Pathogenesis

In a 2004 review by Wiersinga, 23 % of pediatric patients with GD were found to have TED, which is very similar to that seen in adult patients with GD (18 %) [74]. However, TED prevalence rates up to 39 % have been reported in childhood GD [94]. A few small studies have attempted to further characterize the epidemiology of pediatric TED and to identify risk factors for the development of clinically significant TED. Durairaj et al. found that 10.0 % (2/20) of pediatric patients with TED had a family history of TED, and 60.0 % (12/20) had a family history of thyroid dysfunction [95]. Young, however, did not find any specific HLA Ag to be prevalent in patients with TED versus patients without TED [96]. Thus, currently there are no reliable genetic markers for identifying which pediatric patients with GD are at increased risk of developing TED.

According to Gogakos and coauthors, although severe TED is less common in children than adults, the epidemiology overall is similar [102]. Furthermore, TED has a similar female-to-male predominance in both children and adults (87 % and 83 %, respectively), and is associated with more severe thyrotoxicosis at the time of diagnosis in all ages. There is often a 2-year lag between the onset of thyroid dysfunction and TED, and a notable family history of thyroid disease in both children and adults. In late adolescence, the clinical features of TED resemble those of the adults [74, 97]. A 2005 European survey of 23 pediatric and 44 adult endocrinologists suggested that smoking was a potential risk factor for the development of TED, as countries with higher smoking prevalence had a higher prevalence of TED among children and adolescents with GD [84]. Although it is not possible to draw conclusions about causality from a survey study, in adults, smoking is an established risk factor for TED (see Chap. 5). Wiersinga postulates that the lower frequency of smoking in children may at least in part explain the tendency for milder clinical manifestations in pediatric TED [74].

Two studies have examined the severity of TED in a total of 163 prepubertal versus postpubertal children and adolescents with GD. Holt et al. did not find evidence of restrictive strabismus in prepubertal subjects. Severe TED seemed to occur less frequently in prepubertal subjects, but the number of subjects in that group was too small to achieve statistical significance (total $N=41$; subjects with TED $N=6$) [98]. In their prospective study of pediatric patients with GD followed by orbital MRI, Antoniazzi et al. reported a better prognosis in subjects who were prepubertal at the time of diagnosis. The authors hypothesized that increasing orbital volume with advancing age and puberty serves as a physiologic decompression [93].

Differential Diagnosis of Eyelid Retraction and Exophthalmos in Children

The findings of exophthalmos and eyelid retraction should prompt a clinical evaluation for the underlying etiology. The differential diagnosis of exophthalmos and eyelid retraction in children is shown in Table 7.2, and includes neurological causes, endocrinopathies, infection, vascular malformations, and malignancies [99–102].

Definition of exophthalmos in children. Nucci et al. used a Hertel exophthalmometer to measure the degree of ocular protrusion in 852 normal Italian subjects ranging from 3 to 10 years old. In each age group, no statistically significant difference was found between boys and girls or between the right and left eye; in fact, no subject had more than a 2 mm difference in measurement between the eyes [103]. Eha et al. suggested that the 97th percentile value may be used to define the upper limit of normal, and by extension, the cutoff for the definition of exophthalmos in pediatric patients [104]; however, this may not be generalizable across all populations (Table 7.3). Quant and Woo found that exophthalmos cutoffs

Table 7.2 Differential diagnosis of exophthalmos and eyelid retraction in children [99–102]

Neurological	• Congenital aberrant innervation of the third cranial nerve • Marcus Gunn jaw-winking • Optic nerve abnormalities • Cyclic oculomotor spasm
Dorsal midbrain syndrome	• Hydrocephalus
Craniofacial	• Craniosynostosis (shallow orbits) • Trisomy 21
Muscular	• Levator muscle fibrosis
Endocrinopathies	• Thyrotoxicosis • Hashimoto's thyroiditis • Cushing's disease • Acromegaly
Malformations	• Vascular malformations (including hemangioma)
Infection	• Orbital cellulitis
Malignancies	• Histiocytosis X (Hand-Schüller-Christian syndrome) • Neuroblastoma • Rhabdomyosarcoma
Other	• Retro-orbital hemorrhage

Table 7.3 Definition of exophthalmos based on ocular protrusion >97th percentile for age, in Italian children [108]

Age (Years)	Ocular Protrusion >97th Percentile (mm)
3–5	>14
6–7	>14
8–10	>15

were higher in Chinese children from Hong Kong compared to Black, Caucasian, or other Chinese children [105].

Gerber et al. reported normal exophthalmometric values in children age 10–14 years ($N=482$) according to age and sexual maturity staging. The authors found that exophthalmometry measurements had a tendency to increase with age and sexual maturity [106]. Because of concerns that normal exophthalmometry values in children over 10 years old may not be reliable due to the significant variability in onset and progression of puberty, some authors have proposed arbitrary definitions of exophthalmos using Hertel exophthalmometers such as >19 or >20 mm, akin to the definition of exophthalmos in adults [78, 93, 104].

Clinical Presentation of Pediatric TED

Characterization of the features of pediatric TED is based on a limited number of retrospective case series and cross-sectional studies. Results of the published studies are shown in Table 7.4.

The most common ocular findings in pediatric TED are proptosis, soft tissue involvement, upper eyelid retraction, stare, and eyelid lag [96, 107]. Extraocular muscle involvement is much less common in pediatric patients compared to adults, and optic nerve involvement has not been reported in pediatric TED. Corneal involvement and exposure keratopathy have been reported in pediatric TED. Of note, one study reported a high frequency of punctate epithelial erosions in Chinese children [108]. Most authors have concluded that pediatric TED is in general less severe than adult TED, and that it usually improves with local, supportive therapy and restoration of normal thyroid function [78, 95, 96, 109, 110]. Only the study reported by Eha and coauthors found that proptosis did not improve with restoration of euthyroidism [104].

Correlation of Pediatric TED with TSI/TRAb Levels

In a retrospective study of South Korean GD children up to 18 years ($n=80$), Lee et al. evaluated risk factors for TED in childhood GD [94]. Multivariate regression analysis indicated that TPO Ab positivity was associated with TED ($p=0.048$). Mean TBII titers and Tg Ab positivity were not statistically significantly different between the GD only versus the GD plus TED groups. In a retrospective review of all patients at Texas Children's Hospital with newly diagnosed GD between 2000 and 2006 ($N=49$), Acuna and coauthors found a significant association between TSI levels at the time of diagnosis and the occurrence of TED ($\chi^2=6.94$, $P=0.029$). The authors concluded that elevated TSI titers may represent a reliable predictor for the development of TED in pediatric patients with GD [109]. Kubo et al. reported a case of a 3-year-old female with GD complicated by TED. The patient was noted to have exophthalmos, with eyelid erythema, lacrimation, lower eyelid entropion, and punctate keratopathy. Her TSI (3,287 %) value was elevated at baseline. Despite initiating anti-TD therapy

Table 7.4 Frequency of eye signs and symptoms in patients with pediatric thyroid eye disease

	Retrospective case studies (*N*=141) [78, 95, 98, 104, 107, 109]	Cross-sectional studies (*N*=100) [96, 108, 110]
Soft tissue involvement	10 (7.1 %)	
Proptosis	91 (64.5 %)	32 (42.7 %)
Extraocular muscle involvement	15 (10.6 %)	1 (1.3 %)
Corneal involvement/exposure keratitis	20 (14.2 %)	11 (14.7 %)
Optic nerve involvement	0 (0 %)	0 (0 %)
Lid lag	53 (37.6 %)	
Lid retraction	89 (63.1 %)	32 (42.7 %)

and achieving euthyroidism within 3 weeks, the TED did not improve. Pulse therapy with methylprednisolone induced a modest and temporary improvement in clinical signs and symptoms and a mild decrease in antibody titers. A year later, the eye disease persisted and the TSI (3,667 %) value was similar to pretreatment. The authors proposed that TSI may represent a predictor of severity and prognosis of TED, and suggested that it be followed longitudinally [111]. Antoniazzi et al. followed pediatric patients with GD (*N*=26) prospectively utilizing orbital MRI. TRAb levels were significantly higher in hyperthyroid patients with TED compared to those without TED both at the time of diagnosis and at the time of follow-up (2–10 years after achieving euthyroidism). The authors suggest a TRAb titer level of >201.7 U/L as a threshold predicting a higher risk of TED in pediatric GD [93]. Overall, the very limited published literature suggests that TSI and TRAb levels may be useful predictors of the risk of development and severity of TED.

Imaging Techniques for Evaluation and Monitoring

There are few published studies in the pediatric literature describing imaging in pediatric TED. Young reported that out of 5 youths who underwent orbital B scan ultrasonography for ocular changes associated with GD, 4 of them demonstrated extraocular muscle thickening. The fifth patient had a normal ultrasound study [96]. Antoniazzi et al. prospectively followed orbital volumes of pediatric patients with GD up to the age of 21. In pediatric patients with TED, the only MRI finding was enlargement of the extraocular muscles, which is consistent with the early, active, edematous stage of eye disease, as opposed to the later fibrotic stage sometimes seen in adults. MRI only confirmed regression of TED that was observed clinically, so it did not appear to add additional information [93].

Effect of GD Treatment on TED

Effect of anti-TDs. Three fourths of pediatric patients on anti-TDs show an improvement of TED; only 1 % experience worsening [112]. In contrast, anti-TDs do not generally alter the course of TED in adult patients [113].

Radioactive iodine. Two randomized, controlled trials have demonstrated that 15 % of adults experienced worsening of TED following RAI ablation for GD [41, 114]. Progression of TED in children following ^{131}I therapy has been reported in only up to 3 % of children, with 90 % showing improvement post RAI therapy, and the remainder experiencing no change in TED [115–118]. A systematic review of the literature found no significant difference between RAI therapy and anti-TD therapy in TED onset or worsening in pediatric patients [115]. However, adolescents with TED, like adults, may benefit from a prophylactic 1- to 3-month oral glucocorticoid taper starting a day after RAI administration [75, 118].

Thyroidectomy. Sherman et al. retrospectively reviewed thyroidectomies performed in pediatric GD subjects. Thirty-four of the 78 total subjects had TED, of which 85 % percent showed improvement in TED postoperatively. One patient (3 %) showed worsening of TED, ultimately requiring orbital decompression. On the other hand, 2 of the 44 patients (5 %) without TED at the time of surgery later developed TED, with a time course that was unlikely to be related to thyroidectomy [80]. Of 16 pediatric TED cases that Gruters retrospectively reviewed, only 1 patient (6 %) exhibited worsening of TED after anti-TD therapy followed by total thyroidectomy [78]. In a study of adult and adolescent GD patients ($n=80$ total), Miccoli et al. found that among those with mild eye disease ($n=40$), 3 out of 32 patients (9 %) who underwent subtotal thyroidectomy experienced worsening of TED, in contrast to none of the 8 patients who underwent total thyroidectomy [119]. However, this study did not report the results for adult patients versus children. Based on the scant data available, a majority of pediatric patients with TED may experience improvement of ocular symptoms post thyroidectomy; however, worsening of symptoms remains a distinct possibility in a minority of individuals.

Treatment of TED

Our review of the pediatric literature suggests that patients should be considered for specific TED treatment only if they have persistence and/or progression of TED after achieving stable euthyroidism [74, 84, 97].

Medical Treatment

Corticosteroids. As mentioned previously, anti-TDs are first-line therapy for pediatric GD. Even in the presence of TED, 94 % of pediatric and adult endocrinologists in Europe would treat with anti-TDs initially, and 66 % would use anti-TDs again in the event of a recurrence after a period of remission [84]. However, if TED remains active despite achieving euthyroidism, or worsens after 4 months of anti-TD therapy, two-thirds of the endocrinologists surveyed would pursue specific treatment for TED. Most (57 %) would opt to use corticosteroids in that situation [84]. In children, the risks of long-term prednisone therapy include weight gain, immunosuppression, and growth failure [91]. Gogakos and coauthors suggest starting with a dose of 5–20 mg of prednisone per day for 4–6 weeks to observe efficacy, followed by a slow taper over 1–3 months as clinically tolerated [80].

Orbital octreotide scintigraphy. Orbital octreotide scintigraphy has been proposed as a useful tool to identify patients with active TED, based on adult studies. A positive orbital octreoscan (i.e., [^{111}In-DPTA-D-Phe] octreotide scintigraphy) could indicate active TED, and thus may be useful for selecting patients that would benefit from immunosuppressive therapy, while a negative initial scan may be consistent with end-stage fibrotic TED, and would predict lack of efficacy of immunosuppressive therapy. After initiating therapy, a follow-up scan showing decreased orbital octreotide uptake would suggest suppression of inflammation and disease activity as a result of anti-inflammatory therapy, thereby serving as a potentially useful tool for following response to therapy [120–124]. However, the octreotide scan has not achieved widespread use, since it is technically challenging to perform, lacks specificity, involves radiation exposure to the patient, and is expensive. Moreover, this technique has not yet been validated in the pediatric population.

Somatostatin analogs. In theory, somatostatin analogs should be efficacious for TED given that retro-ocular tissues display all five somatostatin receptor subtypes (SSTs 1–5), and octreotide has an inhibitory effect on the immune system and fibroblasts via targeting of SSTs 2,3,5 [74, 125, 126]. Initial, uncontrolled studies using octreotide in adults with TED showed a positive effect, likely the result of the natural history of the disease as described by Rundle [127]. Likewise, in the pediatric literature, Krassas treated 3 adolescent patients who were euthyroid on anti-TDs but exhibited moderate-to-severe TED with monthly octreotide for 4 months (Sandostatin LAR 20 mg intramuscularly). All 3 adolescents showed significant improvement in their TED signs and symptoms, and improved their clinical activity scores [97]. Several subsequent randomized, controlled clinical trials in the adult literature have not demonstrated improvement of

TED in adults [61–63, 121, 128, 129]. Newer generation somatostatin analogs such as SOM 230 have affinity for a wider range of somatostatin receptors and thus may prove more effective for the treatment of TED [74, 97].

Rituximab, azathioprine, and selenium. Alternative therapies that have been attempted in adults with TED include rituximab, azathioprine, and selenium. There are no reports of rituximab, azathioprine, or selenium use in pediatric TED. However, these therapeutic agents have been used in pediatric subjects with other conditions such as post-transplant, juvenile idiopathic arthritis, and microscopic polyangiitis. Rituximab, an anti-B cell drug, blocks the CD20 receptor, and has been shown to reduce inflammation. Rituximab appears to be safe for pediatric patients when used short-term, but the long-term effects are not yet known [130]. Clinical reports suggest that studies are needed to explore the potential benefits of rituximab for TED [131, 132]. One randomized double-blind, placebo-controlled trial thus far found no effect of rituximab in adults with TED [133], while additional randomized controlled trials are underway [132]. Azathioprine inhibits enzymes required for DNA and RNA synthesis, thereby suppressing rapidly dividing cells, such as B- and T-lymphocytes [134], but has not been effective in alleviating TED [135]. Rituximab and azathioprine should only be considered as salvage therapy for pediatric patients who have failed conventional treatments. Selenium is known to have antioxidant properties, and has been shown to help improve cases of mild TED in adults [59]. Selenium supplementation appears to be safe for use in pediatric patients, and has been shown to reduce thyroid volume in euthyroid pediatric patients with early autoimmune thyroiditis [136]. The effect of selenium on pediatric TED is unknown.

Orbital irradiation. Although orbital irradiation for TED has been used in adults with controversial therapeutic benefits, it has not been utilized in pediatric patients due to the theoretical concerns of potential radiation-related tumorigenesis [74, 97].

Surgical Treatment

Orbital decompression. Specific surgical management of pediatric TED has rarely been reported, likely due to the generally mild presentation and benign natural history of the disease. Orbital growth continues after the age of 7, and evaluation with serial orbital imaging suggests that prepubertal patients will have physiologic decompression during puberty, when expansion of orbital volume occurs naturally [74, 80, 93, 95, 97].

Summary

Severe, clinically significant pediatric TED appears to be a rare occurrence. Most cases of childhood TED significantly improve or resolve once the patient is rendered euthyroid. Although anti-TDs are the mainstay of therapy for pediatric GD, they are not without risk, and years of treatment may not lead to lasting remission. Significantly elevated TSI and TRAb titers may represent a good predictor of severe and/or persistent TED. Alternatively, definitive therapy (i.e., thyroidectomy or RAI ablation) for GD may be considered, and may secondarily improve or resolve the pediatric patient's TED as well. In general, thyroidectomy in the hands of an experienced surgeon is a better definitive treatment option for children less than 10 years of age, but RAI with the goal of thyroid ablation seems to be a safe and effective alternative for older children and adolescents. A prophylactic 1- to 3-month prednisone taper following radioiodine ablation may prevent potential worsening of TED in children.

References

1. Adams Waldorf KM, Nelson JL. Autoimmune disease during pregnancy and the microchimerism legacy of pregnancy. Immunol Invest. 2008;37(5):631–44.
2. Balucan FS, Morshed SA, Davies TF. Thyroid autoantibodies in pregnancy: their role, regulation and clinical relevance. J Thyroid Res. 2013;2013:182472.

3. Buyon JP. The effects of pregnancy on autoimmune diseases. J Leukoc Biol. 1998;63(3):281–7.
4. Fugazzola L, Cirello V, Beck-Peccoz P. Microchimerism and endocrine disorders. J Clin Endocrinol Metab. 2012;97(5):1452–61.
5. Adams Waldorf KM, Gammill HS, Lucas J, Aydelotte TM, Leisenring WM, Lambert NC, et al. Dynamic changes in fetal microchimerism in maternal peripheral blood mononuclear cells, CD4+ and CD8+ cells in normal pregnancy. Placenta. 2010;31(7):589–94.
6. Williams RH, Larsen PR. Williams textbook of endocrinology. Philadelphia: Saunders; 2003.
7. Schott M, Morgenthaler NG, Fritzen R, Feldkamp J, Willenberg HS, Scherbaum WA, et al. Levels of autoantibodies against human TSH receptor predict relapse of hyperthyroidism in Graves' disease. Horm Metab Res. 2004;36(2):92–6.
8. Klintschar M, Schwaiger P, Mannweiler S, Regauer S, Kleiber M. Evidence of fetal microchimerism in Hashimoto's thyroiditis. J Clin Endocrinol Metab. 2001;86(6):2494–8.
9. Klintschar M, Immel UD, Kehlen A, Schwaiger P, Mustafa T, Mannweiler S, et al. Fetal microchimerism in Hashimoto's thyroiditis: a quantitative approach. Eur J Endocrinol. 2006;154(2):237–41.
10. Renne C, Ramos Lopez E, Steimle-Grauer SA, Ziolkowski P, Pani MA, Luther C, et al. Thyroid fetal male microchimerisms in mothers with thyroid disorders: presence of Y-chromosomal immunofluorescence in thyroid-infiltrating lymphocytes is more prevalent in Hashimoto's thyroiditis and Graves' disease than in follicular adenomas. J Clin Endocrinol Metab. 2004;89(11):5810–4.
11. Walsh JP, Bremner AP, Bulsara MK, O'Leary P, Leedman PJ, Feddema P, et al. Parity and the risk of autoimmune thyroid disease: a community-based study. J Clin Endocrinol Metab. 2005;90(9):5309–12.
12. Chan GW, Mandel SJ. Therapy insight: management of Graves' disease during pregnancy. Nat Clin Pract Endocrinol Metab. 2007;3(6):470–8.
13. Abalovich M, Amino N, Barbour LA, Cobin RH, De Groot LJ, Glinoer D, et al. Management of thyroid dysfunction during pregnancy and postpartum: an Endocrine Society Clinical Practice Guideline. J Clin Endocrinol Metab. 2007;92(8 Suppl):S1–47.
14. Krajewski DA, Burman KD. Thyroid disorders in pregnancy. Endocrinol Metab Clin North Am. 2011; 40(4):739–63.
15. Patil-Sisodia K, Mestman JH. Graves hyperthyroidism and pregnancy: a clinical update. Endocr Pract. 2010;16(1):118–29.
16. Brent GA. Clinical practice. Graves' disease. N Engl J Med. 2008;358(24):2594–605.
17. Weetman AP. Graves' disease. N Engl J Med. 2000; 343(17):1236–48.
18. Smith BHR. Thyroid-stimulating immunoglobulins in Graves' disease. Lancet. 1974;304(7878):427–30.
19. Stagnaro-Green A. Clinical review 152: postpartum thyroiditis. J Clin Endocrinol Metab. 2002;87(9): 4042–7.
20. Fitzpatrick DL, Russell MA. Diagnosis and management of thyroid disease in pregnancy. Obstet Gynecol Clin North Am. 2010;37(2):173–93.
21. Stagnaro-Green A, Abalovich M, Alexander E, Azizi F, Mestman J, Negro R, et al. Guidelines of the American Thyroid Association for the diagnosis and management of thyroid disease during pregnancy and postpartum. Thyroid. 2011;21(10):1081–125.
22. Glinoer D. The regulation of thyroid function in pregnancy: pathways of endocrine adaptation from physiology to pathology. Endocr Rev. 1997;18(3):404–33.
23. Gonzalez-Jimenez A, Fernandez-Soto ML, Escobar-Jimenez F, Glinoer D, Navarrete L. Thyroid function parameters and TSH-receptor antibodies in healthy subjects and Graves' disease patients: a sequential study before, during and after pregnancy. Thyroidology. 1993;5(1):13–20.
24. Kamijo K. TSH-receptor antibodies determined by the first, second and third generation assays and thyroid-stimulating antibody in pregnant patients with Graves' disease. Endocr J. 2007;54(4):619–24.
25. Tamaki H, Amino N, Iwatani Y, Tachi J, Mitsuda N, Tanizawa O, et al. Discordant changes in serum anti-TSH receptor antibody and antithyroid microsomal antibody during pregnancy in autoimmune thyroid diseases. Thyroidology. 1989;1(2):73–7.
26. Amino N, Kuro R, Tanizawa O, Tanaka F, Hayashi C, Kotani K, et al. Changes of serum anti-thyroid antibodies during and after pregnancy in autoimmune thyroid diseases. Clin Exp Immunol. 1978;31(1):30–7.
27. Lacey B, Chang W, Rootman J. Nonthyroid causes of extraocular muscle disease. Surv Ophthalmol. 1999;44(3):187–213.
28. Patrinely JR, Osborn AG, Anderson RL, Whiting AS. Computed tomographic features of nonthyroid extraocular muscle enlargement. Ophthalmology. 1989;96(7):1038–47.
29. Germain S, Saha S, Nelson-Piercy C, Stanford M, Carroll P. Severe sight-threatening thyroid eye disease presenting de novo in an euthyroid pregnant woman. Endocr Abstracts. 2008;15:393.
30. Stafford IP, Dildy III GA, Miller Jr JM. Severe Graves' ophthalmopathy in pregnancy. Obstet Gynecol. 2005;105(5 Pt 2):1221–3.
31. Abbouda A, Trimboli P, Bruscolini A. A mild Grave's ophthalmopathy during pregnancy. Semin Ophthalmol. 2014;29(1):8–10.
32. Nüßgens Z, Roggenkämper P, Schweikert HU. Endocrine orbitopathy unusual deterioration during pregnancy. Klin Monatsbl Augenheilkd. 1993;202(02):130–3.
33. Burch HB, Wartofsky L. Graves' ophthalmopathy: current concepts regarding pathogenesis and management. Endocr Rev. 1993;14(6):747–93.
34. Dickinson J, Perros P. Thyroid-associated orbitopathy: who and how to treat. Endocrinol Metab Clin North Am. 2009;38(2):373–88, ix.
35. Meriggioli MN, Sanders DB. Autoimmune myasthenia gravis: emerging clinical and biological heterogeneity. Lancet Neurol. 2009;8(5):475–90.

36. Batocchi AP, Majolini L, Evoli A, Lino MM, Minisci C, Tonali P. Course and treatment of myasthenia gravis during pregnancy. Neurology. 1999;52(3):447–52.
37. Marino M, Ricciardi R, Pinchera A, Barbesino G, Manetti L, Chiovato L, et al. Mild clinical expression of myasthenia gravis associated with autoimmune thyroid diseases. J Clin Endocrinol Metab. 1997;82(2):438–43.
38. Gold R, Schneider-Gold C. Current and future standards in treatment of myasthenia gravis. Neurotherapeutics. 2008;5(4):535–41.
39. Cummings CW, Flint PW. Cummings otolaryngology head & neck surgery, Vol. 3. Philadelphia: Mosby Elsevier; 2010.
40. Bartalena L, Pinchera A, Marcocci C. Management of Graves' ophthalmopathy: reality and perspectives. Endocr Rev. 2000;21(2):168–99.
41. Tallstedt L, Lundell G, Torring O, Wallin G, Ljunggren JG, Blomgren H, et al. Occurrence of ophthalmopathy after treatment for Graves' hyperthyroidism. The Thyroid Study Group. N Engl J Med. 1992;326(26):1733–8.
42. Stan MN, Garrity JA, Bahn RS. The evaluation and treatment of graves ophthalmopathy. Med Clin North Am. 2012;96(2):311–28.
43. Bartalena L, Baldeschi L, Dickinson AJ, Eckstein A, Kendall-Taylor P, Marcocci C, et al. Consensus statement of the European group on Graves' orbitopathy (EUGOGO) on management of Graves' orbitopathy. Thyroid. 2008;18(3):333–46.
44. Clementi M, Di Gianantonio E, Cassina M, Leoncini E, Botto LD, Mastroiacovo P. Treatment of hyperthyroidism in pregnancy and birth defects. J Clin Endocrinol Metab. 2010;95(11):E337–41.
45. Heufelder AE, Bahn RS, Smith TJ. Regulation by glucocorticoids of interferon gamma-induced HLA-DR antigen expression in cultured human orbital fibroblasts. Clin Endocrinol (Oxf). 1992;37(1):59–63.
46. Meyer KC, Decker C, Baughman R. Toxicity and monitoring of immunosuppressive therapy used in systemic autoimmune diseases. Clin Chest Med. 2010;31(3):565–88.
47. Kahaly GJ, Pitz S, Hommel G, Dittmar M. Randomized, single blind trial of intravenous versus oral steroid monotherapy in Graves' orbitopathy. J Clin Endocrinol Metab. 2005;90(9):5234–40.
48. Carmichael SL, Shaw GM, Ma C, Werler MM, Rasmussen SA, Lammer EJ. Maternal corticosteroid use and orofacial clefts. Am J Obstet Gynecol. 2007;197(6):585.e1–7, discussion 683–4.e1–7.
49. Park-Wyllie L, Mazzotta P, Pastuszak A, Moretti ME, Beique L, Hunnisett L, et al. Birth defects after maternal exposure to corticosteroids: prospective cohort study and meta-analysis of epidemiological studies. Teratology. 2000;62(6):385–92.
50. Chen KK, Powrie RO. Approach to the use of Glucocorticoids in Pregnancy for Nonobstetric Indications. 2010:736–41.
51. Ostensen M, Khamashta M, Lockshin M, Parke A, Brucato A, Carp H, et al. Anti-inflammatory and immunosuppressive drugs and reproduction. Arthritis Res Ther. 2006;8(3):209.
52. Guller S, Kong L, Wozniak R, Lockwood CJ. Reduction of extracellular matrix protein expression in human amnion epithelial cells by glucocorticoids: a potential role in preterm rupture of the fetal membranes. J Clin Endocrinol Metab. 1995;80(7):2244–50.
53. Lockwood CJ, Radunovic N, Nastic D, Petkovic S, Aigner S, Berkowitz GS. Corticotropin-releasing hormone and related pituitary-adrenal axis hormones in fetal and maternal blood during the second half of pregnancy. J Perinat Med. 1996; 24(3):243–51.
54. Tegethoff M, Pryce C, Meinlschmidt G. Effects of intrauterine exposure to synthetic glucocorticoids on fetal, newborn, and infant hypothalamic-pituitary-adrenal axis function in humans: a systematic review. Endocr Rev. 2009;30(7):753–89.
55. Lunghi L, Pavan B, Biondi C, Paolillo R, Valerio A, Vesce F, et al. Use of glucocorticoids in pregnancy. Curr Pharm Des. 2010;16(32):3616–37.
56. Kurtoglu S, Sarici D, Akin MA, Daar G, Korkmaz L, Memur S. Fetal adrenal suppression due to maternal corticosteroid use: case report. J Clin Res Pediatr Endocrinol. 2011;3(3):160–2.
57. Briggs GG, Freeman RK, Yaffe SJ. Drugs in pregnancy and lactation: a reference guide to fetal and neonatal risk. Philadelphia: Lippincott Williams & Wilkins; 2005.
58. National Heart Lung, Blood Institute, National Asthma Education and Prevention Program, Third Expert Panel on the Diagnosis and Management of Asthma. Expert Panel report 3 guidelines for the diagnosis and management of asthma. Bethesda: U.S. Department of Health and Human Services, National Institutes of Health, National Heart, Lung, and Blood Institute; 2007. Available from: http://purl.access.gpo.gov/GPO/LPS93946
59. Marcocci C, Kahaly GJ, Krassas GE, Bartalena L, Prummel M, Stahl M, et al. Selenium and the course of mild Graves' orbitopathy. N Engl J Med. 2011;364(20):1920–31.
60. Chang TC, Liao SL. Slow-release lanreotide in Graves' ophthalmopathy: a double-blind randomized, placebo-controlled clinical trial. J Endocrinol Invest. 2006;29(5):413–22.
61. Dickinson AJ, Vaidya B, Miller M, Coulthard A, Perros P, Baister E, et al. Double-blind, placebo-controlled trial of octreotide long-acting repeatable (LAR) in thyroid-associated ophthalmopathy. J Clin Endocrinol Metab. 2004;89(12):5910–5.
62. Stan MN, Garrity JA, Bradley EA, Woog JJ, Bahn MM, Brennan MD, et al. Randomized, double-blind, placebo-controlled trial of long-acting release octreotide for treatment of Graves' ophthalmopathy. J Clin Endocrinol Metab. 2006;91(12):4817–24.
63. Wemeau JL, Caron P, Beckers A, Rohmer V, Orgiazzi J, Borson-Chazot F, et al. Octreotide (long-acting release formulation) treatment in patients with graves' orbitopathy: clinical results of a

four-month, randomized, placebo-controlled, double-blind study. J Clin Endocrinol Metab. 2005; 90(2):841–8.
64. de Menis E, Billeci D, Marton E, Gussoni G. Uneventful pregnancy in an acromegalic patient treated with slow-release lanreotide: a case report. J Clin Endocrinol Metab. 1999;84(4):1489.
65. Mikhail N. Octreotide treatment of acromegaly during pregnancy. Mayo Clin Proc. 2002;77(3):297–8.
66. Neal JM. Successful pregnancy in a woman with acromegaly treated with octreotide. Endocr Pract. 2000;6(2):148–50.
67. Wakelkamp IM, Baldeschi L, Saeed P, Mourits MP, Prummel MF, Wiersinga WM. Surgical or medical decompression as a first-line treatment of optic neuropathy in Graves' ophthalmopathy? A randomized controlled trial. Clin Endocrinol (Oxf). 2005;63(3): 323–8.
68. ACOG Committee opinion. Nonobstetric surgery in pregnancy. Number 284, August 2003. Int J Gynaecol Obstet. 2003;83(1):135.
69. Rojansky N, Reubinoff BE, Shapira SC, Weinstein D. Safety of surgical intervention during the second trimester of pregnancy. A case report. J Reprod Med. 1994;39(10):821–4.
70. Fernandez Sanchez JR, Rosell Pradas J, Carazo Martinez O, Torres Vela E, Escobar Jimenez F, Garbin Fuentes I, et al. Graves' ophthalmopathy after subtotal thyroidectomy and radioiodine therapy. Br J Surg. 1993;80(9):1134–6.
71. Winsa B, Rastad J, Akerstrom G, Johansson H, Westermark K, Karlsson FA. Retrospective evaluation of subtotal and total thyroidectomy in Graves' disease with and without endocrine ophthalmopathy. Eur J Endocrinol. 1995;132(4):406–12.
72. Werner SC, Ingbar SH, Braverman LE, Cooper DS. Werner & Ingbar's the thyroid : a fundamental and clinical text. Philadelphia, Pa.; London: Lippincott Williams & Wilkins; 2012.
73. Watkins MG, Dejkhamron P, Huo J, Vazquez DM, Menon RK. Persistent neonatal thyrotoxicosis in a neonate secondary to a rare thyroid-stimulating hormone receptor activating mutation: case report and literature review. Endocr Pract. 2008;14(4):479–83.
74. Wiersinga WM. Thyroid associated ophthalmopathy: pediatric and endocrine aspects. Pediatr Endocrinol Rev. 2004;1 Suppl 3:513–7.
75. Bauer AJ. Approach to the pediatric patient with Graves' disease: when is definitive therapy warranted? J Clin Endocrinol Metab. 2011;96(3):580–8.
76. Segni M, Leonardi E, Mazzoncini B, Pucarelli I, Pasquino AM. Special features of Graves' disease in early childhood. Thyroid. 1999;9(9):871–7.
77. Gruneiro-Papendieck L, Chiesa A, Finkielstain G, Heinrich JJ. Pediatric Graves' disease: outcome and treatment. J Pediatr Endocrinol Metab. 2003;16(9): 1249–55.
78. Gruters A. Ocular manifestations in children and adolescents with thyrotoxicosis. Exp Clin Endocrinol Diabetes. 1999;107 Suppl 5:S172–4.
79. Bartley GB, Gorman CA. Diagnostic criteria for Graves' ophthalmopathy. Am J Ophthalmol. 1995; 119(6):792–5.
80. Sherman J, Thompson GB, Lteif A, Schwenk II WF, van Heerden J, Farley DR, et al. Surgical management of Graves disease in childhood and adolescence: an institutional experience. Surgery. 2006;140(6):1056–61, discussion 1061–2.
81. Kaguelidou F, Alberti C, Castanet M, Guitteny MA, Czernichow P, Leger J. Predictors of autoimmune hyperthyroidism relapse in children after discontinuation of antithyroid drug treatment. J Clin Endocrinol Metab. 2008;93(10):3817–26.
82. Leger J, Gelwane G, Kaguelidou F, Benmerad M, Alberti C. Positive impact of long-term antithyroid drug treatment on the outcome of children with Graves' disease: national long-term cohort study. J Clin Endocrinol Metab. 2012;97(1):110–9.
83. Segni M, Gorman CA. The aftermath of childhood hyperthyroidism. J Pediatr Endocrinol Metab. 2001;14 Suppl 5:1277–82, discussion 1297–8.
84. Krassas GE, Segni M, Wiersinga WM. Childhood Graves' ophthalmopathy: results of a European questionnaire study. Eur J Endocrinol. 2005;153(4): 515–21.
85. Gorton C, Sadeghi-Nejad A, Senior B. Remission in children with hyperthyroidism treated with propylthiouracil. Long-term results. Am J Dis Child. 1987; 141(10):1084–6.
86. Hamburger JI. Management of hyperthyroidism in children and adolescents. J Clin Endocrinol Metab. 1985;60(5):1019–24.
87. Kaguelidou F, Carel JC, Leger J. Graves' disease in childhood: advances in management with antithyroid drug therapy. Horm Res. 2009;71(6):310–7.
88. Weetman AP. Graves' hyperthyroidism: how long should antithyroid drug therapy be continued to achieve remission? Nat Clin Pract Endocrinol Metab. 2006;2(1):2–3.
89. Nikiforov Y, Gnepp DR, Fagin JA. Thyroid lesions in children and adolescents after the Chernobyl disaster: implications for the study of radiation tumorigenesis. J Clin Endocrinol Metab. 1996;81(1):9–14.
90. Read Jr CH, Tansey MJ, Menda Y. A 36-year retrospective analysis of the efficacy and safety of radioactive iodine in treating young Graves' patients. J Clin Endocrinol Metab. 2004;89(9):4229–33.
91. Rivkees SA, Sklar C, Freemark M. Clinical review 99: the management of Graves' disease in children, with special emphasis on radioiodine treatment. J Clin Endocrinol Metab. 1998;83(11):3767–76.
92. Safa AM, Schumacher OP. Letter: follow-up of children treated with 131-I. N Engl J Med. 1976; 294(1):54.
93. Antoniazzi F, Zamboni G, Cerini R, Lauriola S, Dall'Agnola A, Tato L. Graves' ophthalmopathy evolution studied by MRI during childhood and adolescence. J Pediatr. 2004;144(4):527–31.
94. Lee JH, Park SH, Koh DG, Suh BK. Thyroid peroxidase antibody positivity and triiodothyronine levels

are associated with pediatric Graves' ophthalmopathy. World J Pediatr. 2014;10(2):155–9.

95. Durairaj VD, Bartley GB, Garrity JA. Clinical features and treatment of graves ophthalmopathy in pediatric patients. Ophthal Plast Reconstr Surg. 2006;22(1):7–12.
96. Young LA. Dysthyroid ophthalmopathy in children. J Pediatr Ophthalmol Strabismus. 1979;16(2):105–7.
97. Gogakos AI, Boboridis K, Krassas GE. Pediatric aspects in Graves' orbitopathy. Pediatr Endocrinol Rev. 2010;7 Suppl 2:234–44.
98. Holt H, Hunter DG, Smith J, Dagi LR. Pediatric Graves' ophthalmopathy: the pre- and postpubertal experience. J AAPOS. 2008;12(4):357–60.
99. Bale Jr JF, Bonkowsky JL, Filloux FM, Hedlund GL, Larsen PD, Nielsen DM. Pediatric neurology. London: Manson; 2011. Available from: http://public.eblib.com/EBLPublic/PublicView.do?ptiID=619351
100. Black EH. Smith and Nesi's ophthalmic plastic and reconstructive surgery. New York: Springer; 2012. Available from: http://dx.doi.org/10.1007/978-1-4614-0971-7
101. Sindhu K, Downie J, Ghabrial R, Martin F. Aetiology of childhood proptosis. J Paediatr Child Health. 1998;34(4):374–6.
102. Stout AU, Borchert M. Etiology of eyelid retraction in children: a retrospective study. J Pediatr Ophthalmol Strabismus. 1993;30(2):96–9.
103. Nucci P, Brancato R, Bandello F, Alfarano R, Bianchi S. Normal exophthalmometric values in children. Am J Ophthalmol. 1989;108(5):582–4.
104. Eha J, Pitz S, Pohlenz J. Clinical features of pediatric Graves' orbitopathy. Int Ophthalmol. 2010;30(6): 717–21.
105. Quant JR, Woo GC. Normal values of eye position and head size in Chinese children from Hong Kong. Optom Vis Sci. 1993;70(8):668–71.
106. Gerber FR, Taylor FH, DeLevie M, Drash AL, Kenny FM. Normal standards for exophthalmometry in children 10 to 14 years of age: relation to age, height, weight, and sexual maturation. J Pediatr. 1972;81(2):327–9.
107. Goldstein SM, Katowitz WR, Moshang T, Katowitz JA. Pediatric thyroid-associated orbitopathy: the Children's Hospital of Philadelphia experience and literature review. Thyroid. 2008;18(9):997–9.
108. Chan W, Wong GW, Fan DS, Cheng AC, Lam DS, Ng JS. Ophthalmopathy in childhood Graves' disease. Br J Ophthalmol. 2002;86(7):740–2.
109. Acuna OM, Athannassaki I, Paysse EA. Association between thyroid-stimulating immunoglobulin levels and ocular findings in pediatric patients with Graves disease. Trans Am Ophthalmol Soc. 2007;105:146–50, discussion 150–1.
110. Uretsky SH, Kennerdell JS, Gutai JP. Graves' ophthalmopathy in childhood and adolescence. Arch Ophthalmol. 1980;98(11):1963–4.
111. Kubo T, Shimizu J, Furujo M, Takeuchi A, Yoshioka-Iwaso H, Eguchi N, et al. An infant case of Graves' disease with ophthalmopathy. Endocr J. 2005;52(5): 647–50.
112. Barnes HV, Blizzard RM. Antithyroid drug therapy for toxic diffuse goiter (Graves disease): thirty years experience in children and adolescents. J Pediatr. 1977;91(2):313–20.
113. Hegedus L, Bonnema SJ, Smith TJ, Brix TH. Treating the thyroid in the presence of Graves' ophthalmopathy. Best Pract Res Clin Endocrinol Metab. 2012;26(3):313–24.
114. Bartalena L, Marcocci C, Bogazzi F, Panicucci M, Lepri A, Pinchera A. Use of corticosteroids to prevent progression of Graves' ophthalmopathy after radioiodine therapy for hyperthyroidism. N Engl J Med. 1989;321(20):1349–52.
115. Ma C, Kuang A, Xie J, Liu G. Radioiodine treatment for pediatric Graves' disease. Cochrane Database Syst Rev. 2008;(3):Cd006294.
116. McCormack S, Mitchell DM, Woo M, Levitsky LL, Ross DS, Misra M. Radioactive iodine for hyperthyroidism in children and adolescents: referral rate and response to treatment. Clin Endocrinol (Oxf). 2009; 71(6):884–91.
117. Rivkees SA, Dinauer C. An optimal treatment for pediatric Graves' disease is radioiodine. J Clin Endocrinol Metab. 2007;92(3):797–800.
118. Tallstedt L, Lundell G. Radioiodine treatment, ablation, and ophthalmopathy: a balanced perspective. Thyroid. 1997;7(2):241–5.
119. Miccoli P, Vitti P, Rago T, Iacconi P, Bartalena L, Bogazzi F, et al. Surgical treatment of Graves' disease: subtotal or total thyroidectomy? Surgery. 1996;120(6):1020–4, discussion 1024–5.
120. Kahaly G, Diaz M, Just M, Beyer J, Lieb W. Role of octreoscan and correlation with MR imaging in Graves' ophthalmopathy. Thyroid. 1995;5(2):107–11.
121. Krassas GE, Dumas A, Pontikides N, Kaltsas T. Somatostatin receptor scintigraphy and octreotide treatment in patients with thyroid eye disease. Clin Endocrinol (Oxf). 1995;42(6):571–80.
122. Moncayo R, Baldissera I, Decristoforo C, Kendler D, Donnemiller E. Evaluation of immunological mechanisms mediating thyroid-associated ophthalmopathy by radionuclide imaging using the somatostatin analog 111In-octreotide. Thyroid. 1997;7(1):21–9.
123. Postema PT, Krenning EP, Wijngaarde R, Kooy PP, Oei HY, van den Bosch WA, et al. [111In-DTPA-D-Phe1] octreotide scintigraphy in thyroidal and orbital Graves' disease: a parameter for disease activity? J Clin Endocrinol Metab. 1994;79(6):1845–51.
124. Wiersinga WM, Gerding MN, Prummel MF, Krenning EP. Octreotide scintigraphy in thyroidal and orbital Graves' disease. Thyroid. 1998;8(5): 433–6.
125. Pasquali D, Notaro A, Bonavolonta G, Vassallo P, Bellastella A, Sinisi AA. Somatostatin receptor genes are expressed in lymphocytes from retroorbital tissues in Graves' disease. J Clin Endocrinol Metab. 2002;87(11):5125–9.
126. Pasquali D, Vassallo P, Esposito D, Bonavolonta G, Bellastella A, Sinisi AA. Somatostatin receptor gene expression and inhibitory effects of octreotide on

primary cultures of orbital fibroblasts from Graves' ophthalmopathy. J Mol Endocrinol. 2000;25(1): 63–71.
127. Update on thyroid eye disease and management. Dove Press; 2009. Available from: http://www.dovepress.com/getfile.php?fileID=5369
128. Krassas GE, Kaltsas T, Dumas A, Pontikides N, Tolis G. Lanreotide in the treatment of patients with thyroid eye disease. Eur J Endocrinol. 1997;136(4): 416–22.
129. Kung AW, Michon J, Tai KS, Chan FL. The effect of somatostatin versus corticosteroid in the treatment of Graves' ophthalmopathy. Thyroid. 1996;6(5):381–4.
130. Otukesh H, Hoseini R, Rahimzadeh N, Fazel M. Rituximab in the treatment of nephrotic syndrome: a systematic review. Iran J Kidney Dis. 2013;7(4): 249–56.
131. Minakaran N, Ezra DG. Rituximab for thyroid-associated ophthalmopathy. Cochrane Database Syst Rev. 2013;(5):Cd009226.
132. Salvi M, Vannucchi G, Beck-Peccoz P. Potential utility of rituximab for Graves' orbitopathy. J Clin Endocrinol Metab. 2013;98(11):4291–9.
133. Stan MN, Garrity JA, Thapa P, Bradley EA, Bahn RS. Randomized Double-Blind. Placebo-controlled Trial of rituximab for treatment of Graves' ophthalmopathy. Presentation in the 83rd annual meeting of the American Thyroid Association, San Juan; 2013.
134. Kapadia MK, Rubin PA. The emerging use of TNF-alpha inhibitors in orbital inflammatory disease. Int Ophthalmol Clin. 2006;46(2):165–81.
135. Perros P, Weightman DR, Crombie AL, Kendall-Taylor P. Azathioprine in the treatment of thyroid-associated ophthalmopathy. Acta Endocrinol. 1990; 122(1):8–12.
136. Onal H, Keskindemirci G, Adal E, Ersen A, Korkmaz O. Effects of selenium supplementation in the early stage of autoimmune thyroiditis in childhood: an open-label pilot study. J Pediatr Endocrinol Metab. 2012;25(7–8):639–44.

Medical Management of Mild and Moderate to Severe Thyroid Eye Disease

8

Lucy Clarke and Petros Perros

Introduction

The distinction between "mild" and "moderate to severe" thyroid eye disease (TED) is blurred and definitions vary. Distinguishing "normal" from "mild" may be even harder. Clinicians who are newcomers to the field of TED are usually surprised by the disparity between the objective clinical findings and the patient's perception, the latter often thought by the observer to be exaggerated. The reverse can also be true, though it is much rarer; in the authors' experience, it tends to be associated with older patients. What is enlightening in every new case of TED is comparison of the present appearance with photographs of the patient prior to the onset of the eye disease. This should be regarded as an essential clinical assessment of no less importance than measuring proptosis or serum levels of thyroid antibodies. The definitions of mild and moderate-to-severe eye disease represent a combination of objective findings and the subjective impact of the disease for that individual [1].

L. Clarke
Newcastle Eye Centre, Royal Victoria Infirmary, Newcastle upon Tyne, UK

P. Perros, B.Sc., M.B.B.S., M.D., F.R.C.P. (✉)
Department of Endocrinology, Royal Victoria Infirmary, Queen Victoria Road, Elliott Building, Newcastle upon Tyne NE1 4LP, UK
e-mail: petros.perros@ncl.ac.uk

The importance of understanding the impact of the disease on the particular individual cannot be overstated. The disease-specific, validated quality of life questionnaire GO-QOL is a useful tool in routine management [2, 3].

Classification of disease severity of patients with TED [1]

Sight-threatening thyroid eye disease

Patients with compressive optic neuropathy (CON) and/or corneal breakdown. This category warrants immediate intervention.

Moderate to severe TED

Patients without sight-threatening disease whose eye disease has sufficient impact on daily life to justify the risks of immunosuppression (if active) or surgical intervention (if inactive). Patients with moderate to severe TED usually have any one or more of the following: lid retraction ≥2 mm, moderate or severe soft tissue involvement, exophthalmos ≥3 mm above normal for race and gender, inconstant or constant diplopia.

Mild TED

Patients whose TED signs and symptoms have only a minor impact on daily life.

(continued)

R.S. Douglas et al. (eds.), *Thyroid Eye Disease*,
DOI 10.1007/978-1-4939-1746-4_8,

(continued)

Patients usually have one or more of the following: minor lid retraction (<2 mm), mild soft tissue involvement, exophthalmos <3 mm above normal for race and gender, transient or no diplopia, and corneal exposure responsive to lubricants.

Clinical Assessment

The pertinent initial questions that need to be addressed include the following:

- Is the diagnosis of TED correct?
- How severe is the disease?
- How active is the disease?
- What is the impact of the disease on the patient?
- Is the patient euthyroid?
- Is the patient a smoker?

The diagnosis of TED is usually obvious, though atypical presentations (Chap. 9) can be challenging. A variety of other diagnoses may masquerade as TED [4]. The severity of the eye disease can be documented on the basis of the NOSPECS classification (Dickinson and Perros, 2001) [5]. Activity is one of the most difficult aspects of TED to quantify. The Clinical Activity Score (CAS) is widely used, especially in Europe (Bartalena et al., 2008) [1]. A CAS score of 4 out of 10 points or more has been associated with a positive predictive value of 80 % of responding to immunosuppressive treatments and a CAS <4 had a 68 % negative predictive value [6]. The VISA classification is used for grading severity and activity and is favored in North America [7]. The effects of the disease on the patient's personal and professional life can be assessed adequately by any skilled clinician who is willing to listen and can ask relevant questions. It may be quantified by several questionnaires, the most validated of which is the GO-QOL [8]. Measuring the serum levels of thyroid hormones easily assesses thyroid status. Inquiring about smoking status is critical for determining the need for smoking cessation as well as the patient's risk for developing more severe disease (Chap. 5)

Initial Management for Patients with Mild and Moderate to Severe TED

The first priority after initial assessment is for the clinician to communicate with the patient. TED is not an easy condition to explain, but it helps patients to understand the disease process and natural history, as well as the objectives of treatment. In order to achieve optimal outcomes, treatments are performed in a carefully choreographed sequence, a process that can be frustrating for patients, as it takes time. Written material and support from patient-led organizations are valuable resources.

Simple Measures

Some simple interventions can relieve troublesome symptoms. Ocular surface symptoms, such as dryness, foreign body sensation, and tearing, should be treated with artificial tear lubricants. Double vision can be managed with Fresnel prisms or occlusion as temporary measures (see Chap. 10). Chapter 13 discusses non-surgical interventions to improve patient symptoms, appearance, and quality of life in greater detail.

Botulinum Toxin

Botulinum toxin is a powerful neurotoxin that blocks the release of acetylcholine at the neuromuscular junction of cholinergic nerves, thereby weakening the force of muscular contraction. It is commercially available and licensed for treatment of a number of conditions characterized by muscle spasm or rigidity. Although the use of botulinum toxin for upper lid retraction in TED is widespread in clinical practice, only several small case series have been published [9, 10]. Both transcutaneous and transconjunctival routes of injection are reported to be efficacious. The mechanism of action is most likely a partial paralytic effect upon Muller's muscle and levator palpebrae superioris.

Common side effects include local bruising and discomfort at the injection site. Ptosis (overcorrection) and diplopia may occur due to the local spread of botulinum to extraocular muscles, most commonly the superior rectus muscle. More severe reactions have been reported, including muscle weakness, dysphagia, and aspiration, occurring rarely with all products that contain botulinum toxin. Extreme caution should be exercised in administering products that contain botulinum toxin to patients who have neurological disorders, or a history of dysphagia or aspiration. Only physicians with appropriate experience should administer products that contain botulinum toxin. Patients should be informed about the risk of spread of toxin and the symptoms, such as dysphagia or respiratory distress, that should prompt urgent medical attention [11].

Avoidance of Risk Factors that Exacerbate TED

Both hyper- and hypothyroidism are detrimental to patients; thus euthyroidism should be established as rapidly as possible and maintained (see Chaps. 1 and 3). Smoking cessation advice and support should be given to patients who smoke (see Chap. 5). The use of anti-oxidant supplements and other potential disease-limiting factors are discussed in detail in Chap. 6.

Watchful Waiting

If the disease has little impact on the patient's quality of life and social/professional activities (a relatively rare scenario), a watchful approach is acceptable and in the majority of cases the disease will improve over several months [12, 13].

Specific Treatments for Mild, Active TED

Selenium plays an important role in health and disease and has antioxidant properties. Selenium supplements have been shown to reduce thyroid autoantibodies in patients with autoimmune thyroid disease [14]. A randomized placebo-controlled study in patients with mild, active TED has shown that 200 μg of sodium selenite daily for 6 months reduced disease severity and activity and improved quality of life [15] (Chap. 6). No side effects were reported. These data suggest that selenium is a disease-modifying treatment in TED. However, the study was conducted in Europe, where selenium deficiency is common. Whether the findings are applicable to selenium replete parts of the world is unclear at present.

Oral or intravenous steroids are effective, but the potential side effects are significant and generally not recommended for patients with mild disease [16]. The most notable exception is for patients who require radioiodine treatment for thyrotoxicosis, when a short course of oral steroids is well tolerated and may prevent worsening or new onset of TED, [17] (Chap. 4).

Orbital irradiation has been used in patients with mild TED and was shown to be more effective than sham irradiation in a randomized study, especially with regards to motility [18]. However, the study found no impact on quality of life and the small, though not negligible, risks of orbital irradiation probably outweigh the benefits. The topic of orbital irradiation is discussed further in the next section.

Specific Treatments for Moderate to Severe, Active TED

Steroids

Systemic steroids are the mainstay of medical treatment for active, moderate to severe eye disease. The mode of administration of steroids is important. Pulses of intravenous steroids are superior to continuous oral steroids [16], both in terms of efficacy and a more favorable side-effect profile. A recent study has shown that the optimal intravenous regimen for moderate to severe TED is weekly doses of 500 mg for 6 weeks followed by 250 mg weekly doses for a further 6 weeks [19]. However this study showed that relapses after completion of treatment were common (about 20 %) and compressive optic neuropathy developed in 7.5 % of patients after completion of treatment. Whether steroids are merely suppressive or disease modifying is an interesting and important question. Evidence in favor of a disease-modifying effect comes from a study of oral steroids in Graves' disease as prophylaxis in patients receiving radioiodine [19] and from a small randomized controlled study [20]. In both of these studies the duration of eye disease prior to steroid treatment was relatively short compared to the study by Bartalena et al. [19] where the effects of steroids were less convincingly disease-modifying. Early intervention may therefore be important for achieving the optimal effect of medical therapies. Cumulative doses of methylprednisolone exceeding 8 g have been associated with acute hepatic failure and this threshold (or equivalent for other glucocorticoids) should not generally be exceeded [16]. If the cumulative steroid dose is less than 8 g of methylprednisolone, and especially if steroids have previously only been given orally, it is appropriate to consider pulses of intravenous methylprednisolone (e.g., starting with weekly 500 mg doses for 4 or 6 weeks). This approach is likely to result in additional anti-inflammatory effects. The response to pulsed intravenous steroid therapy is usually evident after 2–4 weeks, so detailed clinical reassessment soon after commencing this treatment will identify non-responders for whom steroids can be withdrawn in order to avoid unnecessary potential side effects.

Relapse of TED after high dose steroids is a common and difficult problem. The options in this scenario are orbital irradiation (see below), combination treatment with oral steroids, and cyclosporine or watchful waiting. The role of biologics including rituximab is discussed in Chap. 9. The effect of selenium supplements in this scenario is unexplored, though it may be justifiable, given that it is well tolerated.

Orbital Irradiation

Six randomized studies of orbital irradiation have been conducted (reviewed by Kahaly (2010) [21]), including three placebo-controlled trials [18, 22, 23]. Two of the studies showed clinical benefit with irradiation, while the third study did not. The authors' view is that orbital irradiation has a role in patients with moderate to severe, active TED who have restricted motility, which is supported by systematic reviews [24, 25], although this is still debated in North America [26].

Randomized, controlled trials indicate that orbital irradiation in combination with oral steroids seems to be more effective than either alone [27, 28]. The efficacy of intravenous steroids in combination with orbital irradiation has not yet been investigated in a randomized, controlled trial.

One of the principal advantages of orbital irradiation is safety, though there are contraindications. Tumorigenesis is a potential concern, although this risk is very small. In three large follow-up studies involving 574 patients monitored for periods of 11–17 years, no tumors were reported [29–31]. A single case of basal cell carcinoma developing 15 years after orbital irradiation has been reported [32]. It is prudent therefore to reserve this treatment for patients older than 35 years [1]. Diabetes, especially if associated with hypertension and preexisting retinopathy, is a relative contraindication [21].

Management of Inactive Disease

Surgical rehabilitation of inactive TED requires a clear understanding of the desired and achievable outcomes between the patient and the surgeon. The patient should understand the sequence of potential surgeries and the time frame required in order to make informed choices. Because the effect of the preceding operation will influence the subsequent one, it is important to address proptosis, strabismus, and lid retraction in approximately that order, if all are present. It can be counterproductive to achieve perfect fusion or a beautiful upper lid position, only to find motility and lid position changes after orbital decompression. Most patients will not require the full series of operations, but should they be required, the journey can take 1–2 years. A customized approach to surgical rehabilitation of patients with TED is detailed in chapters 11 and 12.

Conclusion

The majority of patients with TED have mild or moderate to severe orbitopathy. Patients with moderate to severe disease are often sufficiently affected to justify medical and surgical treatments. Smoking cessation is critical for patients in any stage of disease process, and selenium supplements may be useful for patients with mild TED. For patients with active, moderate to severe disease, steroids are the first-line medical therapy, and orbital irradiation may be beneficial for non-diabetic patients with strabismus. Biological agents are discussed in the next chapter. A multidisciplinary approach involving the endocrinologist and ophthalmologist, as well as the thyroid surgeon or radiation oncologist as needed, facilitates delivery of optimal care.

References

1. Bartalena L, Baldeschi L, Dickinson A, Eckstein A, et al. Consensus statement of the European Group on Graves' orbitopathy (EUGOGO) on management of GO. Eur J Endocrinol. 2008;158:273–85.
2. Terwee CB, Gerding MN, Dekker FW, Prummel MF, Wiersinga WM. Development of a disease specific quality of life questionnaire for patients with Graves' ophthalmopathy: the GO-QOL. Br J Ophthalmol. 1998;82:773–9.
3. Terwee CB, Dekker FW, Mourits MP, Gerding MN, Baldeschi L, Kalmann R, Prummel MF, Wiersinga WM. Interpretation and validity of changes in scores on the Graves' ophthalmopathy quality of life questionnaire (GO-QOL) after different treatments. Clin Endocrinol (Oxf). 2001;54:391–8.
4. Mourits MP. Diagnosis and differential diagnosis of Graves' orbitopathy. In: Wiersinga WM, Kahaly GJ, editors. Graves' orbitopathy. A multidisciplinary approach-questions and answers. 2nd ed. Basel: Karger; 2010. p. 66–75.
5. Dickinson AJ, Perros P. Controversies in the clinical evaluation of active thyroid-associated orbitopathy: use of a detailed protocol with comparative photographs for objective assessment. Clin Endocrinol (Oxf). 2001;55:283–303.
6. Mourits MP, Prummel MF, Wiersinga WM, Koornneef L. Clinical activity score as a guide in the management of patients with Graves' ophthalmopathy. Clin Endocrinol (Oxf). 1997;47:9–14.
7. Dolman PJ. Evaluating Graves' orbitopathy. Best Pract Res Clin Endocrinol Metab. 2012;26: |229–48.
8. Goldberg RA. The evolving paradigm of orbital decompression surgery. Arch Ophthalmol. 1998;116: 95–6. http://www.eugogo.eu.
9. Uddin J, Davies P. Treatment of upper eyelid retraction associated with thyroid eye disease with subconjunctival botulinum toxin injection. Ophthalmology. 2002;109:1183–7.
10. Shih MJ, Liao SL, Lu HY. A single transcutaneous injection with Botox for dysthyroid lid retraction. Eye (Lond). 2004;18:466–9.
11. MHRA. http://www.mhra.gov.uk/Safetyinformation/DrugSafetyUpdate/CON254816118 (2013)
12. Perros P, Kendall-Taylor P. Natural history of thyroid eye disease. Thyroid. 1998;8:423–5.
13. Menconi F, Profilo MA, Leo M, Sisti E, Altea MA, Rocchi R, Latrofa F, Nardi M, Vitti P, Marcocci C, Marino M. Spontaneous improvement of untreated mild Graves' ophthalmopathy: the Rundle curve revisited. Thyroid. 2014;24:60–6.
14. Schomburg L. Selenium, selenoproteins and the thyroid gland: interactions in health and disease. Nat Rev Endocrinol. 2011;8:160–71.
15. Marcocci C, Kahaly GJ, Krassas GE, Bartalena L, et al. Selenium and the course of mild Graves' orbitopathy. N Engl J Med. 2011;364:1920–31.
16. Zang S, Ponto KA, Kahaly GJ. Clinical review: Intravenous glucocorticoids for Graves' orbitopathy: efficacy and morbidity. J Clin Endocrinol Metab. 2011;96:320–32.
17. Wiersinga WM, Bartalena L. Epidemiology and prevention of Graves' ophthalmopathy. Thyroid. 2002;12: 855–60.
18. Prummel MF, Terwee CB, Gerding MN, Baldeschi L, Mourits MP, Blank L, Dekker FW, Wiersinga WM. A randomized controlled trial of orbital radiotherapy versus sham irradiation in patients with mild Graves' ophthalmopathy. J Clin Endocrinol Metab. 2004; 89:15–20.
19. Bartalena L, Krassas GE, Wiersinga W, Marcocci C, et al. Efficacy and safety of three different cumulative doses of intravenous methylprednisolone for moderate to severe and active Graves' orbitopathy. J Clin Endocrinol Metab. 2013;97:4454–63.
20. van Geest RJ, Sasim IV, Koppeschaar HP, Kalmann R, et al. Methylprednisolone pulse therapy for patients with moderately severe Graves' orbitopathy: a prospective, randomized, placebo-controlled study. Eur J Endocrinol. 2008;158:229–37.
21. Kahaly GJ. Management of moderately severe Graves' orbitopathy. In: Wiersinga WM, Kahaly GJ, editors. Graves' orbitopathy. A multidisciplinary approach-questions and answers. 2nd ed. Basel: Karger; 2010. p. 120–58.
22. Mourits MP, van Kempen-Harteveld ML, García MB, Koppeschaar HP, Tick L, Terwee CB. Radiotherapy for Graves' orbitopathy: randomised placebo-controlled study. Lancet. 2000;355:1505–9.
23. Gorman CA, Garrity JA, Fatourechi V, Bahn RS, et al. A prospective, randomized, double-blind, placebo-controlled study of orbital radiotherapy for Graves' ophthalmopathy. Ophthalmology. 2001;108:1523–34.

24. Stiebel-Kalish H, Robenshtok E, Hasanreisoglu M, Ezrachi D, Shimon I, Leibovici L. Treatment modalities for Graves' ophthalmopathy: systematic review and metaanalysis. J Clin Endocrinol Metab. 2009;94:2708–16.
25. Rajendram R, Bunce C, Lee RW, Morley AM. Orbital radiotherapy for adult thyroid eye disease. Cochrane Database Syst Rev. 2012 Jul 11; 7:CD007114.
26. Bradley EA, Gower EW, Bradley DJ, Meyer DR, Cahill KV, Custer PL, Holck DE, Woog JJ. Orbital radiation for graves ophthalmopathy: a report by the American Academy of Ophthalmology. Ophthalmology. 2008; 115:398–409.
27. Bartalena L, Marcocci C, Chiovato L, Laddaga M, Lepri G, Andreani D, Cavallacci G, Baschieri L, Pinchera A. Orbital cobalt irradiation combined with systemic corticosteroids for Graves' ophthalmopathy: comparison with systemic corticosteroids alone. J Clin Endocrinol Metab. 1983;56:1139–44.
28. Marcocci C, Bartalena L, Bogazzi F, Bruno-Bossio G, Lepri A, Pinchera A. Orbital radiotherapy combined with high dose systemic glucocorticoids for Graves' ophthalmopathy is more effective than radiotherapy alone: results of a prospective randomized study. J Endocrinol Invest. 1991;14:853–60.
29. Kahaly GJ, Rösler HP, Pitz S, Krummenauer F, Hommel G. Radiotherapy for Graves' Ophthalmopathy. J Clin Endocrinol Metab. 2001;86:2327–8.
30. Wakelkamp IM, Tan H, Saeed P, Schlingemann RO, Verbraak FD, Blank LE, Prummel MF, Wiersinga WM. Orbital irradiation for Graves' ophthalmopathy: is it safe? A long-term follow-up study. Ophthalmology. 2004;111:1557–62.
31. Marcocci C, Bartalena L, Rocchi R, Marinò M, et al. Long-term safety of orbital radiotherapy for Graves' ophthalmopathy. J Clin Endocrinol Metab. 2003;88: 3561–6.
32. Haenssle HA, Richter A, Buhl T, Haas E, Holzkamp R, Emmert S, Schön MP. Pigmented basal cell carcinomas 15 years after orbital radiation therapy for Graves ophthalmopathy. Arch Dermatol. 2011;147: 511–2.

Management of Severe Thyroid Eye Disease and Use of Biological Agents

9

Mario Salvi, Richard L. Scawn, Roman Farjardo, Bobby S. Korn, and Don O. Kikkawa

Introduction

Multiple classification and grading systems exist for thyroid eye disease (TED) but for the purpose of this chapter, severe disease broadly includes severe inflammatory orbitopathy, sight-threatening disease, and/or proptosis greater than 25 mm [1, 2]. As orbital edema and inflammation increase, surrounding structures are compressed, including vasculature and the optic nerve. Elevated venous pressure and reduced flow within the superior ophthalmic vein may ensue [3]. The resulting venous vascular congestion may further increase intra-orbital edema and pressure, potentially compounding inflammatory signs and symptoms.

M. Salvi, M.D.
Department of Clinical Sciences and Community Health, Graves Orbitopathy Unit, Fondazione Ca'Granda IRCCS, University of Milan, Milan, Italy

R.L. Scawn, M.B.B.S., F.R.C.Ophth
R. Farjardo, M.D. • B.S. Korn, M.D., Ph.D., F.A.C.S.
D.O. Kikkawa, M.D., F.A.C.S.
Division of Ophthalmic Plastic and Reconstructive Surgery, Department of Ophthalmology, Shiley Eye Center, University of California San Diego, La Jolla, CA, USA
e-mail: dkikkawa@ucsd.edu

Risk Factors

One predictor of disease severity may be the rate at which symptoms progress [4]. Patients with more acutely progressing disease, represented by a steeper slope on Rundle's curve, are more likely to have symptoms of severe disease [4, 5]. The incidence and severity of TED shows significant gender predilections. Although TED is more prevalent in women, the gender preponderance reverses in severe disease, where it occurs four times more often in male patients [6, 7]. Age is also a risk factor for developing severe TED. There is a positive correlation between age and severity, with patients over the age of 60 at risk of more severe disease [2, 8, 9]. In addition, smokers have a higher prevalence of severe TED than non-smokers [10]. This may be related to an increase in connective tissue that correlates with cumulative smoking [11]. More than 4,000 chemicals exist within cigarette smoke; thus, deciphering the precise mechanism by which smoking has a deleterious effect on TED remains elusive (but see Chap. 5). Orbital fibroblasts exposed to cigarette smoke in vitro show increased adipogenesis and hyaluronic acid production, which is proportional to the smoke concentration [11]. Smoking is associated with a modest increase in free T3 and T4, possibly through sympathetic nervous system stimulation [12]. Although smoking cessation is imperative

R.S. Douglas et al. (eds.), *Thyroid Eye Disease*,
DOI 10.1007/978-1-4939-1746-4_9, © Springer Science+Business Media New York 2015

in the optimal management of TED, the success rate in curtailing patient smoking is generally low, with cessation rates ranging from 2 % after a physician's verbal advice to 5–12 % with nicotine replacement [12].

On the molecular level, the TSH receptor antibody (TRAb) continues to be investigated as a predictor of disease severity. One study showed a correlation between serum TRAb concentrations and the severity of TED [13]. Another study showed that after adjusting for known risk factors such as age and smoking, TRAb levels are higher initially and at follow-up in patients with severe TED [14]. However, a consistent relationship between antibodies and disease severity has not been demonstrated, and interestingly smoking is associated with reduction in thyroid peroxidase and thyroglobulin antibodies [13].

Classification

Many grading schemes of TED have been proposed, as detailed in Chap. 1. Grading systems may incorporate clinical signs and symptoms, as well as the patient's perception of disease impact. Different classification systems have been developed over time seeking to balance accuracy and simplicity in the assessment of disease severity. The VISA classification attempts to document both disease severity and activity [15]. **V**ision threatening disease, **I**nflammation, **S**trabismus and patient **A**ppearance are scored up to a maximum of 20 with higher scores corresponding to more severe disease. In addition to the current VISA classification, a quality of life assessment may be added to quantify the patient's perspective of their disease severity [16]. The Clinical Activity Score (CAS) was one of the first validated measures of disease activity. It is often used clinically to assess the response of immunosuppressive therapy within the dynamic phase of the disease. A CAS score of 4 or higher has been shown to have an 80 % positive predictive value and 64 % negative predictive value in regard to the efficacy of corticosteroids [17]. The European Group on Graves' Orbitopathy (EUGOGO)'s severity scales classifies disease severity based on impact on daily life [18]. The most severe classification, termed "sight-threatening," entails optic neuropathy and/or corneal breakdown requiring immediate intervention. Patients in the "moderate-to-severe" category have symptoms that are not sight-threatening but have sufficient impact to justify immunosuppression and/or surgery.

Treatment Options

The management of severe TED may require multiple treatment modalities including a combination of immunosuppression, orbital irradiation, and orbital decompression. The goal of treatment is to control or reverse the disease and rehabilitate the patient using the most conservative measures while minimizing side effects. Patients must be encouraged to stop smoking, because smoking not only increases the risk of severe disease, it also diminishes treatment efficacy, as elaborated in Chap. 5. For instance, the response to high dose oral prednisolone and retrobulbar irradiation was 68 % in smokers versus 94 % in non-smokers [19].

Immunosuppression

Corticosteroids are often the first line of treatment for severe, active disease. Corticosteroids clinically decrease orbital inflammation and congestion. Oral prednisone dosing ranges from 0.5 mg to 1 mg/kg per day, with improvement usually seen within the first week. This is usually tapered to the minimum necessary to maintain improvement. Long-term side effects of corticosteroids, including hepatotoxicity, Cushing's syndrome, osteoporosis, cataracts, glaucoma, and diabetes mellitus, typically preclude extended treatment regimes. While it is not our practice to use an extended course of oral corticosteroids, it is important to consider bisphosphonate use and regular monitoring for steroid-related complications with prolonged therapy.

Some studies suggest that pulsed IV methylprednisolone (MP) is more effective and has an improved side effect profile compared with high dose oral prednisone [20, 21]. In one study of 70 patients with moderate-to-severe TED, 77 % of patients in the IV group responded to treatment compared to 51 % of patients in the oral group. The IV group had statistically significant improvements in visual acuity, chemosis, and quality of life, whereas the oral group suffered from more side effects and adverse events. A 2009 review and meta-analysis of randomized controlled trials concluded that pulsed IV corticosteroids are significantly more effective than oral corticosteroids in reducing CAS in cases of severe TED and were accompanied by a lower rate of adverse events [22].

IV steroids also appear significantly more effective in managing compressive optic neuropathy (CON) with 79 % of patients showing improvement versus 33 % of those on oral treatment [23]. Although the overall incidence of adverse events may be lower in IV steroid delivery, a greater proportion of serious adverse events may occur with IV steroid administration [24]. Serious adverse events include acute hepatic failure, cardiovascular thrombosis, and death. The incidence of fatality with IV corticosteroids has been estimated at 0.6 [24–26]. Although multiple treatment regimes have been reported, current recommendations include not exceeding a cumulative dose of 8 g of MP and avoiding IV doses on consecutive days unless sight-threatening disease is present [21, 23]. In patients with CON, the presence of optic disc swelling and marked visual field defects are predictive of incomplete response to IV MP necessitating orbital decompression to control the disease [27]. IV steroids are usually delivered slowly over 60–90 min with cardiac monitoring [21]. Patients with hepatic dysfunction, poorly controlled diabetes, and cardiovascular disease are not suitable candidates for IV steroids. Treatment monitoring should include liver enzymes and EKG [21]. IV steroid therapy may not be amenable to pure outpatient management. Additional costs in delivery and adverse event monitoring may make it unsuitable for some patients.

For patients with disease refractory or intolerant to corticosteroids, other medical options are available in the management of inflammation. The effects of azathioprine monotherapy were disappointing but it has shown some promise and is being evaluated in the CIRTED trial [28–30]. Oral cyclosporine has been used in combination therapy with steroids and its addition allows reduction of the dose of steroids for comparable efficacy [31]. Biological agents including rituximab (RTX) are discussed separately in this chapter.

Orbital Radiotherapy

Orbital irradiation may be employed as an adjunct in severe TED [32]. Proposed mechanisms for the efficacy of radiation include temporary lymphocyte sterilization, terminal differentiation of fibroblasts, and decreased antigen presentation via the destruction of tissue-bound monocytes [33]. While controlled studies of orbital radiotherapy have shown a modest effect on ocular motility, one clinical trial showed radiation alone may be no more effective than sham irradiation controls; although enrollment of patients late in their disease course may have tempered efficacy [34, 35]. The combination of orbital irradiation and corticosteroids may be more effective than either treatment alone [35, 36].

A common treatment regimen is 20 Gy in 10 divided doses over a 2-week period. Some clinicians have suggested using orbital irradiation to reduce the likelihood of emergent surgical decompression or to increase the effectiveness of surgical decompression [35, 37]. Orbital radiotherapy is well tolerated but contraindicated in patients with active diabetic or hypertensive retinopathy [38]. It is also not recommended for patients younger than 35 years of age due to mutagenic risk. Although cataract development has been associated with orbital radiotherapy, the risk is considered low and more likely related to concurrent steroid use [38].

Orbital Decompression in Severe Disease

Orbital decompression is primarily indicated as an emergent sight saving intervention for CON when medical treatment has failed, and secondarily in the quiescent phase for surgical rehabilitation of patients with disfiguring exophthalmos [30, 39–41]. In addition to apical expansion and proptosis reduction, orbital decompression appears to reduce orbital inflammatory signs (Fig. 9.1) [41].

Orbital decompression appears successful in improving visual functioning in a majority of patients with the rate of visual recovery correlating to the duration of optic neuropathy [29, 42]. Even in long standing optic neuropathy (>6 months) improvements in visual functioning can be seen. For CON with evidence of apical crowding on imaging (Fig. 9.2), orbital decompression is frequently combined with steroids or radiotherapy [41].

Decompression surgery may involve removal of a combination of the lateral wall, medial wall, orbital fat, and orbital floor [44]. In apical compression an adequate decompression should include the posterior medial wall and ethmoid air cells [44]. Although single wall decompression for CON has been described, recurrent optic neuropathy after single wall decompression has been reported [45]. Our approach for apical compression includes maximal decompression to both expand the orbital apex and also reduce proptosis. This approach avoids subsequent decompression for residual proptosis or recurrent CON.

Rituximab and Biological Therapies

RTX is FDA approved in non-Hodgkin's lymphoma, chronic lymphocytic leukemia, rheumatoid arthritis (RA), Wegener's granulomatosis (granulomatosis with polyangiitis), and microscopic polyangiitis but has been used off-label in

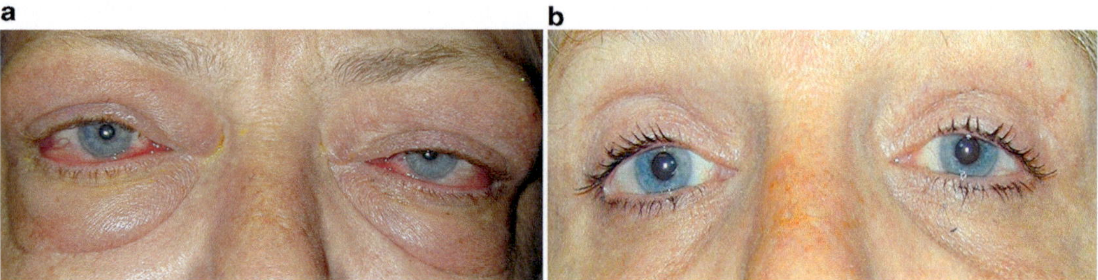

Fig. 9.1 (**a**) A 48-year-old female with severe inflammatory TED. (**b**) Same patient following rehabilitative orbital decompression surgery

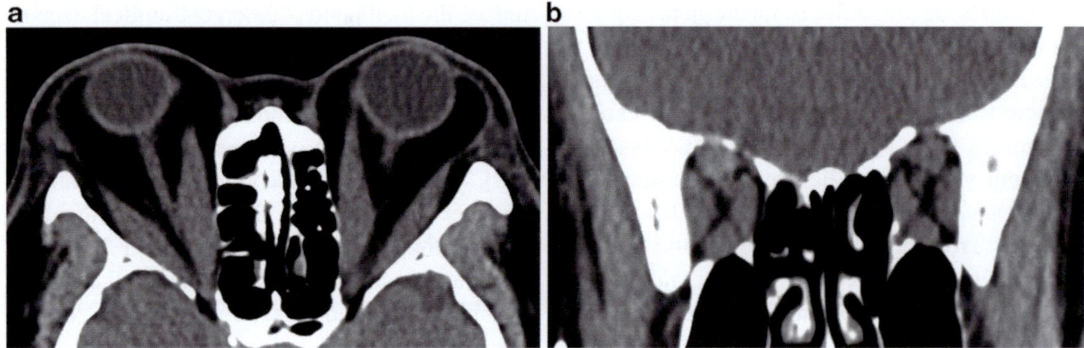

Fig. 9.2 (**a**) Axial CT of patient with severe thyroid eye disease demonstrating proptosis, extraocular muscle enlargement, optic nerve stretch, and fat infiltration. (**b**) Coronal CT of same patient

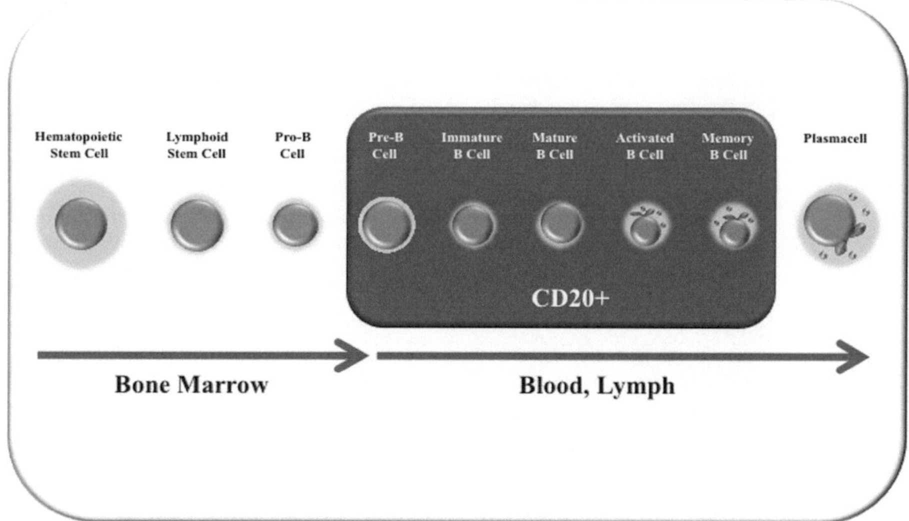

Fig. 9.3 Expression of the CD 20 antigen during B cell differentiation

various autoimmune disorders. RTX is a chimeric mouse-human monoclonal antibody that targets *CD20*, a human B lymphocyte-specific antigen expressed on more than 95 % of B cells from the stages of immature to mature B cells, as well as memory B cells but not on antibody-producing plasma cells [46]. As a consequence, therapy with RTX removes B lymphocytes and short-lived plasma cells (Fig. 9.3), but not long-lived plasma cells. Thus antibody production is maintained over a long period of time and immunoglobulin (Ig) levels tend not to change despite peripheral B cell depletion [47, 48]. RTX depletes more than 95 % of mature B cells in blood and primary lymphoid organs after 2 days by a single RTX treatment in mice. In humans, the mechanism of action of RTX in the treatment of autoimmune diseases remains unclear: response to treatment does not always correlate with complete B cell depletion and RTX might only indirectly affect autoantibody production [49, 50]. Clinical trials of RTX in RA have shown that it is effective in ameliorating the symptoms with improvement usually seen within 8–16 weeks and persisting for the duration of B cell depletion (typically 16–24 weeks) [51]. The rationale for RTX use in TED includes potential blockade of pathogenic autoantibody generation, depletion of B cell antigen-presentation, and inflammatory cytokine production. However an uncontrolled study demonstrated that in patients with TED, RTX does not affect TRAb titers, suggesting that its efficacy may result from its effect on B cell functions other than that of antibody production [52] or another mechanism entirely.

Infusion related reactions are the most frequently reported side effects of RTX [53]. Most patients experience minor allergic reactions during the first RTX infusion, because the drug is a humanized mAb. Reactions are tempered by antihistamine and low dose hydrocortisone prior to infusion and by slowing the rate of IV infusion during the first hour. Major acute infusion reactions, caused by inflammatory cytokine release and complement activation, may be present in about 10 % of patients and are usually reversible.

RTX has been reported to increase the risk of infections, especially Hepatitis B reactivation. The increased risk correlates with dose and duration and occurs more frequently in patients with neoplasia [54, 55]. A recent review of over 3,000 patients with rheumatoid arthritis showed comparable serious infection rates in those treated with RTX versus placebo plus methotrexate (MTX) [56]. No increased risk of malignancy over time was observed. Progressive multifocal

Table 9.1 Characteristics of patients with severe Graves' orbitopathy treated with rituximab

Study (No. of reference)	No. of patients treated	RTX dose	§CAS before therapy	CAS after therapy (16 weeks)	Severity after #RTX	Side effects	GO relapse
Salvi et al. [39]	1	1 g twice with 2 week interval + 1 g at 23 w	7	2	Transient improvement of visual acuity	Minor, infusion related	No
Khanna et al. [40]	6	1 g twice with 2 week interval	5.5	1.3	All improved	2 (minor), 1 (major, cardiac death, likely unrelated to therapy)	No
Krassas et al. [43]	1	1 g twice with 2 week interval	7	7	Worsened	n.r.	Yes
Salvi et al. [44]	3	100 mg single dose	5.3	1.6	All improved	2 (major but transient)	No
Mitchell et al. [42]	5	500 mg or 1 g at 2 week interval	6.5	3	6 pts. improved 3 pt. unchanged	4 (minor)	No

leukoencephalopathy (PML) has been reported in patients receiving RTX, but predominantly in patients with systemic lupus erythematosus (SLE) [57]. More than 40 % of PML cases occurred in patients with SLE, including those on relatively minimal immunosuppression, suggesting that SLE itself may also predispose to PML development [58].

The effects of RTX in patients with active and severe TED have been studied in 13 patients (Table 9.1) in non-controlled studies, although successful therapy has been described in another 30 patients with active moderate-severe TED. One patient with acute CON received two doses of 1,000 mg RTX, 2 weeks apart. A significant but transient clinical response was seen, with the restoration of normal vision for 16 weeks until B cell return in the peripheral blood, at which time visual deterioration recurred [59]. RTX re-treatment resulted in only transient improvement necessitating orbital decompression. In the patient's orbital tissues incomplete B cell depletion was noted, with relatively abundant CD19+5+ lymphocytes, which usually characterize early repopulation and autoreactive B cell clones [60].

The therapeutic efficacy of RTX in active, severe TED unresponsive to glucocorticoids was reported in a series of six patients [45]. RTX therapy was associated with significant decrease of the CAS at 8 weeks and 6 months. Four of these patients improved visual acuity to pre-morbid values, but had no improvement of extraocular motility or proptosis. In this study, 1,000 mg IV RTX was administered 2 weeks apart in combination with steroid therapy, which was subsequently tapered off without relapse of inflammation. Minor side effects were described in two patients, but a fatal cardiac event, not attributed to RTX, occurred in one patient. TED improvement and stabilization was associated with abundant peripheral CD25 cells (T_{regs}), which have been reported to be predictive of successful RTX therapy in RA [61]. RTX treatment was studied in a series of patients with steroid-refractory TED, of whom five had CON. The dose of RTX was varied from 500 to 1,000 mg every 2 weeks, based on attainment of peripheral B cell depletion [62]. All the patients in this series improved their NOSPECS score from grade 6 to grade 4. Failure of RTX in preventing active TED progression to CON was described in one patient who was also unresponsive to IV MP [62]. Proposed reasons for therapeutic failure include: RTX was administered too late in the disease course or RTX might have induced increased soft tissue edema and apical optic nerve compression, as a consequence of orbital cytokine release. This effect has been reported in two patients with TED, who experienced transient visual deterioration within an hour from RTX infusion, but spontaneous recovery to normal visual acuity 3–4 h later [63].

Although prospective studies designed to assess the effectiveness of RTX in patients with severe TED are needed, the data available suggest a potential benefit in some. The evidence is mainly based on studies conducted in patients with active, moderate-severe disease, which show that RTX is acting as a disease modifying agent. Recent preliminary data of a randomized controlled trial in these patients seem to show that RTX is more effective than steroids in the inactivation of TED and in preventing relapses of disease, usually observed in 20–30 % [64]. Further data are needed before considering RTX treatment suitable for the most severe forms of disease.

Other biological therapies used in TED include etanercept and infliximab, but data on clinical efficacy is limited [65]. The biologic agent, tocilizumab has shown early promise in a recent retrospective series of TED patients refractive to IV steroid therapy [66]. Tocilizumab is an FDA approved humanized monoclonal IgG1 antibody to the interleukin-6 (IL-6) receptor for use in active moderate to severe rheumatoid arthritis. Of eighteen patients treated, 14 had a CAS score greater than 6, one had optic neuropathy, and one failed previous biological therapy. CAS improved in all 18 patients, proptosis reduced in 13/18, and ocular motility improved in 15/18. The patients with CON improved without the need for orbital decompression. These positive preliminary results were achieved despite half the patients being active smokers, but further clinical trials are warranted [66].

Conclusion

Severe TED management typically requires a multidisciplinary approach involving endocrinologists, orbital surgeons, strabismus specialists, and neuro-ophthalmologists. After severe sight-threatening orbitopathy has been controlled, rehabilitation with decompression, strabismus, and eyelid surgery can restore function, aesthetics, and quality of life [67, 68].

References

1. Kalmann R, Mourits MP, van der Pol JP, Koornneef L. Coronal approach for rehabilitative orbital decompression in Graves' ophthalmopathy. Br J Ophthalmol. 1997;81(1):41–5.
2. Burch HB, Wartofsky L. Graves' ophthalmopathy: current concepts regarding pathogenesis and management. Endocr Rev. 1993;14(6):747.
3. Somer D, Ozkan SB, Ozdemir H, Atilla S, Soylev MF, Duman S. Colour Doppler imaging of superior ophthalmic vein in thyroid-associated eye disease. Jpn J Ophthalmol. 2002;46(3):341–5.
4. Dolman PJ, Rootman J. Predictors of disease severity in thyroid-related orbitopathy. (chap 18) Orbital disease. Present status and future challenges. Boca Raton: Taylor and Francis; 2005.
5. Rundle FF. Management of exophthalmos and related ocular changes in Graves' disease. Metabolism. 1957;6(1):36–48.
6. Dolman PJ. Evaluating Graves' orbitopathy. Best Pract Res Clin Endocrinol Metab. 2012;26(3):229–48.
7. Bartley GB, Fatourechi V, Kadrmas EF, Jacobsen SJ, Ilstrup DM, Garrity JA, Gorman CA. The incidence of Graves' ophthalmopathy in Olmsted County, Minnesota. Am J Ophthalmol. 1995;120(4):511.
8. Wiersinga WM, Bartalena L. Epidemiology and prevention of Graves' ophthalmopathy. Thyroid. 2002; 12(10):855–60.
9. Perros P, Crombie AL, Matthews JN, Kendall-Taylor P. Age and gender influence the severity of thyroid-associated ophthalmopathy: a study of 101 patients attending a combined thyroid-eye clinic. Clin Endocrinol (Oxf). 1993;38(4):367.
10. Prummel MF, Wiersinga WM. Smoking and risk of Graves' disease. JAMA. 1993;269(4):479.
11. Szucs-Farkas Z, Toth J, Kollar J, Galuska L, Burman KD, Boda J, Leovey A, Varga J, Ujhelyi B, Szabo J, Berta A, Nagy EV. Volume changes in intra- and extra-orbital compartments in patients with Graves' ophthalmopathy: effect of smoking. Thyroid. 2005;15(2):146.
12. Cawood TJ, Moriarty P, O'Farrelly C, O'Shea D. Smoking and thyroid-associated ophthalmopathy: a novel explanation of the biological link. J Clin Endocrinol Metab. 2007;92(1):59–64.
13. Wiersinga WM. Smoking and thyroid. Clin Endocrinol (Oxf). 2013;79:145–51.
14. Eckstein AK, Plicht M, Lax H, Neuhauser M, Mann K, Lederbogen S, Heckmann C, Esser J, Morgenthaler NG. Thyrotropin receptor autoantibodies are independent risk factors for Graves' ophthalmopathy and help to predict severity and outcome of the disease. J Clin Endocrinol Metab. 2006;91(9):3464.
15. Dolman PJ, Rootman J. VISA Classification for Graves' orbitopathy. Ophthal Plast Reconstr Surg. 2006;22(5):319–24.
16. Fayers T, Dolman PJ. Validity and reliability of the TED-QOL: a new three-item questionnaire to assess quality of life in thyroid eye disease. Br J Ophthalmol. 2011;95(12):1670–4.
17. Mourits MP, Prummel MF, Wiersinga WM, Koornneef L. Clinical activity score as a guide in the management of patients with Graves' ophthalmopathy. Clin Endocrinol (Oxf). 1997;47(1):9–14.
18. EUGOGO website. www.eugogo.eu
19. Bartalena L, Marcocci C, Tanda ML, Manetti L, Del'Unto E, Batolomei MP, Nardi M, Martino E, Pinchera A. Cigarette smoking and treatment outcomes in Graves' ophthalmopathy. Ann Intern Med. 1998; 129:632–5.

20. Kahaly GJ, Pitz S, Hommel G, Dittmar M. Randomized, single blind trial of intravenous versus oral steroid monotherapy in Graves' orbitopathy. J Clin Endocrinol Metab. 2005;90(9):5234–40.
21. Marcocci C, Marinò M. Treatment of mild, moderate-to-severe and very severe Graves' orbitopathy. Best Pract Res Clin Endocrinol Metab. 2012;26(3):325–37.
22. Stiebel-Kalish H, Robenshtok E, Hasanreisoglu M, Ezrachi D, Shimon I, Leibovici L. Treatment modalities for Graves' ophthalmopathy: systematic review and metaanalysis. J Clin Endocrinol Metab. 2009;94(8):2708–16.
23. Marcocci C, Bartalena L, Tanda ML, Manetti L, Dell'Unto E, Rocchi R, Barbesino G, Mazzi B, Bartolomei MP, Lepri P, Cartei F, Nardi M, Pinchera A. Comparison of the effectiveness and tolerability of intravenous or oral glucocorticoids associated with orbital radiotherapy in the management of severe Graves' ophthalmopathy: results of a prospective, single-blind, randomized study. J Clin Endocrinol Metab. 2001;86(8):3562–7.
24. Marcocci C, Watt T, Altea MA, Rasmussen AK, Feldt-Rasmussen U, Orgiazzi J, Bartalena L, European Group of Graves' Orbitopathy. Fatal and non-fatal adverse events of glucocorticoid therapy for Graves' orbitopathy: a questionnaire survey among members of the European Thyroid Association. Eur J Endocrinol. 2012;166(2):247–53.
25. Zang S, Ponto KA, Kahaly GJ. Clinical review: intravenous glucocorticoids for Graves' orbitopathy: efficacy and morbidity. J Clin Endocrinol Metab. 2011;96(2):320–32.
26. Bartalena L, Krassas GE, Wiersinga W, Marcocci C, Salvi M, Daumerie C, Bournaud C, Stahl M, Sassi L, Veronesi G, Azzolini C, Boboridis KG, Mourits MP, Soeters MR, Baldeschi L, Nardi M, Currò N, Boschi A, Bernard M, von Arx G, European Group on Graves' Orbitopathy. Efficacy and safety of three different cumulative doses of intravenous methylprednisolone for moderate to severe and active Graves' orbitopathy. J Clin Endocrinol Metab. 2012;97(12):4454–63.
27. Currò N, Covelli D, Vannucchi G, Campi I, Pirola G, Simonetta S, Dazzi D, Guastella C, Pignataro L, Beck-Peccoz P, Ratiglia R, Salvi M. Therapeutic outcomes of high dose intravenous steroids in the treatment of dysthyroid optic neuropathy. Thyroid. 2014;24:897–905.
28. Perros P, Weightman DR, Crombie AL, Kendall-Taylor P. Azathioprine in the treatment of thyroid-associated ophthalmopathy. Acta Endocrinol (Copenh). 1990;122(1):8–12.
29. Claridge KG, Ghabrial R, Davis G, Tomlinson M, Goodman S, Harrad RA, Potts MJ. Combined radiotherapy and medical immunosuppression in the management of thyroid eye disease. Eye (Lond). 1997;11(Pt 5):717–22.
30. Verity DH, Rose GE. Acute thyroid eye disease (TED): principles of medical and surgical management. Eye (Lond). 2013;27(3):308–19.
31. Wiersinga WM. Graves' orbitopathy: management of difficult cases. Indian J Endocrinol Metab. 2012;16 Suppl 2:S150–2.
32. Tanda ML, Bartalena L. Efficacy and safety of orbital radiotherapy for graves' orbitopathy. J Clin Endocrinol Metab. 2012;97(11):3857–65.
33. Trott KR, Kamprad F. Radiobiological mechanisms of anti-inflammatory radiotherapy. Radiother Oncol. 1999;51(3):197–203.
34. Mourits MP, van Kempen-Harteveld ML, Garcia MB, Koppeschaar HP, Tick L, Terwee CB. Radiotherapy for Graves' orbitopathy: randomised placebo-controlled study. Lancet. 2000;355(9214):1505–9.
35. Dolman PJ, Rath S. Orbital radiotherapy for thyroid eye disease. Curr Opin Ophthalmol. 2012;23(5):427–32.
36. Rajendram R, Bunce C, Lee RW, Morley AM. Orbital radiotherapy for adult thyroid eye disease. Cochrane Database Syst Rev. 2012 Jul 11; 7.
37. Kazim M, Trokel S, Moore S. Treatment of acute Graves orbitopathy. Ophthalmology. 1991;98(9):1443–8.
38. Wakelkamp IM, Tan H, Saeed P, Schlingemann RO, Verbraak FD, Blank LE, Prummel MF, Wiersinga WM. Orbital irradiation for Graves' ophthalmopathy: is it safe? A long-term follow-up study. Ophthalmology. 2004;111(8):1557–62.
39. Lyons CJ, Rootman J. Orbital decompression for disfiguring exophthalmos in thyroid orbitopathy. Ophthalmology. 1994;101(2):223–30.
40. Baldeschi L, Wakelkamp IM, Lindeboom R, Prummel MF, Wiersinga WM. Early versus late orbital decompression in Graves' orbitopathy: a retrospective study in 125 patients. Ophthalmology. 2006;113(5):874–8.
41. Wakelkamp IM, Baldeschi L, Saeed P, Mourits MP, Prummel MF, Wiersinga WM. Surgical or medical decompression as a first-line treatment of optic neuropathy in Graves' ophthalmopathy? A randomized controlled trial. Clin Endocrinol (Oxf). 2005;63(3):323–8.
42. Oh SR, Tung JD, Priel A, Levi L, Granet DB, Korn BS, Kikkawa DO. Reduction of orbital inflammation following decompression for thyroid-related orbitopathy. Biomed Res Int. 2013;2013:794984.
43. Jeon C, Shin JH, Woo KI, Kim YD. Clinical profile and visual outcomes after treatment in patients with dysthyroid optic neuropathy. Korean J Ophthalmol. 2012;26(2):73–9.
44. Korn B, Kikkawa DO. Video Atlas of Oculofacial plastic and reconstructive surgery. Saunders: Elsevier; 2011. p. 160.
45. Khanna D, Chong KK, Afifiyan NF, Hwang CJ, Lee DK, Garneau HC, Goldberg RA, Darwin CH, Smith TJ, Douglas RS. Rituximab treatment of patients with severe, corticosteroid-resistant thyroid-associated ophthalmopathy. Ophthalmology. 2010;117(1):133–9.
46. Stashenko P, Nadler LM, Hardy R, Schlossman SF. Characterization of a human B lymphocyte-specific antigen. J Immunol. 1980;125:1678–85.

47. Ahuja A, Anderson SM, Khalil A, Shlomchik MJ. Maintenance of the plasma cell pool is independent of memory B cells. Proc Natl Acad Sci U S A. 2008;105:4802–7.
48. Avivi I, Stroopinsky D, Katz T. Anti-CD20 monoclonal antibodies: beyond B cells. Blood Rev. 2013; 27:217–23.
49. Edwards JC, Szczepanski L, Szechinski J, Filipowicz-Sosnowska A, Emery P, Close DR, Stevens RM, Shaw T. Efficacy of B-cell-targeted therapy with rituximab in patients with rheumatoid arthritis. N Engl J Med. 2004;350:2572–81.
50. Thurlings RM, Vos K, Wijbrandts CA, Zwinderman AH, Gerlag DM, Tak PP. Synovial tissue response to rituximab: mechanism of action and identification of biomarkers of response. Ann Rheum Dis. 2004;67: 917–25.
51. Popa MJ, Leandro G, Cambridge JC, Edwards W. Repeated B lymphocyte depletion with rituximab in rheumatoid arthritis over 7 yrs. Rheumatology. 2007;46:626–30.
52. Vannucchi G, Campi I, Bonomi M, Covelli D, Dazzi D, Currò N, Simonetta S, Bonara P, Persani L, Guastella C, Wall J, Beck-Peccoz P, Salvi M. Rituximab treatment in patients with active Graves' orbitopathy: effects on proinflammatory and humoral immune reactions. Clin Exp Immunol. 2010;161:436–43.
53. Descotes J. Immunotoxicity of monoclonal antibodies. MAbs. 2009;1:104–11.
54. Yx K, Tan DS, Tan IB, Tao M, Lim ST. Hepatitis B virus reactivation in a patient with resolved hepatitis B virus infection receiving maintenance rituximab for malignant B-cell lymphoma. Ann Intern Med. 2009;150:655–6.
55. Evens AM, Jovanovic BD, Su YC, Raisch DW, Ganger D, Belknap SM, et al. Rituximab-associated hepatitis B virus (HBV) reactivation in lymphoproliferative diseases: meta-analysis and examination of FDA safety reports. Ann Oncol. 2011;22:1170–80.
56. Van Vollenhoven RF, Emery P, Bingham CO, Keystone EC, Fleischmann RM, Furst DE, Tyson N, Collinson N, Lehane PB. Long-term safety of rituximab in rheumatoid arthritis: 9.5-year follow-up of the global clinical trial programme with a focus on adverse events of interest in RA patients. Ann Rheum Dis. 2013;72:1496–502. doi:10.1136/annrheumdis-2012-201956.
57. Food and Drug Administration. FDA Public Health Advisory: life-threatening brain infection in patients with systemic lupus erythematosus after Rituxan (rituximab) treatment. http://www.fda.gov/cder/drug/ (2006).
58. Molloy ES, Calabrese LH. Progressive multifocal leukoencephalopathy in patients with rheumatic diseases: are patients with systemic lupus erythematosus at particular risk? Autoimmun Rev. 2008;8:144–416.
59. Salvi M, Vannucchi G, Campi I, Currò N, Simonetta S, Covelli D, Pignataro L, Guastella C, Rossi S, Bonara P, Dazzi D, Ratiglia R, Beck-Peccoz P. Rituximab treatment in a patient with severe thyroid-associated ophthalmopathy: effects on orbital lymphocytic infiltrates. Clin Immunol. 2009;131:360–5.
60. Boissier MC, Assier E, Biton J, Denys A, Falgarone G, Bessis N. Regulatory T cells (Treg) in rheumatoid arthritis. Joint Bone Spine. 2009;76:10–4.
61. Mitchell AL, Gan EH, Morris M, Johnson K, Neoh C, Dickinson AJ, Perros P, Pearce SH. The effect of B cell depletion therapy on anti-TSH receptor antibodies and clinical outcome in glucocorticoid refractory Graves' orbitopathy. Clin Endocrinol (Oxf). 2013;79:437–42.
62. Krassas GE, Stafilidou A, Boboridis KG. Failure of rituximab treatment in a case of severe thyroid ophthalmopathy unresponsive to steroids. Clin Endocrinol (Oxf). 2010;72:853–5.
63. Salvi M, Vannucchi G, Currò N, Introna M, Rossi S, Bonara P, Covelli D, Dazzi D, Guastella C, Pignataro L, Ratiglia R, Golay J, Beck-Peccoz P. A small dose of rituximab may be sufficient to treat Graves' orbitopathy: new insights into the mechanism of action. Arch Ophthalmol. 2012;130:122–4.
64. Salvi M, Vannucchi G, Campi I, Covelli D, Currò N, Dazzi D, Avignone S, Sina C, Beck-Peccoz P. Double blind Randomized controlled study of rituximab and intravenous steroid treatment in Graves' orbitopathy (GO): analysis of the primary endpoint at 24 weeks. 37th Annual Meeting, Leiden, The Netherlands, 7–11 September 2013.
65. Bhatt R, Nelson CC, Douglas RS. Thyroid-associated orbitopathy: current insights into the pathophysiology, immunology and management. Saudi J Ophthalmol. 2011;25(1):15–20.
66. Pérez-Moreiras JV, Alvarez-López A, Gómez EC. Treatment of active corticosteroid-resistant graves' orbitopathy. Ophthal Plast Reconstr Surg. 2014;30:162–7.
67. Wiersinga WM. Combined thyroid eye clinic: the importance of a multidisciplinary health care in patients with Graves' orbitopathy. Pediatr Endocrinol Rev. 2010;7 Suppl 2:250–3.
68. European Group on Graves' Orbitopathy (EUGOGO). Outcome of orbital decompression for disfiguring proptosis in patients with Graves' orbitopathy using various surgical procedures. Br J Ophthalmol. 2009;93(11):1518–23.

10 Strabismus in Thyroid Eye Disease

Bokkwan Jun and Prem S. Subramanian

Pathophysiology of Extraocular Muscle Change

Graves' disease is the most common dysthyroid state associated with orbitopathy, and it may be defined as the triad of hyperthyroidism with diffuse thyroid enlargement, orbitopathy, and pretibial myxedema. Thyroid eye disease (TED) is an inflammatory autoimmune disorder of the orbit that is probably caused by immune cross-reactivity between orbital and thyroid antigens. The onset of TED occasionally may precede or follow that of hyperthyroidism by several years and approximately 40 % of Graves' disease patients have or will develop orbitopathy within 18 months [1]. As discussed elsewhere in this textbook, the close relationship between Graves' disease and TED has suggested that both conditions derive from a single systemic pathologic process and share the thyrotropin receptor (TSHR) as a common autoantigen that is expressed both in thyroid follicular cells and orbital fibroblasts. Circulating thyrotropin receptor autoantibodies activate this receptor on orbital fibroblasts and this results in their increased secretion of hyaluronic acid and the differentiation into mature adipocytes (enhanced adipogenesis) [1–4]. Cytokines and other mediators of inflammation, produced by infiltrating mononuclear cells and macrophages, accumulate within the orbit and contribute to the local inflammatory process [2–4]. Activated CD4+ and CD8+ T cells infiltrate perivascularly and diffusely in the orbit, and interact with autoreactive B cells, plasma cells, and macrophages and secrete proinflammatory cytokines. This cellular process leads to enlargement of the extraocular muscles (EOM), expansion of the orbital adipose tissue, and orbital inflammation characteristic of the disease. Relevant to this chapter, the inflammation and glycosaminoglycan deposition in the soft tissues, including the EOM, can cause the edema of the tissue in early, acute phase and eventual fibrosis in the chronic phase.

During the early, inflammatory stages of TED, before restrictive strabismus is noted, microscopic examination of the EOM reveals infiltration between the muscle fibers with mononuclear inflammatory cells [5]. Interfibrillar spaces are enlarged and contain an amorphous material rich in hyaluronic acid. Acute muscle enlargement may also be mediated by raised muscle tension secondary to transition from slow to fast muscle types induced by the hyperthyroid state [6].

B. Jun, M.D., Ph.D.
Division of Neuro-Ophthalmology, Department of Ophthalmology, Wilmer Eye Institute, The Johns Hopkins Hospital, Johns Hopkins University School of Medicine, 600 N. Wolfe Street, Woods 457, Baltimore, MD 21287, USA

P.S. Subramanian, M.D., Ph.D. (✉)
Department of Ophthalmology, Neurology, and Neurosurgery, The Johns Hopkins Hospital, Johns Hopkins University School of Medicine, 600 N. Wolfe Street, Woods 457, Baltimore, MD 21287, USA
e-mail: psubram1@jhmi.edu

R.S. Douglas et al. (eds.), *Thyroid Eye Disease*,
DOI 10.1007/978-1-4939-1746-4_10, © Springer Science+Business Media New York 2015

Following infiltration of the endomysial space of the muscle by lymphocytes, macrophages, and neutrophils, muscle cells decrease in numbers, and the contractile properties of the affected muscles may be compromised. Nonetheless, restriction rather than paresis seems to result in both the acute and chronic phases of disease. Stimulated fibroblasts produce increased levels of glycosaminoglycans, which attract water osmotically, contributing to interstitial edema [5]. At the cellular level, there is a marked expansion of the endomysial space in the EOM of patients with recently inactive TED [7]. Collagen synthesis and deposition occur in interfascicular membranes and extraocular muscle sheaths [8]. In the healing phase of TED, the muscles become fibrotic and inelastic, resulting in permanently restricted eye movement.

Histologic studies of TED have focused on EOM, owing to their obvious enlargement in patients with the disease (Fig. 10.1). Electron microscopy reveals intact extraocular muscle fibers that are widely separated by an amorphous accumulation of granular material consisting primarily of collagen fibrils and glycosaminoglycans, among which hyaluronan predominates [7]. The polyanionic charge and high osmotic pressure of this matrix substance make it extremely hydrophilic and capable of binding many times its weight in water. Consequently, the muscle bodies become edematous and may enlarge to many times their normal size. In the inactive stage, atrophy and fibrosis of muscle bundles are evident, with extension of fibrous strands into adjacent adipose tissues. Histologic features of thyroid dermopathy are similar to those seen in the orbit, with hyaluronan accumulation in the reticular dermis, although with less abundant lymphocytic infiltration and no evidence of fat expansion [9].

After orbital decompression surgery, volumetric changes of EOM have been observed. Increased medial rectus muscle volume has been shown postoperatively in patients with stable TED, in whom there were clinical signs of recurrent orbital inflammation [10, 11]. The etiology of postoperative extraocular muscle volumetric changes is still unclear. If the disease process is still active at the time of decompression surgery, progression of extraocular muscle enlargement with and without compressive optic neuropathy could occur as a continuation of the process. However, this should not occur in the context of

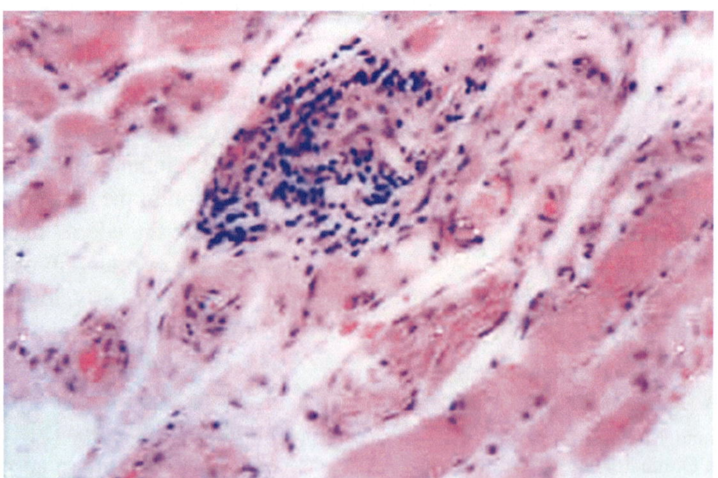

Fig. 10.1 Histologic appearance of extraocular muscle in Graves' ophthalmopathy (hematoxylin and eosin). The focal and perivascular interstitial inflammatory mononuclear cell infiltrate is in close association with intact striated extraocular muscle fibers widely separated by amorphous granular material. From Bahn RS. Graves' ophthalmopathy. N Engl J Med. 2010;362:726–38.

inactive disease [12]. There are several hypotheses regarding the cause of these changes. It could be reactivation of TED after orbital decompression that may have been induced by activation of antigen presenting cells and fibroblasts in the T-cell mediated inflammatory process incited by the surgery. Even a subclinical inflammatory reaction postoperatively could play a role in the early postoperative period. Alternatively, hydrostatic pressure change within the orbit and muscle secondary to the expanded orbital volume and relatively reduced intraorbital and intramuscular pressures could allow for muscle volume expansion. Glycosaminoglycans, known to be present in extraocular muscles during the inactive phase of TED by transmission electron microscopy, may be the driving force behind these changes in muscle size [7].

Imaging Findings

Neuroimaging of TED plays an important role in the differential diagnosis and interdisciplinary management of patients with TED and is required in patients with asymmetric ptosis, in suspected compressive optic neuropathy and prior to decompression surgery. Orbital imaging, such as magnetic resonance imaging (MRI), computed tomography (CT), and ultrasound show enlargement of the EOM, an increase in orbital fat tissue volume and enlargement of the lacrimal glands. Orbital MRI with fat saturation and gadolinium should be considered in a patient with decreased vision to evaluate for compressive optic nerve changes and to differentiate them from non-compressive neuropathy, in determining the appropriate intervention, and to monitor the progress or response to medical or surgical treatment. Orbital CT is the modality of choice for planning orbital decompression surgery since it provides precise imaging of the orbital apex especially of the osseous structures and it also may be considered when MRI is not available. MRI is preferred for studies assessing disease activity because of its better performance in the evaluation in soft tissues. Usually MRI is considered as both quantitative and qualitative rather than CT, which is considered as only quantitative. Orbital ultrasound offers the advantage of availability in most offices, but it has a high inter-observer variability. Orbital tissue edema, enlargement of extraocular muscles, and increase of retrobulbar fat volume are usually observed [13]. The classic morphological findings in TED are spindle-shaped expansion of typically more than one of the extraocular muscles (>4 mm) without involvement of the corresponding tendon, seen best on axial views of either imaging modality. Additionally, presentation of preferential muscle involvement, starting with early involvement of the inferior rectus followed by the medial rectus, the superior rectus, and finally the lateral rectus muscle is a characteristic finding, seen best on coronal views. In the case of long-lasting TED, a spontaneous bony decompression is noted with an impression of the normally parallel laminae papyraceae leading to the so-called "Coca Cola sign".

MRI

MRI may help to detect disease activity and to predict the response of medical therapy. Increased T2 signal in the EOM is associated with a good response to orbital irradiation (Fig. 10.2), and STIR (Short T1 Inversion Recovery) imaging, an inversion recovery pulse sequence with specific timing to suppress the fat signal, is useful for predicting the outcome of immunosuppressive therapy. High signal intensity in T2 also is associated with a good response to methylprednisolone pulse therapy. Exophthalmos from the increase in fat tissue volume is observed more in young female patients and exophthalmos from enlargement of EOM is more typical in older male patients. Because prolonged T2 relaxation time theoretically reflects free water content as a manifestation of inflammation in the tissue, an increase of T2 signal intensity may indicate the active stage with swelling in the enlarged eye muscles. The appearance of low T2 signal intensity may indicate the progress of fibrotic changes in EOM with subsequent adhesion of the muscles to the retro-ocular tissues [14].

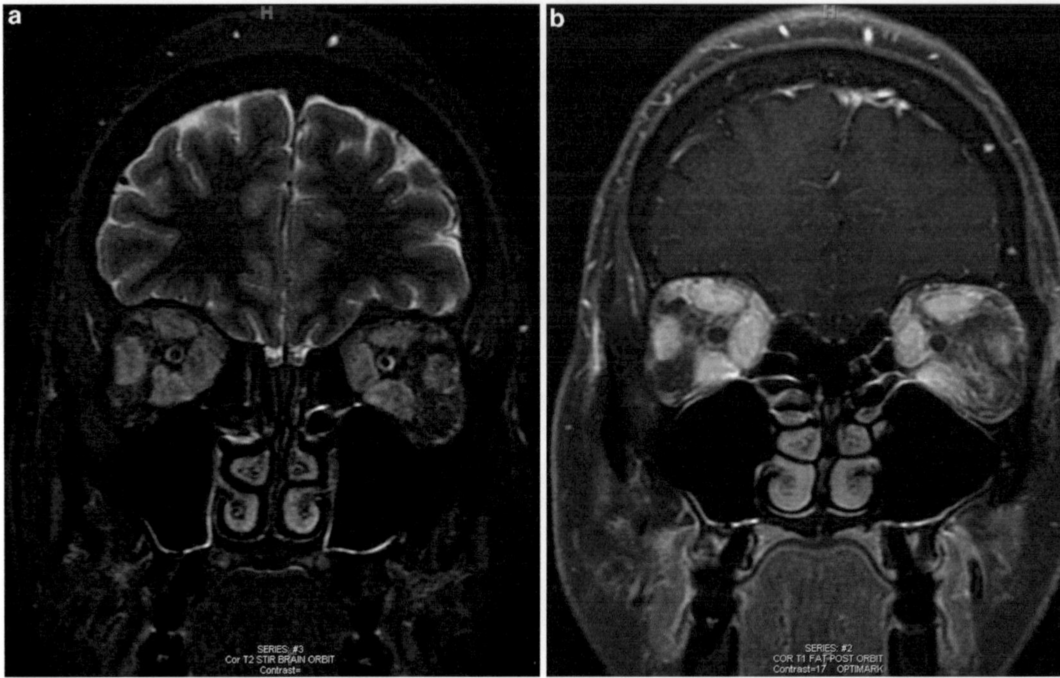

Fig. 10.2 Magnetic resonance imaging of orbit in a patient with strabismus. (**a**) Coronal T2 STIR, (**b**) Coronal T1 fat suppression postcontrast MRI, marked enlargement of the extraocular muscles bilaterally, with greatest involvement of the superior, medial, and inferior recti. There is heterogeneity within the orbital fat

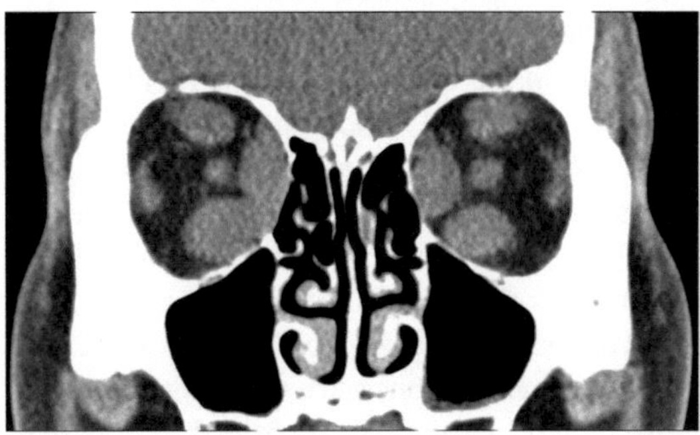

Fig. 10.3 Computed tomographic findings in a patient with strabismus from thyroid ophthalmopathy. Coronal view, soft tissue window, showing marked enlargement of the medial and inferior rectus muscles with moderate enlargement of the superior rectus muscles. There is relative sparing of the lateral rectus muscles

CT

CT is generally the preferred imaging modality for the initial diagnosis of patients with TED because of its ability to visualize bone and soft tissues in the orbit (Fig. 10.3). It also aids the evaluation of the orbital walls, sinuses, cribriform plate, and orbital fat in planning for decompression surgery. Compared to MRI, CT is less efficient in the evaluation of soft tissue changes. CT findings in TED may include bone changes, especially in the lamina papyracea of the ethmoid, with medial bowing resulting from chronic mechanical pressure by enlarged EOM. Lacrimal gland displacement and enlargement, exophthalmos, anterior soft tissue swelling and superior ophthalmic vein dilation may also be observed. In chronic disease, fatty degeneration of the extraocular muscles might be detected as hypo-attenuated areas on CT. CT imaging may be useful in deciding whether recession and/or resection can be considered. For example, if patients have greater proptosis and larger superior rectus muscles on imaging preoperatively, they are more likely to develop late overcorrection after inferior rectus muscle recession for restrictive hypotropia. Therefore, combined superior and inferior rectus muscle recession may be considered. If the muscle is not enlarged or inflamed on imaging, resection of EOM, especially the lateral rectus muscle, may be performed.

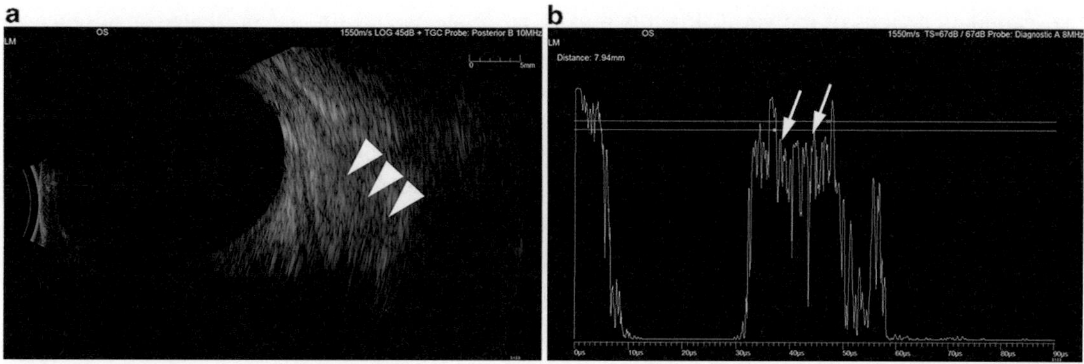

Fig. 10.4 Echographic findings. (**a**) B-scan ultrasound image shows enlarged EOM in retrobulbar space (*arrowhead*). (**b**) A-scan demonstrates high internal reflectivity (*arrows*) characteristic of thyroid ophthalmopathy

Ultrasound

Both A-scan and B-scan echography are performed for evaluation of TED (Fig. 10.4). Interpretation of the images can be challenging and requires clinical expertise of a certified orbital echographer. Normal extraocular muscle has relatively lower internal reflectivity than surrounding tissue since it has homogeneous arrangement of muscle fibers. A-scans are used to assess these tissue characteristics and are particularly sensitive for identifying thickening or thinning of the muscles and for differentiating underlying pathologies. However, it is easier to visualize the orbital structures using B-scan techniques, and B-scans are very helpful in topographic evaluations and in the initial identification of individual rectus muscle enlargement. The internal reflectivity of the EOM may change as a result of tissue swelling and cellular infiltration. In the active phase, the EOM have a lower internal reflectivity, due to swelling, whereas in the inactive, chronic phase, the muscles tend to show irregular high reflectivity from the echogenic fibrotic scar tissue.

Timing of Onset of Strabismus

The incidence of strabismus in TED is somewhat variable depending on the population and timing. Between 15 and 51 % of TED patients develop strabismus, and it is most commonly secondary to restriction of extraocular motility from inflammatory and fibrotic changes [15–18]. Data from a large cohort of TED patients demonstrate that 9.2 % of patients required strabismus surgery; in comparison, 6.7 % underwent decompression procedures [19]. Most patients with TED and strabismus have a history of hyperthyroidism; however they may be euthyroid, or even hypothyroid at the time of presentation. In a large cohort of patients with TED, appearance of diplopia was seen up to 11 years after diagnosis of TED based on other orbital or eyelid findings [20]. Other signs and symptoms of TED typically start 2 years prior to the onset of diplopia. Exophthalmos, when present, usually precedes diplopia. Subclinical eye involvement is common in nearly 70 % of adult patients with Graves' hyperthyroidism, with extraocular enlargement detected on MRI or CT [21].

As noted above, the effect of hyperthyroidism on the EOM occurs in two stages. The inflammatory phase, characterized by a lymphocytic infiltrate of the EOM and orbital tissues, may result in strabismus that changes when EOM fibrosis causes restriction of extraocular motility. Because the inferior rectus and medial rectus muscles are most often involved, hypotropia and esotropia result. Any of the rectus muscles may be involved, and recent data demonstrate more frequent involvement of the oblique muscles (particularly the inferior oblique) than previously recognized [22, 23]. Patients are often bothered by diplopia in primary gaze at distance because of common involvement of inferior rectus and medial rectus muscles. Torsional changes may also be noted because of the secondary actions of the vertical rectus muscles in addition to oblique muscle tightness.

Differential diagnosis of acquired strabismus in an adult includes cranial nerve palsies, orbital inflammatory conditions such as myositis and orbital pseudotumor, and extraocular muscle involvement with a systemic disease such as myasthenia gravis or chronic progressive external ophthalmoplegia. Graves' disease may occur in approximately 5–10 % of patients with myasthenia gravis, and myasthenia gravis has been reported in 0.2 % of patients with Graves' disease. Myasthenia gravis often presents with a history of variability and worsening of symptoms with fatigue. In order to differentiate these acquired strabismic conditions, orbital imaging with CT or MRI can be done to assess the extraocular muscles. In TED, the inferior and medical rectus muscles are most commonly involved. Classically, there is an enlargement of the muscle belly with sparing of the muscle tendon, which is in contrast to myositis where there is diffuse enlargement of the muscle from the origin to the tendon. Laboratory tests including thyroid hormone levels (TSH, T3, free T4, thyroid-stimulating immunoglobulin, TSH receptor antibodies) as well as acetylcholine receptor antibody tests need to be considered to evaluate for myasthenia gravis in conjunction with Graves' disease.

Typical Findings

Over 90 % of patients with TED develop upper eyelid retraction, which is a typical and highly sensitive sign and is seen mostly in the hyperthyroid state. Proposed mechanisms for lid abnormalities in TED include increased circulating catecholamines, overaction of the levator palpebrae superioris, and superior rectus muscles to compensate for inferior rectus restriction, or inflammation and scarring of the levator complex. Similarly, lower eyelid retraction, or inferior scleral show, is associated with inferior rectus tightness. Thus, the eyelid signs should prompt the clinician to evaluate extraocular motility and alignment carefully, even if strabismus is not readily apparent and/or diplopia is not reported. Proptosis is the second most common finding in TED, but it does not correlate well with the presence or absence of extraocular motility disturbances. Lower lid retraction may be exacerbated by increasing proptosis. A tight inferior rectus muscle, which impairs the normal Bell phenomenon, together with lower eyelid retraction may worsen the corneal exposure and eye irritation that results from proptosis. The resulting blurred vision also may impair normal fusion and can induce diplopia by unmasking an underlying phoria. EOM engorgement may result from crowding at the orbital apex, and secondary orbital venous hypertension can cause conjunctival redness and caruncular swelling. It is important to distinguish this type of redness and swelling from the signs associated with active orbitopathy, as the former will not respond to typical anti-inflammatory therapies.

Any type of strabismus is possible in TED. Common patterns of strabismus in TED are hypotropia secondary to inferior rectus restriction, esotropia secondary to medial rectus restriction, and hypertropia secondary to superior rectus restriction (Fig. 10.5). Because medial rectus tightness is far more common than lateral rectus involvement, manifest exotropia should raise suspicion for an additional or alternative etiology to TED-related strabismus, such as myasthenia gravis. However, presence of a vertical heterotropia may unmask a preexisting and unrelated exophoria, and full horizontal motility may help establish this possibility although it does not exclude myasthenia. Similarly, hypertropia and A-pattern exotropia with intorsion after recession of the inferior rectus may occur. The strabismus of TED is tremendously variable with regard to presentation, findings, and response to treatment. Intraocular pressure may increase especially in upgaze and it is usually secondary to inferior rectus restriction or orbital congestion. Because this is a mechanical form of increased intraocular pressure, topical drops for lowering the intraocular pressure are often ineffective. Optic neuropathy occurs in approximately 5 % of patients with TED and it is due to compression of the optic nerve by large indurated muscles at the orbital apex. The clinical risk factors for the development of TED-related compressive optic neuropathy include medial rectus enlargement and diplopia,

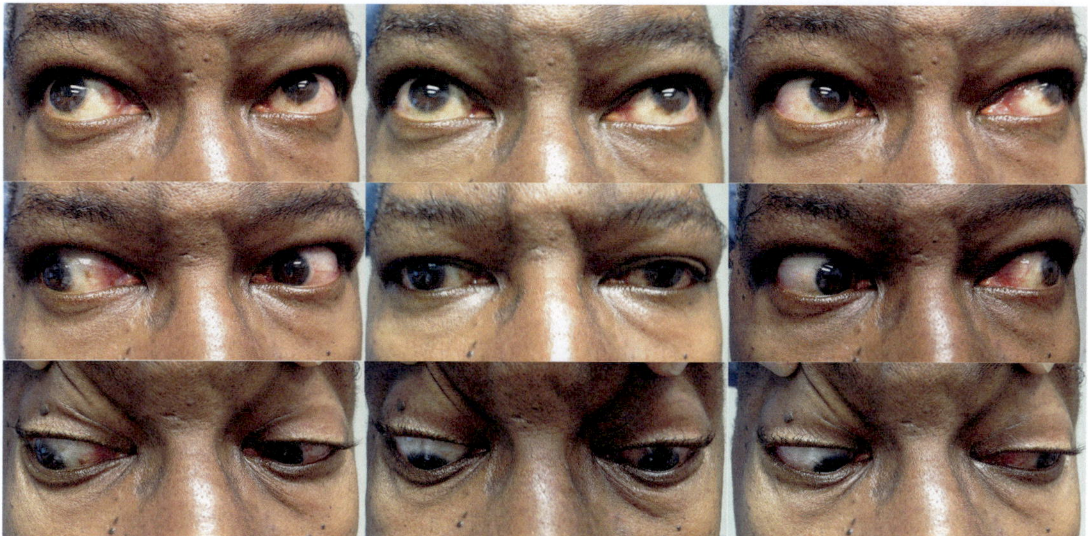

Fig. 10.5 Photograph of a patient with restrictive strabismus in the 9 cardinal gaze positions. The patient noted vertical diplopia, consistent with the asymmetric limitation of left eye depression and right eye elevation. Eyelid retraction is present as well

and careful examination of the optic disc and evaluation of automated perimetry should be performed in patients with TED-associated diplopia.

Initial Workup

As discussed elsewhere in this text, the diagnosis of TED is based on recognition of clinical features and may be supported by serologic tests of thyroid function and immune testing, and orbital imaging. Specialized diagnostic tests are usually not required for bilateral eye disease in the presence of autoimmune thyroid disease. If a patient presents with symptoms and signs of TED without a history of systemic thyroid disease, endocrinologic investigation including thyroid-stimulating immunoglobulin (TSI) and thyroid-stimulating hormone (TSH) levels may be required to detect any thyroid dysfunction. Abnormalities in thyroid hormonal tests (T3, free T4, and TSH) and/or the presence of thyroid specific antibodies (anti-thyroglobulin, anti-thyroid peroxidase and anti-TSH receptor) help to support the diagnosis, but they are not essential, and their absence does not exclude the diagnosis. Orbital imaging should be performed if the diagnosis is not certain from the clinical and laboratory data, or when optic neuropathy is suspected or surgical intervention is considered.

Natural History

As described in Chap. 2, TED follows a biphasic course, with a progressive or active inflammatory phase followed by a stable or inactive phase. The initial inflammatory phase may be progressive and generally lasts for 6–18 months before a plateau phase is reached. This is followed by resolution of inflammation and the final inactive "burnt out" stage [24, 25]. Graves' ophthalmopathy activity, as judged by inflammatory signs and symptoms, is slightly separated from the curve of severity, usually evaluated based on degree of proptosis, eyelid aperture, diplopia, and visual acuity [26, 27]. According to this model, the activity peak would precede the severity peak by a few months [28].

Overall, TED improves spontaneously in approximately 60 % of cases, remains stable in 25 %, and deteriorates in about 15 % [10, 11, 28]. Congestive changes are more likely to improve than ocular myopathic changes. Extraocular muscle fibrosis may happen early in the inflammatory process, and thus patients who develop moderate to severe restriction of eye muscle function and globe excursion are less likely to experience spontaneous recovery of single binocular vision. It is our experience that the course of TED is to a large degree independent of the thyroid status but tends to be more severe in patients with poorly controlled hyperthyroidism and those rendered hypothyroid. The role of orbital decompression in the onset of diplopia remains debated. Clearly, there is an immediate postoperative onset of diplopia in a percentage of patients undergoing decompression surgery, and the incidence will vary depending upon the decompression technique used [12, 29–32]. However, the natural history of diplopia in TED would indicate that a certain number of these cases were likely to develop whether or not the patient had a decompression early in the course of their disease. The average age of patients experiencing diplopia in TED is 50, which is higher than the average age of overall TED incidence. Older patients, white males, and cigarette smokers tend to have a more severe course of the disease [7, 33–35]. Younger patients tend to have more orbital symptoms and signs and are less likely to develop strabismus with TED, while older patients tend to have more extraocular muscle involvement rather than orbital swelling [13, 36, 37].

Management

General management of TED applies to the treatment of patients with diplopia and strabismus as well; they should stop smoking and work with their endocrinologist or primary care physician to achieve a euthyroid state, although correction of dysfunction is known to have little direct effect on the progression of thyroid strabismus. Cigarette smoking adversely affects the ocular signs of TED and is correlated with diplopia in a dose-dependent manner [14, 38]. Smoking status also correlates with likelihood of needing strabismus surgery [15–18, 39]. As it is a modifiable risk factor, all patients with Graves' disease should be advised strongly to stop smoking and have this counseling clearly documented in the medical record.

Medical Management

Systemic Corticosteroids (IV or Oral)

Moderate to severe, active, inflammatory phase of TED often responds to the systemic administration of corticosteroids particularly in cases of reduced visual acuity, visual field deficits, color deficits, or afferent pupillary defects. Systemic corticosteroids may be given orally or intravenously and may improve orbital congestion, acute ocular misalignment, and optic neuropathy. Prolonged steroid therapy is not indicated because of the risks of long-term steroid use. The best evidence points to the use of pulsed intravenous corticosteroid rather than daily oral dosing [40]. A recent randomized prospective study of IV corticosteroid dosing found that the greatest improvement in overall ophthalmic status and quality of life was observed with a regimen of 830 mg weekly for 6 weeks followed by 415 mg weekly for 6 weeks (cumulative dose 7.47 g); a lower dose scheme of 540 mg for 6 weeks and then 270 mg for 6 weeks (total dose 4.98 g) was nearly as effective and carried lower risk. However, neither regimen resulted in ocular motility improvement in the majority of treated patients, and one-third of patients in the lower dose cohort progressed despite treatment [41]. Oral prednisone at a dose of 60–80 mg/day followed by dose reduction every 2 weeks for a total treatment duration of 4–6 months is known to be as effective as IV methylprednisolone infusion twice weekly for 6 weeks, but the oral steroid may be more frequently associated with side effects [42]. We recommend using corticosteroids for diplopia when there is objective worsening of strabismus (progressive limitation of ductions) with other clinical signs and symptoms (chemosis, pain, periorbital swelling) or radiographic evidence (EOM hyperintensity on T2 MRI) of active disease. We favor intravenous steroid treatment because of the side effect profile. However, strabismus may still worsen if a fibrotic response to the inflammatory phase begins prior to the treatment taking effect.

Orbital Radiotherapy

Radiation therapy (RT) has also been used as a treatment for TED-associated strabismus. Orbital irradiation is usually given over 10–12 sessions (200 cGy each session) for a total dose of 2,000–2,200 cGy. It should not be repeated because of the risk of additive radiation, and many experts avoid radiation in patients who smoke or have other vasculopathic risk factors (e.g., diabetes mellitus). It is only indicated in patients who are in the inflammatory phase. There is controversy about the role and efficacy of orbital irradiation. It remains as a viable option for patients who cannot tolerate systemic corticosteroid therapy. The efficacy of orbital XRT for strabismus was called into question by a prospective, masked trial comparing one radiated orbit in a patient to the fellow, sham-irradiated, control orbit. In this study, no difference was observed between the two sides [43]. However, improved ocular motility, specifically with attempted elevation, has been demonstrated in other prospective studies [44]. A recent meta-analysis of available data also indicates that it may be effective in the stabilization of progressive external ophthalmoplegia. The treating physician should be aware that radiation therapy frequently has a significant lag of several weeks before any anti-inflammatory effect is seen.

Other Agents Including Biologics

Limited data on the use of biologic agents in the management of refractory TED have appeared recently in the literature. The physician must be cautioned at this juncture about recommending such therapy to patients with typical TED, given the limited power of these studies with limited patient numbers, the lack of a clear understanding regarding dosage, duration of treatment for TED, and the potential systemic side effects. The biologic agents targeting the underlying molecular basis of TED may be considered as a potential alternative therapy for TED patients who are unable to tolerate corticosteroids. Rituximab is a monoclonal chimeric antibody against CD20, a transmembrane protein present on immature and mature B cells but not plasma cells. It is approved for the treatment of non-Hodgkin lymphomas, chronic lymphocytic leukemia, and rheumatoid arthritis. Rituximab effectively depletes the CD20 B-cell population for 6–9 months. Rituximab for TED has shown improvement in the clinical activity score and sustained efficacy for >18 months [45]. Optimal dosing is not yet determined and published doses have ranged from 100 mg in a single infusion to 1,000 mg per infusion for 3–4 infusions. Most patients in published studies were treated for compressive optic neuropathy, and while available data suggest that existing strabismus did not change [46], it is possible that its anti-inflammatory effect could prevent later strabismus in patients with active TED and extraocular muscle edema rather than fibrosis.

Insulin-like growth factor 1 receptor (IGF-1R) has been suggested to play an important role in regulating the autoimmune response [47]. Graves' autoantibodies interact directly with IGF-1R expressed on orbital fibroblasts. IGF-1R and proteins involved in IGF-1R signaling are upregulated/dysregulated in orbital fibroblasts of TED patients [48]. Graves' autoantibodies reproduce key pathophysiological responses, specifically in orbital fibroblasts from TED patients and these responses are mimicked by IGF-1 [3]. IGF-1R and thyrotropin receptor, the two main autoantigens implicated in TED, are physically and functionally coupled in orbital fibroblasts. Inhibiting IGF-1R completely blocks pathophysiological responses in orbital fibroblasts of TED patients. The applicability of this pathway to EOM changes is not yet certain. However, it is tempting to speculate that medications that can prevent or thwart the auto-inflammatory cascades leading to extraocular muscle fibrosis would also prevent TED-related strabismus.

Conservative/Temporizing Measures

Observation may be appropriate in TED, if the strabismus is not stable and the patient does not complain of double vision in primary gaze or reading position. The patient also may choose observation when informed of the data regarding low to moderate efficacy of medical treatment to improve diplopia. If the patient is considering orbital decompression surgery for proptosis or for treatment of compressive optic neuropathy, then specific treatment of the strabismus should be deferred until decompression has been performed and orthoptic measurements are stable. One of the common complications of orbital decompression is the development or worsening of diplopia, but because the onset or worsening is frequently temporary, nonsurgical management of diplopia may be desirable. The strabismus in TED is often highly incomitant because of extraocular muscle restriction, and it may not follow specific patterns (such as worsening in gaze directed away from the tight muscle) because of multiple muscle involvement.

Prisms have been used successfully in such patients, and even high power (over 20 PD) prisms may be tolerated [49]. Press-on (Fresnel) prisms are preferable to ground-in prism when the strabismus is unstable. A properly positioned Fresnel prism can offer relief of diplopia in primary gaze and down gaze. In some patients, the degree of misalignment is too large or unstable for prism use. Other nonsurgical management options include occlusion of part or all of one spectacle lens and botulinum toxin injections into EOM. The primary goal of this management is to relieve double vision in primary and/or reading position. Occlusion with Scotch satin tape or with Bagolini filters can provide excellent and discrete relief of diplopia, compared with pirate patches [50]. Botulinum toxin may be injected into the superior rectus for the treatment of hypertropia, with a long-lasting mean reduction of 10 PD achieved after two or three injections [51]. However, post-injection ptosis is common, and patients must be aware of the high likelihood of this temporary iatrogenic ptosis.

Surgery

Principles of Surgery

Surgeries in TED usually progress in a staged, sequential fashion. Orbital abnormalities (proptosis, fat herniation) are addressed first, and they are followed by strabismus correction and eyelid repair. Not all patients require each step, of course, but the order must be considered to maximize predictability of the final results. The overall goals of surgical therapy in TED are improvement of function, reduction or elimination of diplopia, reversal of ocular surface damage, reversal of vision loss, and reduction in disfiguring proptosis and lid retraction. Successful elective surgery should be performed after appropriate medical control of hyperthyroidism or hypothyroidism with abstinence of smoking and when orbital disease has been stable [52]. The goal of strabismus surgery is to establish single binocular vision in primary gaze and reading position, to restore and maintain good fusion, and to create the largest possible field of single binocular vision. In almost all cases, surgery for thyroid-related strabismus consists of recessions of restricted rectus muscles. One of the particular challenges of strabismus surgery for TED is choosing the amount of recession to perform. In cases of a small angle strabismus, recession of a tight muscle by dosing table amounts may not have as much effect as expected because restriction is not relieved adequately. On the other hand, larger recessions can give even more effect than expected because of the combined effect of relief of the restriction and muscle retroplacement. The general concept for recession of tight muscles in TED is that larger than expected recessions are needed for small deviations and smaller than expected recession are needed for large deviations, sometimes summarized as "more is less, and less is more." When planning surgery for vertical deviations, the effect on both primary position and down gaze for reading must be considered for optimal postoperative visual function. For hypotropia, bilateral asymmetric inferior rectus recession or placement of a posterior fixation suture on the contralateral inferior rectus may reduce the chance of overcorrection in downgaze. In other cases, if forced duction reveals the involved muscle to be too tight to prevent overcorrection, then the recession of contralateral inferior rectus muscle may be performed. Recent studies have demonstrated that selective resection of rectus muscles may be possible without creating more globe restriction [53]. Inferior oblique surgery also may be useful, as pathogenic involvement of this muscle may be more frequent than generally recognized [23].

Surgery may be performed under general anesthesia or after retrobulbar or peribulbar block; unless there is a significant contraindication, general anesthesia is preferred to allow for proper forced duction testing. Correcting restrictive strabismus caused by TED is challenging because of higher unpredictability than with other forms of acquired adult strabismus, such as cranial nerve palsy. Although the surgical dosing tables are helpful in treating strabismus in children and adults without TED, they do not seem to be as effective in cases of TED-associated strabismus. Surgical success rates in the literature range from 43 to 100 %, and reoperation rates range from 17 to 45 % [54–57]. Reoperation rates in cases of early surgical intervention during the active phase of TED are as high as 50 %, and although long-term success has been reported in a select group of patients, there is a greater risk of complications if surgery is performed at such a time [58–60]. Most surgeons will defer operating until the strabismus has been stable for at least 6 months; however, the restrictive process may continue to evolve years after resolution of active inflammation. There are several variables that should be considered prior to surgery, which include preoperative motility restriction, misalignment in primary gaze and reading position and in the direction opposite the restricted muscle(s), and intraoperative forced ductions. Based on the findings, the surgical approach may entail operation on the (often uninvolved) contralateral superior rectus muscle, contralateral inferior rectus muscle, and ipsilateral inferior rectus muscle in cases of hypotropia, for example. Progressive overcorrection after inferior rectus muscle recessions has been reported and is more frequent than in nonthyroid strabismus [61]. Several theories exist regarding the etiology of overcorrection with inferior rectus recessions, including scarring of Lockwood's ligament with continued posterior tension on the recessed muscle, and continued increased stimulation of the superior rectus muscle in the eye with the weakened inferior rectus muscle as a result of Hering's law, with the contralateral superior rectus muscle maintaining increased stimulation against a restricted inferior rectus muscle.

Methods

The rectus muscles are often extremely tight in TED, and severe restriction can make exposure of the eye muscles difficult because the globe does not rotate easily. During the manipulation of restricted EOM, caution must be taken to avoid pulling too hard on a tight muscle to prevent injury or pulled-in-two syndrome [62]. Conjunctival dissection can be challenging because of friable tissue from the disease and/or prior orbital radiation. Especially during forced duction testing, the conjunctiva can be easily damaged and may bleed, thus obscuring surgical landmarks. Several surgical pearls are important in these cases. In order to prevent postoperative lower eyelid retraction when the patient requires inferior rectus muscle recession, an adjustable suture can be applied to the lower eyelid retractors after they are dissected free of their attachment to the inferior rectus muscle and gently divided to allow lower eyelid elevation independent of the rectus muscle. Disinserting a very tight muscle from the globe carries an elevated risk of globe perforation because the tight muscle may elevate the sclera. The surgeon must ensure excellent visualization of the muscle and the adjacent sclera.

Because of the difficulty in predicting the dose of surgery, adjustable suture surgery has been advocated by many surgeons [63, 64]. However, adjustable suture use may be associated with a higher rate of late slippage of a tight rectus muscle (especially the inferior rectus) after recession with adjustable suture [61]. Success rates of strabismus surgery in TED patients vary between 38 and 80 % with fixed suture techniques and between 64 and 82 % with adjustable sutures [20, 65]. Techniques including "relaxed" EOM positioning, where correction of the restricted duction and not the deviation is performed, have been studied and show efficacy as well [59, 66, 67]. In this method, preoperative duction testing and forced duction testing under general anesthesia are necessary to confirm which muscles were restricted and need to be recessed. After proper dissection and disinsertion of the restricted muscle(s), forced ductions are repeated to ensure free movement of the globe. The disinserted muscle then is allowed to rest freely on the globe without tension with the anteroposterior axis of the eye perpendicular to the frontal plane, and the position at which the disinserted tendon rests against the sclera is marked. The tendon is then sutured to the sclera at the site of the mark.

Table 10.1 Comparison of outcomes in published studies of adjustable and nonadjustable suture strabismus surgery in TED patients (data from ref. [68])

	Better in adjustable suture	Better in nonadjustable suture	Equally as effective
Accuracy of long-term ocular alignment	Awadein (2008), Broniarczyk (2003), Tripathi (2003)	Correa (1998), Vazquez (1999)	Altintas (2006), Bishop (2004), Kono (2000), Kraus (1993), Mohan (1998), Park (2009), Yanovitch (2009)
Patient satisfaction	Tripathi (2003)		
Relief from diplopia	Broniarczyk (2003), Tripathi (2003)		

Table 10.2 Published outcomes of EOM recession for strabismus in TED

	Kraus et al. [65]	Skov et al. [17]	Kushner [63]	Trokel et al. [64]	Total
Success rates without prisms					
Nonadjustable	38 % (10/26)	100 % (2/2)	75 % (6/8)	43 % (21/49)	46 % (39/85)
Adjustable	64 % (7/11)	50 % (1/2)	92 % (24/26)	40 % (2/5)	77 % (34/44)
P value	0.279	1.0	0.483	1.0	<0.001
Reoperation rates					
Nonadjustable	35 % (9/26)	0 % (0/2)	25 % (2/8)	29 % (14/49)	29 % (25/85)
Adjustable	9 % (1/11)	0 % (0/2)	8 % (2/26)	40 % (2/5)	11 % (5/44)
P value	0.224	1.0	0.483	0.985	0.021

Prospective, randomized studies comparing the various techniques have not been conducted, and most published series include retrospective analysis of only one technique performed by a single surgeon or very small group of surgeons (Table 10.1). So far there have been no reliable data regarding which technique produces a more accurate long-term ocular alignment following strabismus surgery, or in which specific situation one technique is definitely superior to the others [68]. Many surgeons still favor adjustable suture strabismus surgery because of the perceived control it provides in the immediate postoperative period (Table 10.2).

Inferior oblique surgery, by balancing the overall excursion of EOM, may produce binocularity in primary position and down reading gaze. The amount of vertical correction from inferior oblique surgery alone is limited, often requiring ipsilateral superior or contralateral inferior rectus surgery. Inferior oblique surgery likely increases the area of binocular single vision and decreases the incidence of overcorrection [23].

Surgical treatment of TED typically involves recession rather than resection of the affected muscles because of concern both for severe inflammation and increased restriction of tight EOM. As noted above, resections may be considered in select cases, including functionally monocular patients who refuse bilateral surgery, patients with residual under corrections after maximal rectus muscle recession, and patients with a residual deviation and no restriction to ocular rotations [19, 53].

Complications

As in all strabismus surgeries, the following complications should be considered and discussed with patients prior the operation. Misidentification of a muscle, damage to adjacent structures, scleral perforation, retinal detachment, anterior segment ischemia, orbital inflammation or infection, slipped or lost EOM, and undesirable alignment changes all may occur. Surgical errors in ophthalmology include procedures performed on the wrong eye or on the wrong muscle [69]. This occurrence may be even more likely in TED strabismus because of the dependence of the surgical plan on intraoperative forced duction testing results. Surgeons are advised to anticipate the findings and create appropriate plans preoperatively which may be referenced during surgery.

Damage to adjacent structures during dissection may occur, resulting in orbital hemorrhage from a vortex vein, damage to the sclera or optic nerve, or fat adherence from perforation of Tenon's capsule. Scleral perforation may occur especially during the muscle disinsertion. Anterior segment ischemia may occur when two or more rectus muscles are operated in the same eye. Because TED strabismus patients are often older than other strabismus patients, an iris fluorescein angiogram should be considered in cases where ischemic risk is higher (systemic vascular disease, prior strabismus surgery, etc.). Orbital inflammation or infection may present typically 1–3 days postoperatively. Slipped or lost muscles may occur during and after operation and it is most commonly encountered with the medial rectus muscle and is most severe if the muscle is tight. Wound irregularities and scarring may develop. Undesirable alignment changes should be kept in mind after any strabismus surgeries and especially in restrictive strabismus. Undercorrections are generally easier for patients to accept; overcorrections, especially with loss of rotations or postoperative diplopia, are more problematic. Unfortunately, it is not unusual for undesirable alignments after surgery for TED strabismus to require reoperation. Patients should be made aware that the frequency of reoperation in all adults with strabismus is as high as 21 %, and specifically in adults with TED it is as high as 50 % [70]. Many patients with TED have strabismus that may change over time, even when preoperative alignment seems to be stable. Surgical outcome can be less predictable because of varying amounts of restriction and fibrosis that occur during postoperative healing in muscles affected by thyroid ophthalmopathy. Therefore, for the TED patient before surgery, it is important to emphasize the possibility of additional surgery and to inform that the goal of the surgery is to eliminate double vision in primary gaze and reading position, not complete relief of double vision in all directions. Most frustrating to the strabismus surgeon is the frequency with which variable and seemingly unpredictable responses occur with surgical treatment. Surgery of the inferior rectus has proven particularly challenging with regard to variable outcomes. Superior oblique muscle involvement may be masked by coexistent inferior rectus muscle involvement and if not identified and addressed at the time of the first surgery may result in symptomatic intorsion and A-pattern exotropia [22]. Intraoperative assessment of torsion and superior oblique tension may also help identify patients at risk. Superior oblique tendon recession simultaneously with inferior rectus muscle recession may prevent development of a postoperative A-pattern exotropia and intorsion [22]. In rare cases, extraocular muscle surgery may reactivate TED [71]. Proptosis often increases after rectus muscle surgery [72] and should be anticipated when planning customized orbital decompression (see Chap. 11). Exposure keratopathy may worsen acutely with recession of an extremely tight vertical rectus muscle despite efforts to minimize lid position change and may require urgent eyelid retractor recession to prevent corneal ulceration.

Conclusions

Strabismus may arise as the sole manifestation of thyroid ophthalmopathy, but it is seen more commonly with other signs and symptoms of the disease, such as proptosis and optic neuropathy with vision loss. In the acute or active phase of disease, it may improve with corticosteroid administration or orbital radiotherapy, and a substantial number of patients improve spontaneously, as evidenced by the fact that fewer than 10 % of TED patients require strabismus surgery. Surgical outcomes remain unpredictable regardless of the method employed, and further clinical trials are needed to identify the best way to address this complex medical problem that carries significant visual morbidity.

References

1. Wiersinga WM, Smit T, van der Gaag R, Koornneef L. Temporal relationship between onset of Graves "ophthalmopathy and onset of thyroidal Graves" disease. J Endocrinol Invest. 1988;11(8):615–9.
2. Rapoport B, Alsabeh R, Aftergood D, McLachlan SM. Elephantiasic pretibial myxedema: insight into

and a hypothesis regarding the pathogenesis of the extrathyroidal manifestations of Graves' disease. Thyroid. 2000;10(8):685–92.

3. Kumar S, Iyer S, Bauer H, Coenen M, Bahn RS. A stimulatory thyrotropin receptor antibody enhances hyaluronic acid synthesis in graves' orbital fibroblasts: inhibition by an IGF-I receptor blocking antibody. J Clin Endocrinol Metab. 2012;97(5):1681–7.
4. van Zeijl CJJ, Fliers E, van Koppen CJ, Surovtseva OV, de Gooyer ME, Mourits MP, et al. Thyrotropin receptor-stimulating Graves "disease immunoglobulins induce hyaluronan synthesis by differentiated orbital fibroblasts from patients with Graves" ophthalmopathy not only via cyclic adenosine monophosphate signaling pathways. Thyroid. 2011;21(2):169–76.
5. Fells P, Kousoulides L, Pappa A, Munro P, Lawson J. Extraocular muscle problems in thyroid eye disease. Eye (Lond). 1994;8(Pt 5):497–505.
6. Simonsz HJ, Kommerell G. Increased muscle tension and reduced elasticity of affected muscles in recent-onset Graves' disease caused primarily by active muscle contraction. Doc Ophthalmol. 1989;72(3–4): 215–24.
7. Pappa A, Jackson P, Stone J, Munro P, Fells P, Pennock C, et al. An ultrastructural and systemic analysis of glycosaminoglycans in thyroid-associated ophthalmopathy. Eye (Lond). 1998;12(Pt 2):237–44.
8. Hansen C, Otto E, Kuhlemann K, Förster G, Kahaly GJ. Glycosaminoglycans in autoimmunity. Clin Exp Rheumatol. 1996;14 Suppl 15:S59–67.
9. Fatourechi V. Pretibial myxedema: pathophysiology and treatment options. Am J Clin Dermatol. 2005; 6(5):295–309.
10. Alsuhaibani AH, Carter KD, Policeni B, Nerad JA. Effect of orbital bony decompression for Graves' orbitopathy on the volume of extraocular muscles. Br J Ophthalmol. 2011;95(9):1255–8.
11. Hu WD, Annunziata CC, Chokthaweesak W, Korn BS, Levi L, Granet DB, et al. Radiographic analysis of extraocular muscle volumetric changes in thyroid-related orbitopathy following orbital decompression. Ophthal Plast Reconstr Surg. 2010;26(1):1–6.
12. Baldeschi L, Lupetti A, Vu P, Wakelkamp IMMJ, Prummel MF, Wiersinga WM. Reactivation of Graves' orbitopathy after rehabilitative orbital decompression. Ophthalmology. 2007;114(7):1395–402.
13. Müller-Forell W, Pitz S, Mann W, Kahaly GJ. Neuroradiological diagnosis in thyroid-associated orbitopathy. Exp Clin Endocrinol Diabetes. 1999;107 Suppl 5:S177–83.
14. Yokoyama N, Nagataki S, Uetani M, Ashizawa K, Eguchi K. Role of magnetic resonance imaging in the assessment of disease activity in thyroid-associated ophthalmopathy. Thyroid. 2002;12(3):223–7.
15. Terwee C, Wakelkamp I, Tan S, Dekker F, Prummel MF, Wiersinga W. Long-term effects of Graves' ophthalmopathy on health-related quality of life. Eur J Endocrinol. 2002;146(6):751–7.
16. Bahn RS. Graves' ophthalmopathy. N Engl J Med. 2010;362(8):726–38.
17. Skov CM, Mazow ML. Managing strabismus in endocrine eye disease. Can J Ophthalmol. 1984;19(6): 269–74.
18. Bartley GB, Fatourechi V, Kadrmas EF, Jacobsen SJ, Ilstrup DM, Garrity JA, et al. Clinical features of Graves' ophthalmopathy in an incidence cohort. Am J Ophthalmol. 1996;121(3):284–90.
19. Bartley GB, Fatourechi V, Kadrmas EF, Jacobsen SJ, Ilstrup DM, Garrity JA, et al. Chronology of Graves' ophthalmopathy in an incidence cohort. Am J Ophthalmol. 1996;121(4):426–34.
20. Flanders M, Hastings M. Diagnosis and surgical management of strabismus associated with thyroid-related orbitopathy. J Pediatr Ophthalmol Strabismus. 1997;34(6):333–40.
21. Enzmann DR, Donaldson SS, Kriss JP. Appearance of Graves' disease on orbital computed tomography. J Comput Assist Tomogr. 1979;3(6):815–9.
22. Holmes JM, Hatt SR, Bradley EA. Identifying masked superior oblique involvement in thyroid eye disease to avoid postoperative A-pattern exotropia and intorsion. J AAPOS. 2012;16(3):280–5.
23. Newman SA. Inferior oblique surgery for restrictive strabismus in patients with thyroid orbitopathy. Trans Am Ophthalmol Soc. 2009;107:72–90.
24. Dickinson AJ, Perros P. Controversies in the clinical evaluation of active thyroid-associated orbitopathy: use of a detailed protocol with comparative photographs for objective assessment. Clin Endocrinol (Oxf). 2001;55(3):283–303.
25. Asman P. Ophthalmological evaluation in thyroid-associated ophthalmopathy. Acta Ophthalmol Scand. 2003;81(5):437–48.
26. Bartley GB. Rundle and his curve. Arch Ophthalmol. 2011;129(3):356–8.
27. Wiersinga WM, Bartalena L. Epidemiology and prevention of Graves' ophthalmopathy. Thyroid. 2002;12(10):855–60.
28. Perros P, Crombie AL, Kendall-Taylor P. Natural history of thyroid associated ophthalmopathy. Clin Endocrinol (Oxf). 1995;42(1):45–50.
29. Ben Simon GJ, Syed HM, Syed AM, Lee S, Wang DY, Schwarcz RM, et al. Strabismus after deep lateral wall orbital decompression in thyroid-related orbitopathy patients using automated hess screen. Ophthalmology. 2006;113(6):1050–5.
30. Roberts CJ, Murphy MF, Adams GG, Lund VJ. Strabismus following endoscopic orbital decompression for thyroid eye disease. Strabismus. 2003; 11(3):163–71.
31. Fabian ID, Rosen N, Ben Simon GJ. Strabismus after inferior-medial wall orbital decompression in thyroid-related orbitopathy. Curr Eye Res. 2013;38(1):204–9.
32. Gilbert J, Dailey RA, Christensen LE. Characteristics and outcomes of strabismus surgery after orbital decompression for thyroid eye disease. J AAPOS. 2005;9(1):26–30.
33. Tellez M, Cooper J, Edmonds C. Graves' ophthalmopathy in relation to cigarette smoking and ethnic origin. Clin Endocrinol (Oxf). 1992;36(3):291–4.

34. Perros P, Crombie AL, Matthews JN, Kendall-Taylor P. Age and gender influence the severity of thyroid-associated ophthalmopathy: a study of 101 patients attending a combined thyroid-eye clinic. Clin Endocrinol (Oxf). 1993;38(4):367–72.
35. Kendler DL, Lippa J, Rootman J. The initial clinical characteristics of Graves' orbitopathy vary with age and sex. Arch Ophthalmol. 1993;111(2):197–201.
36. Metz HS, Woolf PD, Patton ML. Endocrine ophthalmomyopathy in adolescence. J Pediatr Ophthalmol Strabismus. 1982;19(1):58–60.
37. Uretsky SH, Kennerdell JS, Gutai JP. Graves' ophthalmopathy in childhood and adolescence. Arch Ophthalmol. 1980;98(11):1963–4.
38. Pfeilschifter J, Ziegler R. Smoking and endocrine ophthalmopathy: impact of smoking severity and current vs lifetime cigarette consumption. Clin Endocrinol (Oxf). 1996;45(4):477–81.
39. Rajendram R, Bunce C, Adams GGW, Dayan CM, Rose GE. Smoking and strabismus surgery in patients with thyroid eye disease. Ophthalmology. 2011; 118(12):2493–7.
40. Kahaly GJ, Pitz S, Hommel G, Dittmar M. Randomized, single blind trial of intravenous versus oral steroid monotherapy in Graves' orbitopathy. J Clin Endocrinol Metab. 2005;90(9):5234–40.
41. Bartalena L, Krassas GE, Wiersinga W, Marcocci C, Salvi M, Daumerie C, et al. Efficacy and safety of three different cumulative doses of intravenous methylprednisolone for moderate to severe and active Graves' orbitopathy. J Clin Endocrinol Metab. 2012;97(12):4454–63.
42. Macchia PE, Bagattini M, Lupoli G, Vitale M, Vitale G, Fenzi G. High-dose intravenous corticosteroid therapy for Graves' ophthalmopathy. J Endocrinol Invest. 2001;24(3):152–8.
43. Gorman CA, Garrity JA, Fatourechi V, Bahn RS, Petersen IA, Stafford SL, et al. A prospective, randomized, double-blind, placebo-controlled study of orbital radiotherapy for Graves' ophthalmopathy. Ophthalmology. 2001;108(9):1523–34.
44. Kazim M, Garrity JA. Orbital radiation therapy for thyroid eye disease. J Neuroophthalmol. 2012;32(2): 172–6.
45. Salvi M, Vannucchi G, Currò N, Introna M, Rossi S, Bonara P, et al. Small dose of rituximab for graves orbitopathy: new insights into the mechanism of action. Arch Ophthalmol. 2012;130(1):122–4.
46. Khanna D, Chong KKL, Afifiyan NF, Hwang CJ, Lee DK, Garneau HC, et al. Rituximab treatment of patients with severe, corticosteroid-resistant thyroid-associated ophthalmopathy. Ophthalmology. 2010; 117(1):133–9. e2.
47. Weightman DR, Perros P, Sherif IH, Kendall-Taylor P. Autoantibodies to IGF-1 binding sites in thyroid associated ophthalmopathy. Autoimmunity. 1993; 16(4):251–7.
48. Ezra DG, Krell J, Rose GE, Bailly M, Stebbing J, Castellano L. Transcriptome-level microarray expression profiling implicates IGF-1 and Wnt signalling dysregulation in the pathogenesis of thyroid-associated orbitopathy. J Clin Pathol. 2012;65(7): 608–13.
49. Tamhankar MA, Ying G-S, Volpe NJ. Prisms are effective in resolving diplopia from incomitant, large, and combined strabismus. Eur J Ophthalmol. 2012; 22:890–7.
50. De Pool ME, Campbell JP, Broome SO, Guyton DL. The dragged-fovea diplopia syndrome: clinical characteristics, diagnosis, and treatment. Ophthalmology. 2005;112(8):1455–62.
51. Dawson E, Ali N, Lee JP. Botulinum toxin injection into the superior rectus for treatment of strabismus. Strabismus. 2012;20(1):24–5.
52. Borumandi F, Hammer B, Kamer L, von Arx G. How predictable is exophthalmos reduction in Graves' orbitopathy? A review of the literature. Br J Ophthalmol. 2011;95(12):1625–30.
53. Yoo SH, Pineles SL, Goldberg RA, Velez FG. Rectus muscle resection in Graves' ophthalmopathy. J AAPOS. 2013;17(1):9–15.
54. Prendiville P, Chopra M, Gauderman WJ, Feldon SE. The role of restricted motility in determining outcomes for vertical strabismus surgery in Graves' ophthalmology. Ophthalmology. 2000;107(3): 545–9.
55. Nguyen VT, Park DJJ, Levin L, Feldon SE. Correction of restricted extraocular muscle motility in surgical management of strabismus in graves' ophthalmopathy. Ophthalmology. 2002;109(2):384–8.
56. Scott WE, Thalacker JA. Diagnosis and treatment of thyroid myopathy. Ophthalmology. 1981;88(6): 493–8.
57. Evans D, Kennerdell JS. Extraocular muscle surgery for dysthyroid myopathy. Am J Ophthalmol. 1983; 95(6):767–71.
58. Metz HS. Complications following surgery for thyroid ophthalmopathy. J Pediatr Ophthalmol Strabismus. 1984;21(6):220–2.
59. Thomas SM, Cruz OA. Comparison of two different surgical techniques for the treatment of strabismus in dysthyroid ophthalmopathy. J AAPOS. 2007;11(3): 258–61.
60. Coats DK, Paysse EA, Plager DA, Wallace DK. Early strabismus surgery for thyroid ophthalmopathy. Ophthalmology. 1999;106(2):324–9.
61. Peragallo JH, Velez FG, Demer JL, Pineles SL. Postoperative drift in patients with thyroid ophthalmopathy undergoing unilateral inferior rectus muscle recession. Strabismus. 2013;21(1):23–8.
62. Dagi LR, Elliott AT, Roper-Hall G, Cruz OA. Thyroid eye disease: honing your skills to improve outcomes. J AAPOS. 2010;14:425–31.
63. Kushner BJ. Adjustable suture technique in strabismus surgery. Ophthalmol Clin North Am. 1992; 5:93–103.
64. Trokel S, Moore S, Kazim M. Diplopia in Graves' disease. Am Orthopt J. 1988;38:159–67.
65. Kraus DJ, Bullock JD. Treatment of thyroid ocular myopathy with adjustable and nonadjustable suture

strabismus surgery. Trans Am Ophthalmol Soc. 1993; 91:67–79. discussion 79–84.
66. Nicholson BP, De Alba M, Perry JD, Traboulsi EI. Efficacy of the intraoperative relaxed muscle positioning technique in thyroid eye disease and analysis of cases requiring reoperation. J AAPOS. 2011;15(4): 321–5.
67. Dal Canto AJ, Crowe S, Perry JD, Traboulsi EI. Intraoperative relaxed muscle positioning technique for strabismus repair in thyroid eye disease. Ophthalmology. 2006;113(12):2324–30.
68. Haridas A, Sundaram V. Adjustable versus non-adjustable sutures for strabismus. Cochrane Database Syst Rev. 2013;7:CD004240.
69. Shen E, Porco T, Rutar T. Errors in strabismus surgery. JAMA Ophthalmol. 2013;131(1):75–9.
70. Mills MD, Coats DK, Donahue SP, Wheeler DT, American Academy of Ophthalmology. Strabismus surgery for adults: a report by the American Academy of Ophthalmology. Ophthalmology. 2004;111(6):1255–62.
71. Xu L, Glass LRD, Kazim M. Reactivation of thyroid eye disease following extraocular muscle surgery. Ophthal Plast Reconstr Surg. 2014;30:e5–6.
72. Gomi CF, Yang S-W, Granet DB, Kikkawa DO, Langham KA, Banuelos LR, et al. Change in proptosis following extraocular muscle surgery: effects of muscle recession in thyroid-associated orbitopathy. J AAPOS. 2007;11(4):377–80.

Customized Minimally Invasive Orbital Decompression for Thyroid Eye Disease

11

Shivani Gupta, Allison N. McCoy, and Raymond S. Douglas

Introduction

Thyroid eye disease (TED) is the most common orbital disorder in adults. Clinical findings are heterogeneous and include proptosis, eyelid retraction, restrictive strabismus, lagophthalmos, soft tissue expansion, orbital congestion, orbital pain/pressure, eyelid edema and erythema, increased intraocular pressure, conjunctival chemosis, and exposure keratopathy. In less than 5 % of patients, expansion of orbital fat and extraocular muscles may lead to compressive optic neuropathy, which requires urgent intervention [1, 2]. The pathophysiologic changes of muscle and fat expansion, fibrosis of orbital tissues, and restriction of extraocular motility occur in a time dependent but highly heterogeneous fashion. In some patients extraocular muscle enlargement with subsequent fibrosis is the predominant feature characterizing "muscle predominant" disease, in which patients are more likely to experience diplopia and compressive optic neuropathy. In others, adipogenesis predominates, clinically characterizing "fat predominant" disease. Commonly, a combination of these two features is present, as approximately half of patients demonstrate increase in both fat and muscle volume [3]. While the majority of TED patients develop mild, self-limited disease, some may experience disabling strabismus, or severe vision loss from compressive optic neuropathy or exposure keratopathy.

TED is divided into active and stable phases; the active, also described as progressive, phase typically lasts between 6 months and 2 years. Supportive measures to improve ocular surface lubrication and minimize diplopia as well as medical treatments that reduce inflammation are the mainstay of treatment during the progressive phase. When disease is severe, immunomodulatory therapies, as discussed in prior chapters, may be required. However, it remains unclear at this time whether these treatments alter the natural history of TED and halt disease progression. Until such treatments are available which obviate the need for surgery in the stable phase by preventing development or halting progression of disease, surgical rehabilitation remains the mainstay of treatment.

Orbital Decompression

Orbital decompression surgery for TED has historically been reserved for patients with vision-threatening disease (optic neuropathy or severe corneal exposure from exophthalmos) or disfig-

S. Gupta, M.D., M.P.H. (✉) • A.N. McCoy, M.D., Ph.D. • R.S. Douglas, M.D., Ph.D.
Division of Eye Plastic, Orbital, and Facial Cosmetic Surgery, Kellogg Eye Center, University of Michigan, 1000 Wall Street, Ann Arbor, MI 48105, USA
e-mail: shivanig@med.umich.edu; almccoy@med.umich.edu; raydougl@med.umich.edu

R.S. Douglas et al. (eds.), *Thyroid Eye Disease*,
DOI 10.1007/978-1-4939-1746-4_11, © Springer Science+Business Media New York 2015

uring axial proptosis. Initial surgical approaches included coronal and transantral techniques to expose the lateral and inferomedial bony orbit. While providing excellent exposure, these techniques were often fraught with extended recovery times, large incisions, and increased risk of postoperative diplopia. In light of declining morbidity with the evolution of minimally invasive decompression techniques, indications have expanded to include patients suffering from orbital congestion, orbital pain and pressure, aesthetic–functional deformity, and those who will require strabismus surgery. A customized approach evaluating the disease from a multidimensional perspective, including nonaxial globe displacement, eyelid retraction, periocular fat expansion, and facial recontouring, is strongly advocated. Individual surgical techniques have been discussed elsewhere in this book. This chapter will provide a stepwise approach to developing a customized surgical plan for rehabilitation of TED patients.

Surgical rehabilitation is typically performed in the stable phase of disease when signs and symptoms of clinical activity are nonprogressive. Several clinical classification systems exist to monitor disease activity, and have been discussed previously. Preoperative evaluation begins with a detailed patient history. Premorbid photographs assessing disease impact upon the patient's facial morphology is critical for individualized aesthetic-reconstructive planning. Comprehensive ophthalmologic examination is performed with detailed examination of vision, pupillary abnormalities, color vision, and visual fields to assess for compressive optic neuropathy. Exophthalmometry is measured using an exophthalmometer and consistent base, ensuring accurate assessment of globe position relative to the lateral orbital rim and to minimize both intra- and inter-observer variability. Ocular motility and alignment should be evaluated in all fields of gaze, and orthoptic measurements recorded routinely to assess disease progression. Nonaxial changes in globe position such as hyperglobus secondary to inferior rectus enlargement and increased telorism may be subtle but are important for rehabilitation planning. Due to the divergent configuration of the lateral orbital walls, increasing axial proptosis results in increased interpupillary distance (IPD). This may be accentuated by medial rectus muscle enlargement and subsequent lateral globe displacement (increased telorism). Eyelid position and the presence of eyelid retraction are assessed by upper eyelid margin to pupillary light reflex distance (MRD1, upper eyelids) and inferior scleral show (lower eyelids). Expansion of periocular tissues including brow/upper eyelid complex and lower eyelids is a common finding. Fat expansion may simulate soft tissue edema, and should be differentiated. Furthermore, edema resulting from vascular congestion should be discerned from edema due to inflammatory, progressive disease. To aid in the distinction of the latter, patients with stable but congestive features will demonstrate stability (or lack of progression) of clinical parameters such as exophthalmometry, strabismus patterns, and eyelid retraction. Such patients may exhibit prolonged edema of the eyelids, chemosis, or dilation of conjunctival vessels, due to compromised vascular outflow from relative muscle expansion. In these cases, a delay in surgical rehabilitation may result from misinterpretating findings of congestive disease. As will be discussed below, patients with congestive features but no disease progression often benefit from customized decompression that improves vascular outflow, thus alleviating congestive symptoms.

Orbital imaging is recommended in the presurgical planning stages. Non-contrast computed tomography (CT) is the study of choice to detail bony orbital anatomy, extraocular muscle size, presence of apical crowding, and relevant sinus and skull base anatomy. Magnetic resonance imaging (MRI) may be used adjunctively for the assessment of disease activity, for detailed evaluation of the orbital soft tissues and apex, or when other diagnoses are being considered, as discussed in Chap. 10. However, the routine use of MRI for presurgical planning in the stable phase is not generally performed.

Assessment of the goals for each patient will derive from several patient-physician discussions and should be the guidelines for preoperative planning. Each individual's goals for surgery may vary considerably based upon discussions weighing the relative risks and benefits of surgery. Functional and aesthetic concerns are addressed, as they are highly interdependent and both may have significant psychosocial impact and substantially affect quality of life (Chap. 13). For patients without diplopia the discussion of surgical decompression approach(es) and risk of postoperative diplopia is critical. Diplopia can be functionally disabling so the risk must be weighed carefully against the potential benefit for each surgical decompression approach.

Proptosis in TED is recorded as a one-dimensional axial change in globe position, but this does not fully reflect the alterations in orbital and facial anatomy that occur in TED. Unfortunately, surgical planning is often focused solely upon axial proptosis reduction. Nonaxial globe alterations are also prominent for many reasons including heterogeneous extraocular muscle involvement with predilection for inferior rectus enlargement with subsequent hyperglobus, as well as divergence of the lateral orbital walls leading to increased telorism as exophthalmos progresses. The customized approach to orbital decompression described here individualizes aesthetic and functional reconstruction based upon many factors. Besides axial and nonaxial globe alterations, considerations include type of disease (fat vs. muscle predominant), presence of CON, risk of future CON due to apical crowding, restrictive strabismus, orbital congestion, eyelid retraction, soft tissue expansion, prolapse of the lacrimal gland, and premorbid facial anatomic variants. These factors are crucial to optimizing functional and aesthetic rehabilitation and are often not addressed by traditional decompression and reconstruction strategies.

Relevant Anatomy

Decompression of the orbit is performed by removal of bone and/or fat, with the lateral wall, medial wall, and orbital floor being the most common targets for bony decompression. Orbital decompression dates back to Dollinger's description in 1911, which was an adaptation of Kroenlein's orbital approach [4]. Decompression of single and/or multiple orbital walls and fat have since been described using coronal, transantral, lateral cutaneous, lateral transconjunctival, upper eyelid crease, transcaruncular, inferior fornix, and endonasal approaches [5–8]. Besides death or vision loss, both of which are exceedingly rare, one of the most functionally debilitating complications of bony orbital decompression is postoperative diplopia. For example, the transantral approach to the orbital floor and medial wall can incur rates of diplopia up to 60 % [9]. Over the past decade or so, there has been a paradigm shift toward minimally invasive orbital approaches that reduce rates of postoperative diplopia. Herein we focus on minimally invasive fat and bony decompression techniques. Orbital floor decompressions are infrequently performed in the authors' practice due to increased risk of postoperative diplopia and hypoglobus as well as the ability to achieve excellent aesthetic functional results in the vast majority of cases [9].

Lateral wall decompression involves removal of portions of the following bones within the orbit: frontal, zygomatic, and the greater wing of the sphenoid. "Deep" lateral decompression includes removal of the diploe of the greater wing of the sphenoid with substantial reduction in axial proptosis. This approach utilizes a small eyelid crease incision, typically without a lateral marginotomy. Medial orbital wall decompression is graded but includes removal of the ethmoid bone. In cases where maximal proptosis reduction is required or in cases with apical crowding causing optic neuropathy or orbital congestion, the palatine bone and posterior infraorbital strut are also removed. Sparing the anterior strut in these cases allows significant axial proptosis reduction while reducing the risk of postoperative diplopia [10]. Orbital fat may be removed from all four quadrants, but is typically removed from the inferotemporal or inferomedial quadrants, to reduce the risk of damage to vital orbital structures. Fat decompression can be performed in combination with bony decompression or in isolation. While several techniques of fat decompression exist,

Table 11.1 Axial proptosis reduction following graded decompression

First "wall": Orbital fat	2–3 mm
Second wall: Lateral wall	3–6 mm
Third wall: Medial wall	4–7 mm
Fourth wall: Orbital floor	5–9 mm

visualization of orbital structures and hemostasis are keys to maximizing fat removal while minimizing risk. When performed in isolation, fat decompressions are advantageous as they may be performed under monitored anesthesia care with reduced surgical time and postoperative recovery.

Table 11.1 is a general guide to expected postoperative axial proptosis reduction after removal of orbital fat and successive bony orbital walls. There is variability in anticipated outcomes based on each patient's degree of fibrosis, fat expansion, and available bone for decompression. Studies have shown a mean proptosis reduction of 0.93 mm per mL of fat removed, and in our experience orbital fat decompression has become the initial consideration, or "first wall" [11]. The removal of bone is then based on need for additional axial proptosis reduction and also takes into consideration several individualized preoperative factors, which will be elaborated. More recently the concept of "balanced" orbital decompression has become popularized due to the reduced likelihood of consecutive diplopia following removal of the medial and lateral orbital walls. However, a review by Goldberg et al. reported reduced rates of diplopia with lateral and fat decompression as compared to balanced decompression, supporting the stepwise approach that is outlined in the table [12]. When additional decompression is required, the combination of fat decompression and a balanced decompression has been shown to have reduced rates of diplopia compared to 3 wall bony decompression that includes the orbital floor [13]. While Table 11.1 addresses axial proptosis reduction following graded orbital decompression, a broader conceptual framework for customized orbital decompression is presented in Fig. 11.1 taking into consideration several preoperative factors, and will be discussed in further detail below.

Customizing Orbital Decompression

Graded Axial Proptosis Reduction: Type of Disease (Fat vs. Muscle Predominant)

Determination of disease type is the first step in creating a customized plan for orbital decompression. Clinical examination and orbital imaging both aid to categorize a patient's disease as fat or muscle predominant. As stated before, many patients may demonstrate expansion of both tissues. Patients with fat predominant disease typically have more proptosis, and reduced rates of diplopia and compressive optic neuropathy as compared to patients with muscle predominant disease [14]. Furthermore, patients with fat predominant disease generally have reduced resistance to retropulsion. On CT scan, proptosis is observed without substantial enlargement of extraocular muscles. In such patients, isolated fat decompression can significantly reduce axial proptosis with minimal risk of consecutive diplopia. Heterogenous fibrosis of orbital fat may influence the decompressive effect; however, this has not yet been fully elucidated. Figure 11.2 demonstrates the computed tomography (CT) scan of a patient with fat predominant disease. Notably, the extraocular muscles appear to be of normal caliber on imaging. This patient underwent bilateral orbital fat decompression, with significant improvement in proptosis and symptoms of exposure keratopathy. An improvement in inferior scleral show was also noted, thus obviating the need for lower lid retraction repair (Fig. 11.2c, d). In cases where fat decompression alone is not sufficient to achieve the desired degree of proptosis reduction (for example in cases with significant fibrosis of fat or severe proptosis), it can be combined with bony decompression of the lateral orbital wall for additional proptosis reduction with minimal postoperative risk of diplopia.

In cases of muscle predominant disease, fat decompression is rarely used as an isolated procedure to decompress the orbit. This is due to the fact that fat decompression may be more technically challenging due to minimal fat expansion, variable

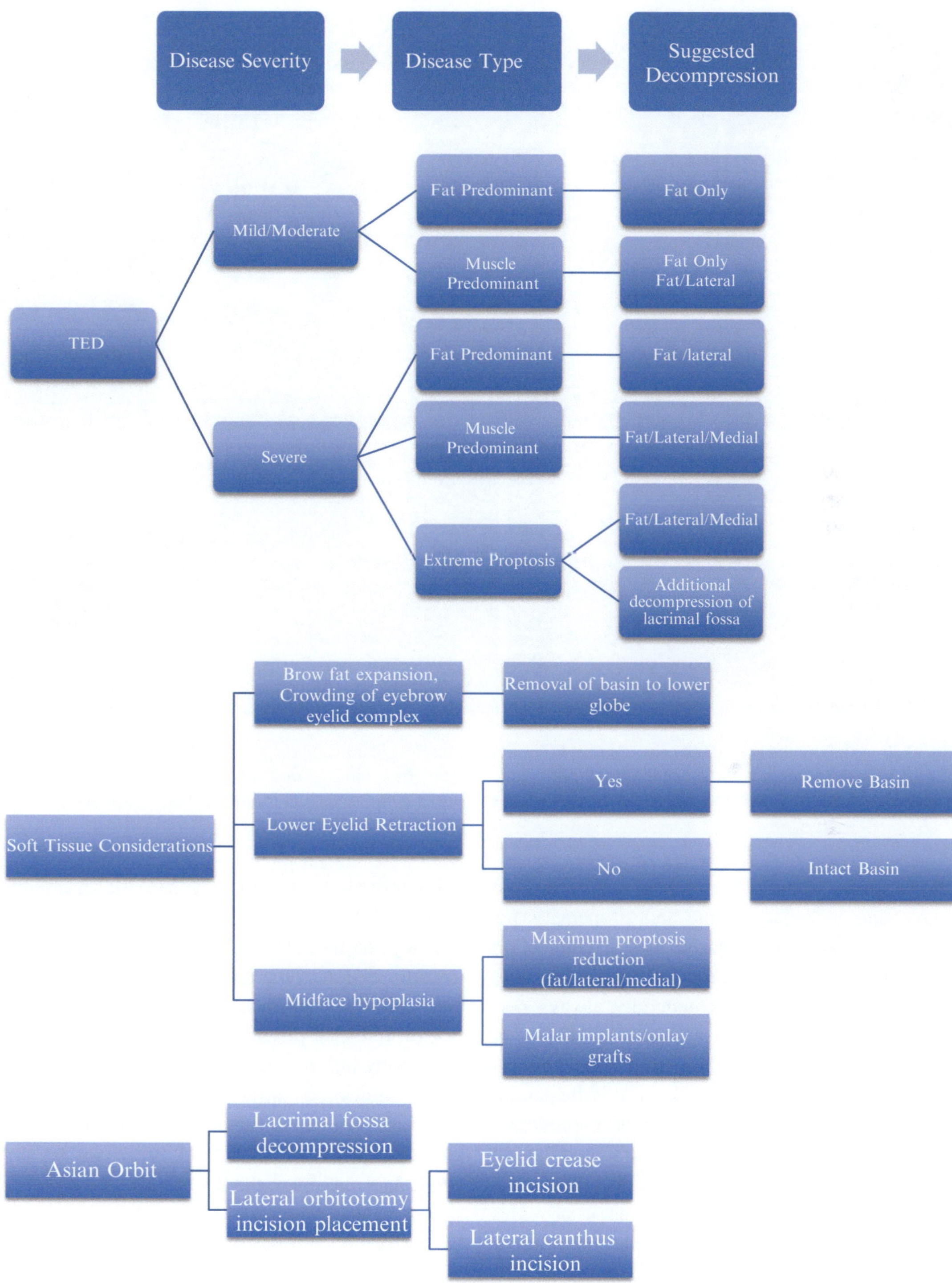

Fig. 11.1 General conceptual frameworks for preoperative planning for TED patients

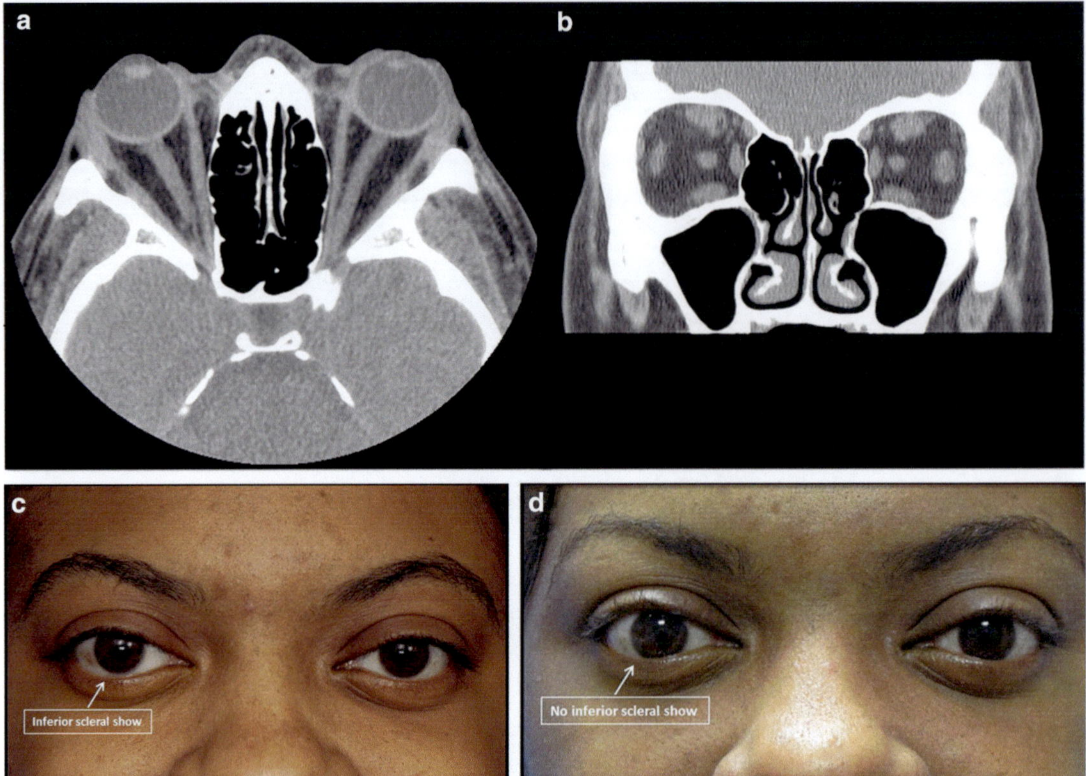

Fig. 11.2 Axial (**a**) and coronal (**b**) non-contrast CT scans of a 27 year-old woman with fat predominant TED. Note proptosis without significant enlargement of extraocular muscles. External photographs of the patient before (**c**) and after (**d**) orbital fat decompression. Note improvement in lower eyelid retraction following decompression

fibrosis of fat, potentially increased risk for muscle injury due to enlargement, and propensity for bleeding related to increased orbital congestion and dilation of vasculature. Therefore in these cases, removal of bone is generally always performed in the stepwise approach as listed in Table 11.1, while also taking into consideration the individualized factors in Fig. 11.1. If the patient has no preoperative diplopia and mild to moderate exophthalmos (less than 6 mm), fat and lateral wall (including deep, lateral orbit) decompression is a preferred surgical approach as it provides excellent proptosis reduction while minimizing postoperative diplopia. In cases of severe exophthalmos (greater than 6 mm) where "maximal" axial proptosis reduction is required, one may consider additional decompression of the medial wall despite the increased risk for diplopia. Although this modified "3 wall" (balanced bone and fat) decompression poses an increased risk for diplopia compared to lateral and fat decompression, the risk appears to be less than traditional 3 wall bony decompression of the orbital floor, medial and lateral walls [13]. Furthermore, sparing of the anterior orbital strut provides a "ledge" for the globe, preventing inferomedial globe dystopia [15].

If additional axial proptosis reduction is required, removal of the deep portion of the frontal bone in the superolateral orbit can be performed to maximize the decompressive effect, as shown in the CT scan in Fig. 11.3. This can also be performed through an eyelid crease incision during standard lateral decompression, obviating the need for craniotomy. In this manner the bone surrounding the superior orbital fissure (greater wing of sphenoid and frontal bones) can be removed in entirety baring dura and substantially expanding orbital volume.

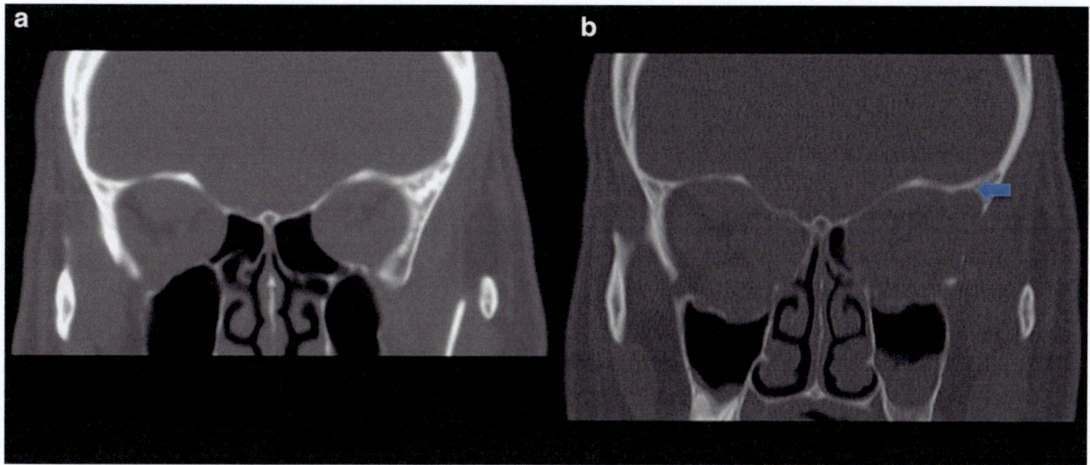

Fig. 11.3 Pre (**a**) and postoperative (**b**) coronal CT scan of a patient with TED. The patient underwent right medial decompression for CON and left lateral and medial wall decompression. Note the removal of bone in the left superolateral quadrant, as marked by the *arrow*

Restrictive Strabismus

As previously discussed, postoperative diplopia is one of the most bothersome complications following orbital decompression. Patients must be counseled regarding the relative risk based upon muscle predominant disease, surgical approach(es), etc. Patients with pre-existing strabismus often require multidisciplinary counseling and planning prior to orbital decompression. A tentative plan for strabismus surgery including the laterality of surgery and the proposed muscles is helpful to plan decompression surgery to ensure symmetry in the final stages. Most commonly, recession of extraocular muscles for TED related restrictive strabismus is performed, though rarely muscles may be resected. Recession of extraocular muscles may lead to worsening axial proptosis [72]; therefore, the surgeon should take into consideration any future plans for muscle recessions, and "over" decompress on the side(s) of the planned strabismus surgery in anticipation of such shifts. In our practice, we generally plan 1–2 mm of additional decompression for patients who will be undergoing recession of extraocular muscles.

Patients with restrictive strabismus typically have muscle predominant disease, most commonly involving the inferior and medial recti muscles. Patients with large muscles exhibit congestive features and often derive substantial benefit from removal of the posteromedial orbit, including the palatine and ethmoid bones during medial wall decompression. Decompression of the posterior orbit yields substantial decompressive effect and has the additional benefit of reducing congestive orbitopathy. Of note, the anterior strut is spared to minimize postoperative globe dystopia and diplopia.

Increased Interpupillary Distance

Widening of the IPD is a subtle, but not uncommon, finding in patients with GD and should not be overlooked as it may contribute to the altered facial morphology of TED. Due to the nonparallel, divergent nature of the lateral orbital walls, axial proptosis is accompanied by increased IPD, an acquired form of hypertelorism. Many astute patients notice the facial alteration especially when accompanied by cheek or buccal fat hypertrophy. Enlargement of the medial rectus muscle may also contribute to lateral globe displacement. Isolated lateral bony decompression often does not adequately address this finding, and therefore careful review of photographs is critical

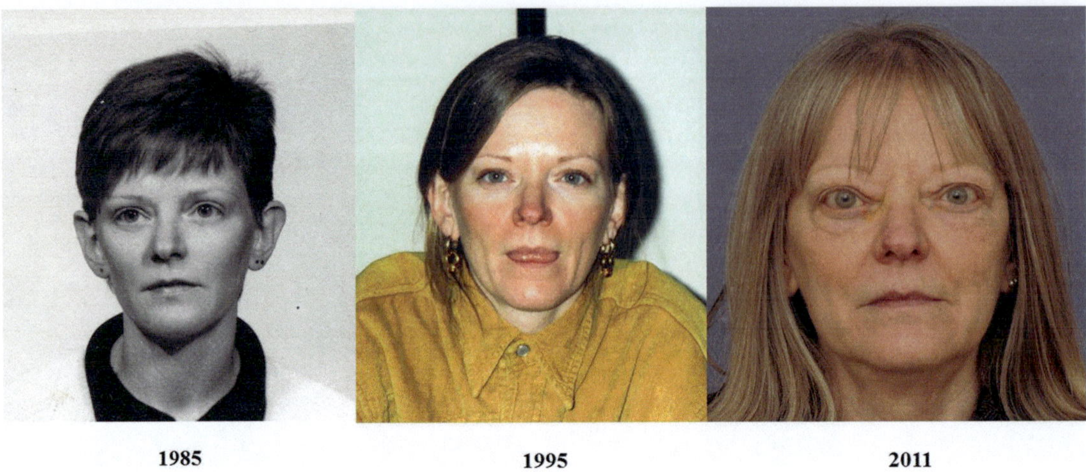

Fig. 11.4 External photograph of a 59 year old woman with TED. Note progressive nonaxial globe displacement (*left* to *right*) leading to increased interpupillary distance

prior to surgery for operative planning (Fig. 11.4). Balanced medial and lateral wall decompression can be considered in such cases, with a nasal shift in globe position achieving a result similar to the patient's pre-morbid appearance [16].

Crowding of the Eyebrow/Lid Complex

Crowding of the upper eyelid and eyebrow complex is common in TED patients due to several factors including expansion of brow and preaponeurotic fat or hyperglobus due to enlargement of the inferior rectus muscle. Additionally, axial proptosis and eyelid retraction leads to widening of the palpebral fissure, causing further crowding of the upper eyelid and brow (Fig. 11.5a). Both histologic and radiographic studies demonstrate expansion of brow and eyelid fat in TED patients, which can lead to significant disfigurement [15, 17]. Removal of the inferior lateral orbit or "basin" of the orbit, as described by Goldberg et al. (Fig. 11.6), repositions the globe inferiorly, thus alleviating the perceived crowding of the eyelid–brow complex [5]. Figure 11.5 demonstrates that significant improvement of the upper eyelid and brow contour can be achieved with decompression surgery alone. Conversely, preservation of the basin should be considered in patients without brow fat expansion, hollow superior sulcus, or normal lower eyelid position relative to the lower limbus.

Lower Eyelid Retraction

Inferior scleral show occurs secondary to proptosis and lower eyelid retraction in TED patients. In many cases, lower eyelid retraction repair is approached with placement of a variety of spacer grafts to augment the middle lamella. Dermis fat, hard palate, ear cartilage, nasal floor mucosa, and acellular collagen matrix grafts such as AlloDerm (LifeCell Corporation, Branchburg, NJ, USA) are commonly used. A recent study, however, demonstrated that surgical decompression alone improves lower eyelid position in patients who do not have subsequent recession of the inferior rectus muscles, and that this effect correlates with degree of proptosis reduction [18]. This suggests that decompression alone can be an effective mechanism to improve lower eyelid retraction and should be integrated into the treatment algorithm for eyelid retraction in patients undergoing surgical rehabilitation. In the authors' experience, this effect is augmented by removal of orbital bone from the "basin" of the orbit, as well as inferior orbital fat decompression. Furthermore in such cases adequate decompression alone often obviates the need for lower eyelid retraction repair.

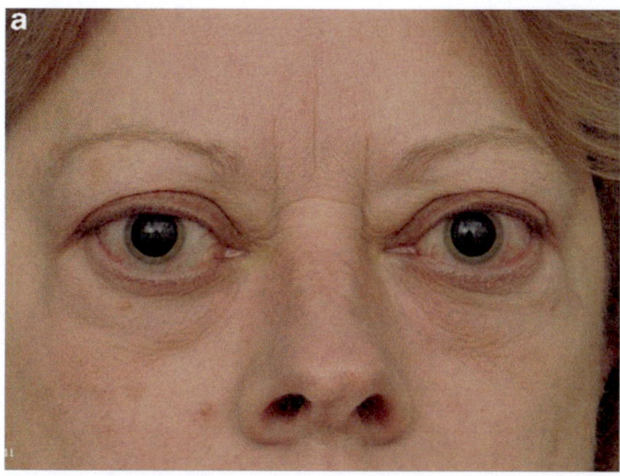

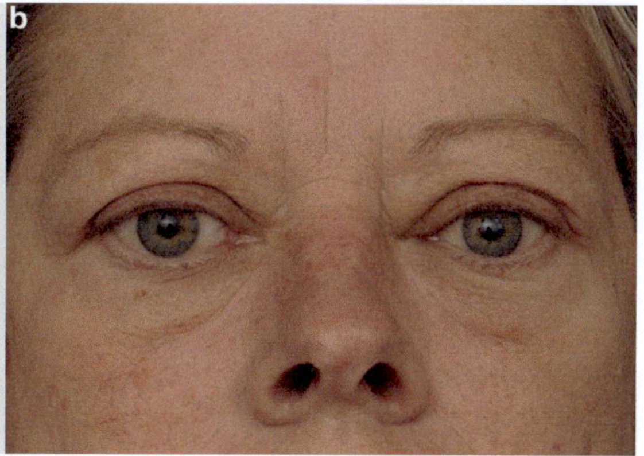

Fig. 11.5 (**a**) Preoperative external photograph of a 57 year old woman with TED demonstrating crowding of the upper eyelid and brow complex due to expansion of brow fat, as well as lower eyelid retraction. (**b**) Postoperative photograph following decompression with focus on removal of the basin. This lowered the globe position and improved the brow and upper eyelid contour. An improvement in lower eyelid retraction can also be noted, without need for lower eyelid surgery

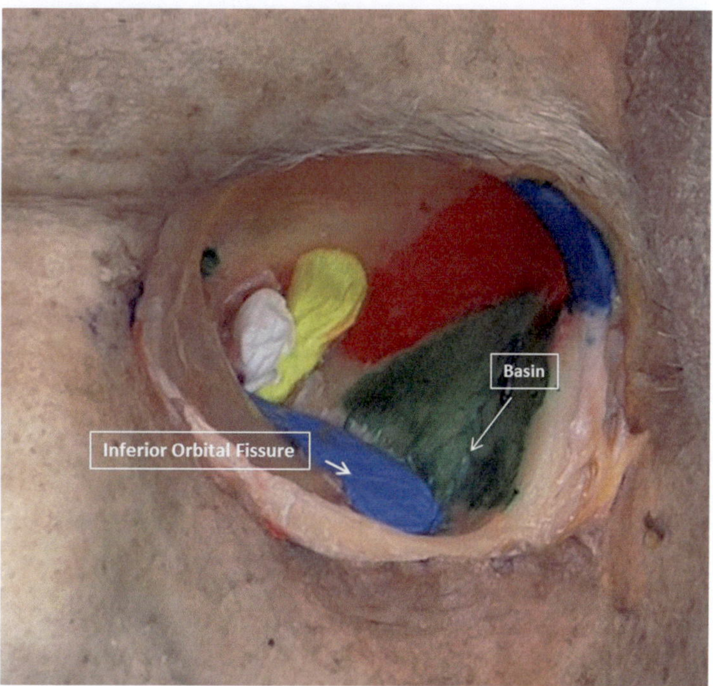

Fig. 11.6 Photograph of a cadaveric orbit. The *green* marking depicts the "basin" of the inferior fissure and orbit

In cases of inferior scleral show due to superior globe dystopia from inferior rectus enlargement, removal of the basin can improve inferior scleral show and globe position while sparing the orbital floor (Fig. 11.7). In patients without lower eyelid retraction, preservation of the basin is recommended to maintain lower eyelid position (Fig. 11.8).

Ethnic Variations

Establishing a customized plan for orbital decompression takes into consideration anatomic differences between patients including bony and soft tissue anatomy. These may vary for a variety of reasons including genetics, gender, age, lifestyle,

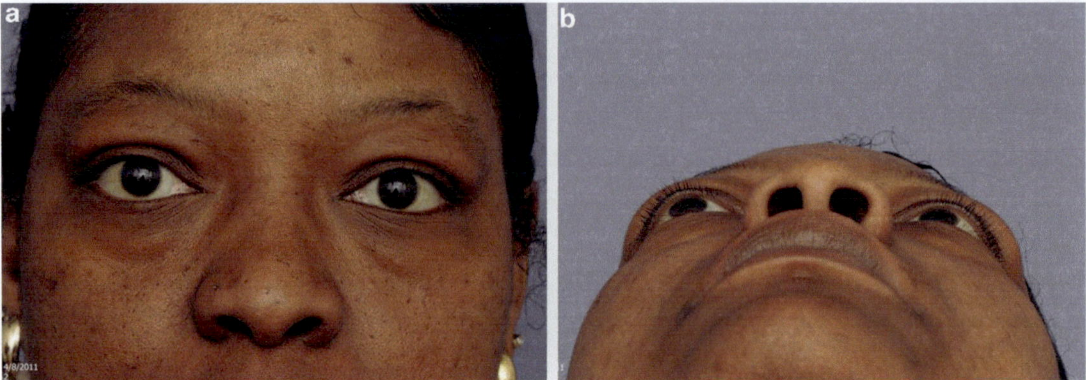

Fig. 11.7 Front (**a**) and worms-eye (**b**) view of a 38 year old woman with right proptosis and hyperglobus from unilateral inferior rectus muscle enlargement

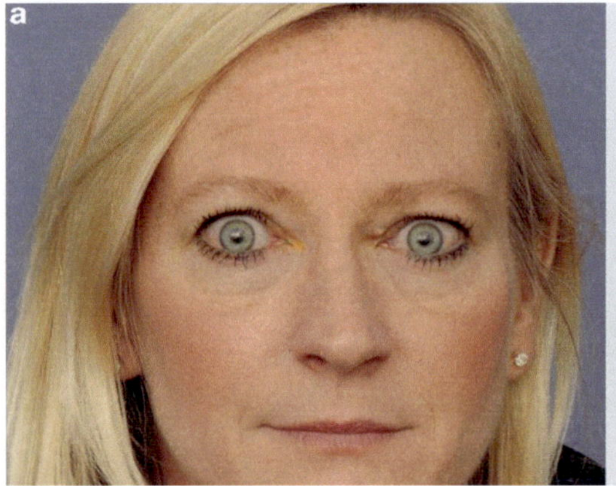

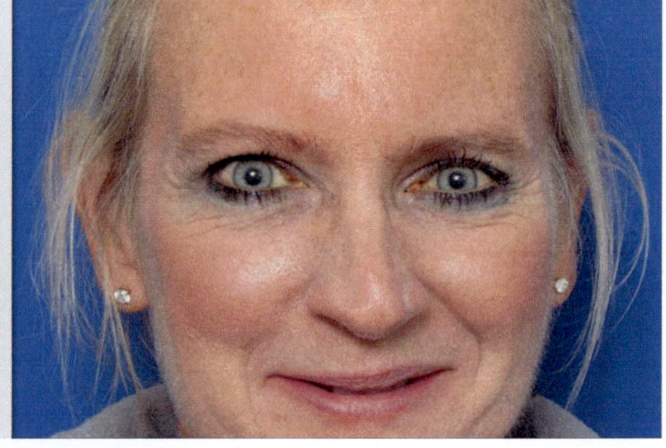

Fig. 11.8 Pre (**a**) and post (**b**) operative external photographs of a 50 year old woman with TED. A bilateral lateral orbital decompression was performed, sparing the basin of the inferior orbital fissure to preserve lower eyelid to limbus relationship

and ethnicity. The goal of axial proptosis reduction should reflect the known anatomic variations in axial globe position between gender and ethnicity, and review of premorbid photographs is essential to establishing the "baseline" for each individual.

Prolapse of the lacrimal gland in TED patients may contribute to facial disfigurement and enhance the effect of periocular fat expansion (Fig. 11.9). Lacrimal gland prolapse is often more visible in Asian and African American patients. In patients with lacrimal gland prolapse, removal of the frontal bone in the superolateral orbit allows adequate volume for retroplacement of the lacrimal gland, and improvement in the upper eyelid contour as well as the eyelid–eyebrow complex. Figure 11.3 depicts the pre- and postoperative CT images of a patient who had right medial wall decompression due to compressive optic neuropathy, and left medial and lateral orbital wall decompression in addition to fat removal for proptosis reduction. The asterisk on the left depicts the removal of bone in the superolateral quadrant, which maximized proptosis reduction while allowing the lacrimal gland to reposition within the orbit.

Nonsurgical Approaches and Extra-Orbital Considerations

A myriad of nonsurgical approaches may be utilized in rehabilitation of TED patients. Patients with eyelid retraction and exposure keratopathy exhibit compensatory depression of their brows

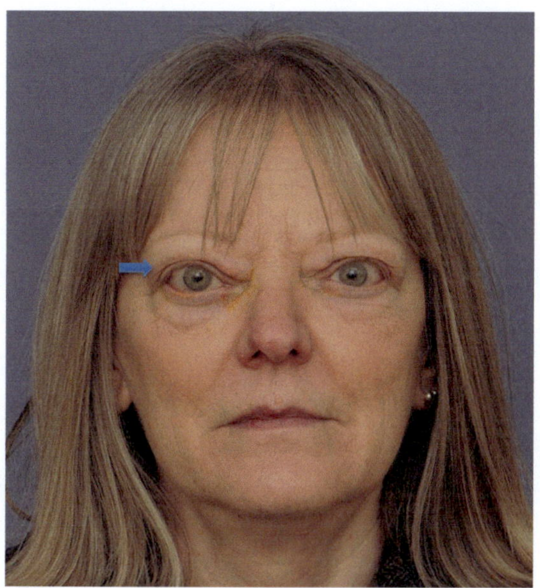

Fig. 11.9 External photograph of a 59 year old woman with TED. Notice the subtle prolapse of the lacrimal gland as marked by the *arrow*

accentuating rhytids. Treatment with neurotoxins such as Botox minimizes the often "angry" look from brow and corrugator overuse, and often relieves the periorbtial ache and discomfort these patients experience. In some patients, proptosis and expansion of the preaponeurotic fat pads may lead to exaggeration of tear trough deformity. Injection of fillers such as hyaluronic acid gels to the lid–cheek junction can result in significant improvement in the lid–cheek contour, and blunting of the typical periocular changes associated with TED. In patients with midface hypoplasia, augmentation of the malar eminence with onlay implants can camouflage exophthalmos or add to the aesthetic improvement with decompression, while providing additional support for the lower eyelid structures.

Conclusions

Techniques in the surgical management of TED have evolved significantly in the past few decades to allow large areas of bone removal through small incisions while minimizing the risks of postoperative, or consecutive, diplopia. During the stable phase of disease, a customized approach to decompression is essential for maximizing functional–aesthetic rehabilitation of each patient.

While significant strides have been made to understand the immunopathogenesis of TED and develop targeted treatments, in the absence of disease modifying therapies, surgical rehabilitation remains the mainstay of treatment.

References

1. Bartley GB, et al. The incidence of Graves' ophthalmopathy in Olmsted County, Minnesota. Am J Ophthalmol. 1995;120(4):511–7.
2. Wiersinga WM, Bartalena L. Epidemiology and prevention of Graves' ophthalmopathy. Thyroid. 2002; 12(10):855–60.
3. Regensburg NI, et al. Do subtypes of graves' orbitopathy exist? Ophthalmology. 2011;118(1):191–6.
4. Dollinger J. Die Druckentlastung der augenhöhle durch entfernung der äuberen orbitalwand bei hochgradigem exophthalmus (morbus Basedowii) und konsekutiver Hornhauterkrankung. Deutsche Medizin Wochenschr. 1911;41:1888–90.
5. Goldberg RA, Kim AJ, Kerivan KM. The lacrimal keyhole, orbital door jamb, and basin of the inferior orbital fissure. Three areas of deep bone in the lateral orbit. Arch Ophthalmol. 1998;116(12): 1618–24.
6. Mourits MP, et al. Orbital decompression for Graves' ophthalmopathy by inferomedial, by inferomedial plus lateral, and by coronal approach. Ophthalmology. 1990;97(5):636–41.
7. Leone Jr CR, Piest KL, Newman RJ. Medial and lateral wall decompression for thyroid ophthalmopathy. Am J Ophthalmol. 1989;108(2):160–6.
8. Kennerdell JS, Maroon JC. An orbital decompression for severe dysthyroid exophthalmos. Ophthalmology. 1982;89(5):467–72.
9. Garrity JA, et al. Results of transantral orbital decompression in 428 patients with severe Graves' ophthalmopathy. Am J Ophthalmol. 1993;116(5): 533–47.
10. Kim JW, Goldberg RA, Shorr N. The inferomedial orbital strut: an anatomic and radiographic study. Ophthal Plast Reconstr Surg. 2002;18(5): 355–64.
11. Wu CH, Chang TC, Liao SL. Results and predictability of fat-removal orbital decompression for disfiguring graves exophthalmos in an Asian patient population. Am J Ophthalmol. 2008;145(4):755–9.
12. Goldberg RA, et al. Strabismus after balanced medial plus lateral wall versus lateral wall only orbital decompression for dysthyroid orbitopathy. Ophthal Plast Reconstr Surg. 2000;16(4):271–7.
13. Unal M, et al. Balanced orbital decompression combined with fat removal in Graves ophthalmopathy: do

we really need to remove the third wall? Ophthal Plast Reconstr Surg. 2003;19(2):112–8.
14. Nunery WR, et al. The risk of diplopia following orbital floor and medial wall decompression in subtypes of ophthalmic Graves' disease. Ophthal Plast Reconstr Surg. 1997;13(3):153–60.
15. Goldberg RA, Shorr N, Cohen MS. The medical orbital strut in the prevention of postdecompression dystopia in dysthyroid ophthalmopathy. Ophthal Plast Reconstr Surg. 1992;8(1):32–4.
16. Alsuhaibani AH, et al. Orbital volume and eye position changes after balanced orbital decompression. Ophthal Plast Reconstr Surg. 2011;27(3):158–63.
17. Papageorgiou KI, et al. Thyroid-associated periorbitopathy: eyebrow fat and soft tissue expansion in patients with thyroid-associated orbitopathy. Arch Ophthalmol. 2012;130(3):319–28.
18. Cho RI, et al. The effect of orbital decompression surgery on lid retraction in thyroid eye disease. Ophthal Plast Reconstr Surg. 2011;27(6):436–8.

12 Noninvasive, Minimally Invasive, and Surgical Pearls for Cosmetic Rejuvenation of the Thyroid Eye Disease Patient

Robert A. Goldberg and Daniel B. Rootman

It is well established that thyroid eye disease (TED) has a significant effect on health related quality of life (QoL) [1–6]. Studies suggest that QoL in TED is similarly impaired to other debilitating chronic diseases such as inflammatory bowel disease and heart failure [2, 3]. Furthermore, this effect is graded, such that individuals with more severe disease tend to have greater impairment in QoL and overall disability [3, 7].

Importantly, functional and cosmetic rehabilitation in TED can have a significant impact [6]. However these interventions are not perfect, and a significant portion of patients will remain unhappy with their appearance and/or function long after they have been "treated" for the disease [8]. While the patient's experience of his or her metamorphosis is certainly central to their sense of well-being [9, 10], positive and negative interactions with the health care system can also play a role in the overall experience [11, 12].

Clinicians should be aware of the transformative effect of TED upon patients' lives, and the role they can play in ameliorating psychological distress. The ability to empathize with patients and provide a supportive environment for care may well be as important as any therapeutic strategy discussed in this textbook.

With this philosophy in mind, the remainder of this chapter will outline pearls for nonsurgical and surgical rehabilitation and cosmetic rejuvenation of patients affected by TED, focusing on minimally invasive techniques.

Noninvasive Techniques to Improve Overall Quality of Life in Patients with Thyroid Eye Disease

Care Environment

The patient experience can be greatly influenced by the environment in which it occurs. Friendly, informative staff set the tone for the encounters that follow, such that a supportive team approach in educating, managing, motivating, and empowering the office staff is an important aspect of patient care.

Mounting evidence suggests that the physical environment in which the care interaction occurs can affect the psychological well-being of patients. Warm, inviting spaces can improve satisfaction with patient–doctor interactions and reduce anxiety [13]. Naturally lit, well-arranged spaces with good air quality can also improve patients' perceptions of their overall care [14]. Ambient additions such as music, art, and fragrances may have a positive effect on a range of

R.A. Goldberg, M.D. (✉) • D.B. Rootman, M.Sc., M.D.
Orbital and Ophthalmic Plastic Surgery,
Jules Stein Eye Institute, 100 Stein Plaza,
Los Angeles, CA 90095, USA
e-mail: Goldberg@jsei.ucla.edu; Rootman@jsei.ucla.edu

R.S. Douglas et al. (eds.), *Thyroid Eye Disease*,
DOI 10.1007/978-1-4939-1746-4_12,

physical and psychological parameters [15]. At the very least, these interventions are unlikely to cause harm and they may reduce stress, improving the subjective patient experience.

Ocular Comfort

During both the inflammatory and post-inflammatory phases of disease, patient comfort can be improved with a range of minimally invasive techniques. Some of the more common and bothersome symptoms for TED patients relate to dry eyes [3, 9]. These symptoms including foreign body sensation, tearing, and ocular pain may result from eyelid malposition and/or orbital congestion. Interventions to improve comfort can range from simple lubricant eyedrops and ointments to more advanced dry eye therapies including topical steroids and topical cyclosporine A, autologous serum tears, specialized contact lenses, as well as temporary or permanent mechanical occlusion of the puncta [16, 17].

In addition to ocular medications and treatments, simple modifications in the home or work environment can be effective, and give the patient some control over their condition. Such modifications include home humidifier use and frequent breaks from the television or computer. Moisture chamber goggles, plastic wrap dressings, and/or eyelid taping at night are more labor-intensive for the patient but can greatly improve comfort, especially for those with nocturnal lagophthalmos.

Single Vision

Strabismus is often cited as the most debilitating and distressing clinical manifestation of TED [3, 7, 18]. Strabismus surgery can provide an adequate field of central single vision in most cases; however, it is often delayed until measurements are stable [19]. During this interval a number of temporizing measures can be offered. Fresnel prisms can correct moderate amounts of deviation, and have the advantage of being temporary and adjustable, such that they can be changed and repositioned as the deviation evolves [20]. Additionally, different prisms can be placed over each bifocal segment if necessary. They do, however, degrade vision at greater strengths, and can be cosmetically unappealing.

Occlusion therapy can be helpful in some patients. Bangerter filters are a reasonable way to titrate the amount of occlusion required [21]. A "pirate patch" of nearly invisible adhesive tape applied to one eyeglass lens can also provide substantial relief from double vision simply and discretely [20, 22].

Botulinum toxin can be also be used in the temporary relief of dysthyroid strabismus. The few studies of this approach support a role for botulinum toxin in cases of acute small to medium angle strabismus [23, 24]. Approximately ¾ of patients will have a significant (>75 %) reduction in the angle of deviation [25]. Although the effect is temporary, lasting only a few months, it can be repeated until definitive therapy can be offered. Additionally, a small group of patients may be maintained on botulinum toxin therapy and avoid strabismus surgery altogether [24, 25].

Psychology

The prevalence of psychiatric disturbances in patients with TED is generally thought to be higher than in the general population, with estimates in the range of 40 % and 20 % for anxiety and depression disorders, respectively [3, 26]. Dysphoric mood states may be even be more prevalent [26, 27].

The presence of mood disturbances in this population requires special attention. Maintaining a positive and holistic doctor–patient relationship is surely beneficial, as may be some of the environmental interventions outlined above. However, many patients may benefit from further evaluation and management by associated services, and it seems prudent to maintain a working relationship with psychiatry and psychology colleagues, as discussed in detail in Chap. 13.

Complementary and alternative medicine can also be helpful. Acupuncture, for instance, is one methodology that has shown benefit to patients with TED. Support groups and patient organizations can additionally be helpful (e.g., http://www.gdatf.org/).

The psychological aspects of the disease are closely tied to self-image and cosmetic appearance, underscoring the importance of cosmetic as well as functional rehabilitation. Rather than considering aesthetic rehabilitation a frivolous or secondary concern, the physician should aim to restore the patient to his or her premorbid appearance as much as technically and financially possible. The restoration of self-image and self-esteem is a great gift to the patient, allowing him or her to resume normal activities and social interactions.

Smoking Cessation

As discussed in previous chapters, patients with Graves' hyperthyroidism who smoke cigarettes have a higher incidence of TED [28]. Additionally, those who develop TED experience more severe disease [28] and a poorer response to therapy [29, 30]. It is clearly in the patients' best interest to quit smoking.

While it is useful for physicians to advise patients to quit smoking [31], the intricacies of pharmacological and behavioral therapies [31–35] are best navigated by professionals who specialize in smoking cessation. It is ideal to refer TED patients who smoke to dedicated programs with experience in managing the bio-psycho-social implications of smoking cessation, or to include such a specialist on the multidisciplinary care team. Smoking cessation is more thoroughly addressed in Chap. 5.

Individualized Approach to the Cosmetic Needs of a Patient with Thyroid Eye Disease

The array of aesthetic changes occurring in individuals affected by TED is vast. Stage and severity of disease play a role in overall appearance; however, clinical scoring systems such as the NO SPECS [36], CAS [37] and VISA classifications [38] tend to focus solely on proptosis, strabismus, and eyelid position. While these clinical entities are also central to the aesthetic assessment of TED, characteristic soft tissue changes in the cheek and brow deserve equal attention [39–41]. TED patients often benefit from aesthetic rejuvenation with botulinum toxin therapy, laser treatment, injectable fillers, and skin care regimens.

Each stage of surgical rehabilitation should focus on the aesthetic outcome, in addition to functional outcomes such as vision and comfort. Paying attention to globe position and interpupillary distance in decompression surgery, lid retraction in strabismus surgery, and eyelid contour in lid lowering surgery are a few examples of this philosophy. Although traditionally orbital decompression was reserved for patients with severe disease, currently even minor degrees of proptosis, asymmetry and/or lid retraction may be indications for minimally invasive surgery in the appropriate patient (see also Chap. 11 and below) [42–44].

Cosmetic Considerations and Minimally Invasive Techniques for Proptosis, Strabismus, Eyelid Position, and Periocular Rejuvenation

Proptosis

Classically orbital decompression was reserved for patients with severe proptosis, corneal exposure, and/or vision loss [42–44]. As surgical techniques have advanced and our ability to provide safe, graded rehabilitation has improved, the indications for surgery have expanded to include more subtle features of congestive and/or cosmetic proptosis.

Cosmetic Considerations in Orbital Decompression: Patient Selection and Technical Pearls

Carriage return over the years a dizzying array of papers have accumulated proposing one technical variation or another for orbital decompression.

Although each group purports the supremacy of their individual technique, there is no evidence or consensus as to which approach is best. Frankly, there are many ways in which an average 3.5–4.5 mm of proptosis reduction can be accomplished [45, 46]. This chapter will therefore focus on the cosmetic implications of the described techniques. These aesthetic considerations can be considered in terms of bony removal (which ones and how much) and soft tissue scarring (where and how extensive).

Incisions

External evidence of surgical intervention can be disturbing to patients. Older large Kroenlein and coronal incisions are unsightly and unnecessary with modern transorbital approaches to the lateral orbit. Approaches that involve removing the temporalis muscle from the bone (including the open coronal approach) can create temporalis wasting, which is a significant cosmetic deformity that worsens with age. Lateral canthal incisions (or variations thereof) are commonly described and do reduce the scar burden considerably compared to larger open procedures. However, splitting the canthus can lead to webbing, eyelid overlap, and poorly camouflaged scars [47]. Furthermore, a lateral canthotomy incision incises the orbicularis fibers perpendicularly and may theoretically result in reduced orbicularis function. A lateral upper eyelid crease incision provides excellent access to the lateral orbit and visualization of the relevant anatomy, while also having the advantage of minimizing damage to orbicularis and leaving an essentially hidden scar. This is our preferred approach to the lateral orbit including the sphenoid diploe.

Along the medial orbit, external Lynch incisions have been appropriately supplanted by transcaruncular techniques [48]. Additionally, endonasal orbitomies are completely concealed postoperatively and offer excellent access to the inferomedial orbit. Both choices provide excellent cosmetic results and ultimately the choice of transcaruncular or transnasal access is likely based on surgeon comfort and preference.

Bony Decompression

Bony removal pattern and extent can also have a significant effect on facial aesthetics beyond the intended proptosis and congestion reduction. Medial and floor decompression that is carried anteriorly to the region of the globe can cause medial and inferior globe dystopia [49]. Particularly in the case of asymmetric surgery, the effect can be significant (Fig. 12.1). Additionally, the incidence of strabismus with anterior decompression can be quite high [50], especially without preserving the inferomedial strut [51].

Thus we choose to avoid opening the medial wall anterior to the anterior ethmoidal foramen and the floor anterior to the maxillary sinus osteum. This approach involves removal of the posterior-inferomedial strut, which is vital for decompression in dysthyroid optic neuropathy, and serves to create space for axial expansion of the orbit posteriorly. There is also a theoretic benefit to maintaining the major normal maxillary and ethmoid sinus

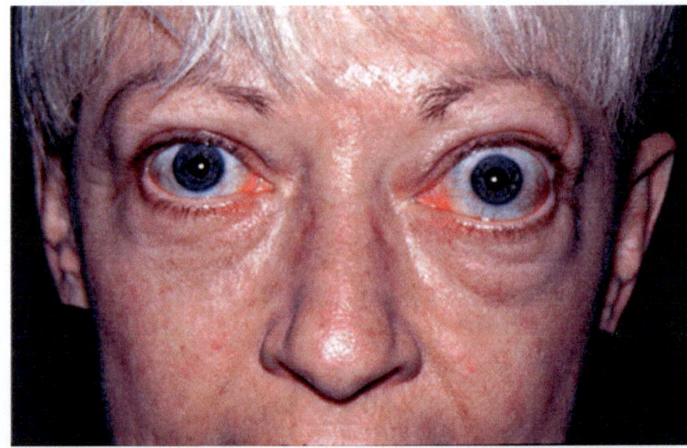

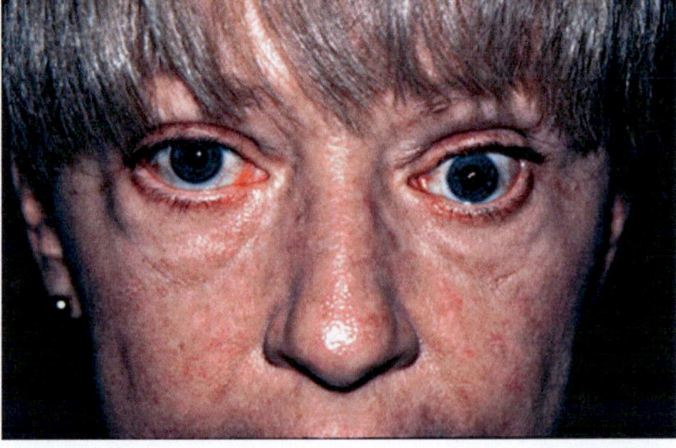

Fig. 12.1 Globe dystopia after aggressive anterior orbital floor decompression

outflow mechanisms, which may reduce the risk of postoperative sinusitis and mucoceles.

The lateral orbit was classically the first to be removed for orbital decompression [52]. Early reports involved removal of the lateral orbital rim and the thin bone overlying the temporalis muscle [53, 54] and this method persists to modern times [55, 56]. However, only limited amounts of proptosis reduction can be achieved in the anterior orbit, where extra-axial globe displacement predominates over axial proptosis reduction. It is advantageous to leave this bone, and rather remove the bone of the deep lateral orbit. The deep bone of the sphenoid diploe lies directly behind globe and allows posterior displacement of the globe in addition to volume expansion.

There is another aesthetic advantage to leaving the anterior lateral wall. The proptosis of TED is associated with some widening of the interpupillary distance, which is part of the disfigurement. Removing the anterior lateral wall can allow the globe to lateralize, widening the interpupillary distance further, which is aesthetically undesirable. Leaving the anterior lateral wall in the area of the equator of the globe minimizes this tendency for expansion of the interpupillary distance. Removing the anterior lateral wall over the temporalis muscle also creates continuity between the orbit and the temporalis fossa, which can induce oscillopsia [55, 57].

Leaving an eggshell of bone over the temporalis muscle and concentrating on the removal of the deep bone of the lateral wall can mitigate these consequences [58]. It is also possible that the deep lateral decompression has a lower incidence of new onset strabismus [59]. These material and theoretic benefits make deep lateral decompression our first choice for decompression requiring moderate amounts of proptosis reduction.

Minimally Invasive Orbital Decompression: Indications and Technique

Patients with even minor amounts of proptosis can have significant congestion that may benefit from orbital decompression (Fig. 12.2). Additionally, holistic cosmetic rejuvenation may warrant 1–3 mm of proptosis reduction in some cases, such that the lid position and periorbital hollows can be optimally managed.

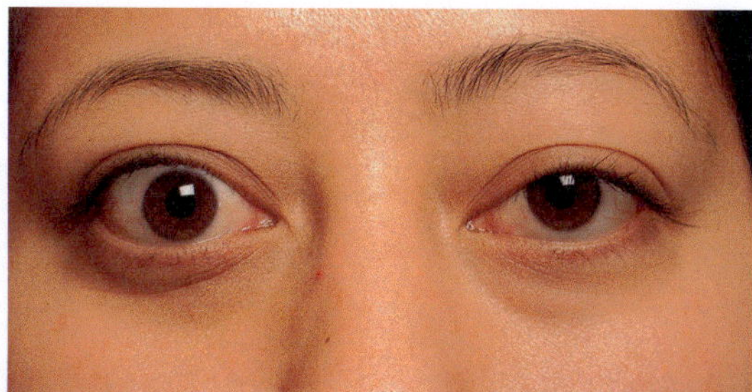
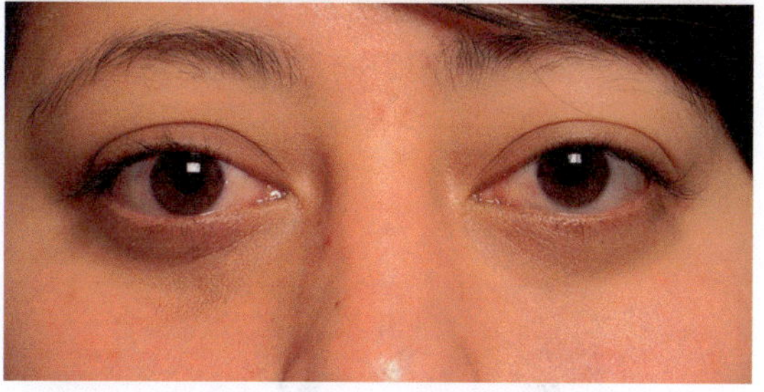

Fig. 12.2 Tense, congested orbit with chemosis and subsequent resolution with symptomatic relief after bilateral decompression

One approach that can be useful involves carving out the basin of the inferior orbital fissure through a transconjunctival incision [60]. This technique entails an inferior transconjunctival approach to the orbital floor. A subperiosteal flap is elevated and the region surrounding the tip of the inferior orbital fissure is exposed. The bone in this region is composed of the thick body of the zygoma and the lateral extent of the maxilla overlying the maxillary sinus (Fig. 12.3). This can be carved with a drill, or if the patient is not sedated, using sharp bone curettes to create a rounding of the lateral orbit (Fig. 12.4). Some opening of the lateral maxillary sinus roof is acceptable in this situation; however opening the central anterior floor can lead to globe dystopia and should be avoided. Fat decompression in the inferior intraconal space can augment proptosis reduction, and both carry low rates of new onset diplopia around 7–8 % [60–64].

In patients with congestion but only mild proptosis, orbital fat removal alone may allow adequate

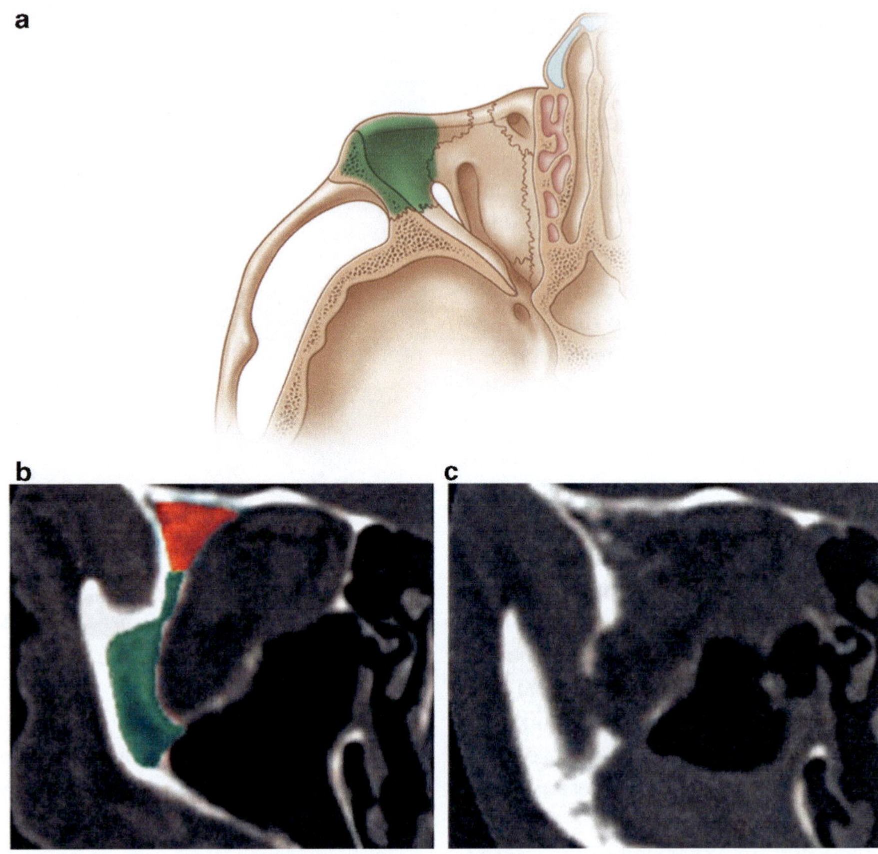

Fig. 12.3 (**a**) The *green* area outlines the thick bone of the inferolateral orbit. The middle frame (**b**) outlines the same bone on coronal computed tomography, and the right pane (**c**) demonstrates the change in volume with decompression of this bone

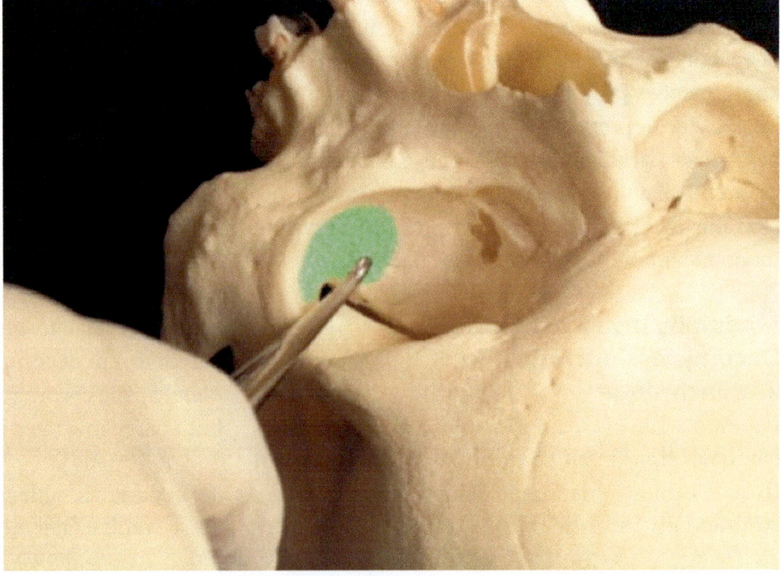

Fig. 12.4 Bone of the lateral orbit that can be accessed with a boney curette

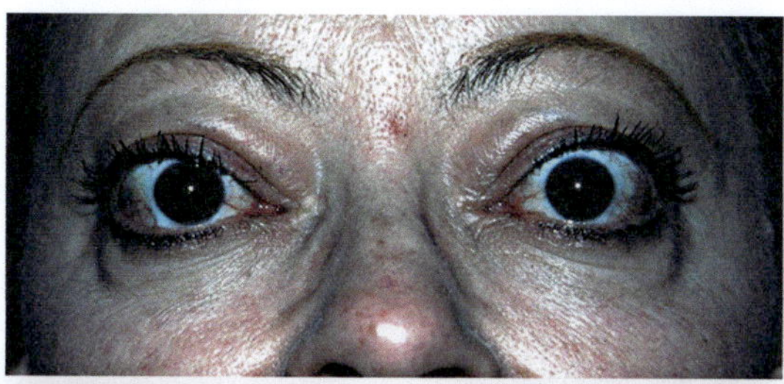

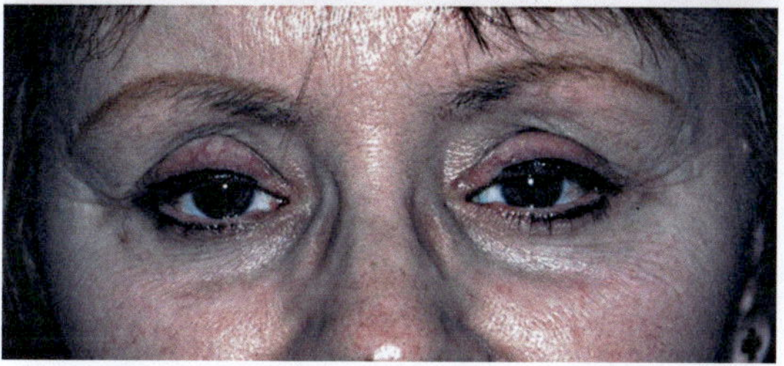

Fig. 12.5 Late overcorrection after aggressive decompression of anterior orbital fat

decongestion and proptosis reduction; through conjunctival approaches, both the inferolateral and inferomedial intraconal pockets can be accessed. A suction cutting technique allows the fat to be gently teased out of the orbit and removed. The fullness of the anterior pads will often improve after removal of intraconal fat, and aggressive removal of the anterior "blepharoplasty" fat can create a hollow appearance (Fig. 12.5). However, if a patient has profound fullness of the anterior fat pads, conservative debulking of these pads can be considered in conjunction with removal of the deeper intraconal fat.

Strabismus

Strabismus surgery has important aesthetic implications. It is well established that manifest strabismus can negatively impact self-perception, social functioning [65], and overall QoL [66]. Studies specifically related to TED have confirmed this relationship, as patients with diplopia are more likely to have symptoms of depression [18], occupational disability [7], and impaired perceptions of their own functional, social, and psychological well-being [3, 5, 12, 67].

Classically staged surgical rehabilitation in TED [19] leaves the patient to suffer the consequences of strabismus often for more than 2 years. However, it is possible to offer minimally and noninvasive measures during this period, as outlined in earlier sections.

When the appropriate time comes for strabismus surgery, TED patients are nearing the end of their facial transformation/rehabilitation cycle. They have often gone through the most significant surgery of the process in decompression. This "home stretch" can be agonizing for patients who have already been through a difficult experience. The implication of this understanding is that any opportunity to combine surgeries and shorten the overall length of rehabilitation will be welcomed.

One strategy that has been employed in this regard is to combine inferior rectus recession surgery with lower lid retractor release [68–70]. This procedure can reduce the amount of retraction caused by inferior rectus recession [71]. We generally prefer to perform it in a minimally invasive en glove fashion [72, 73]. This can be combined with volume augmentation in the form of a dermis fat graft or fat pearl transfer (Fig. 12.6) if necessary. It is also useful to place the lower eyelid on stretch with a Frost suture, which can be loosened in the postoperative area for adjustment of strabismus sutures, and then re-tightened.

Eyelid Retraction

Lid retraction is one of the most common and earliest signs of TED. It is cosmetically unappealing to patients and can contribute to ocular irritation in the form of exposure keratopathy. Classically and definitively, the treatment for retraction is surgical, and a wide range of techniques for both the upper and lower eyelids have been described. Surgery is typically deferred until the post-inflammatory stage of disease, after decompression and strabismus correction have been performed. This time period can be condensed with temporizing measures and by combining

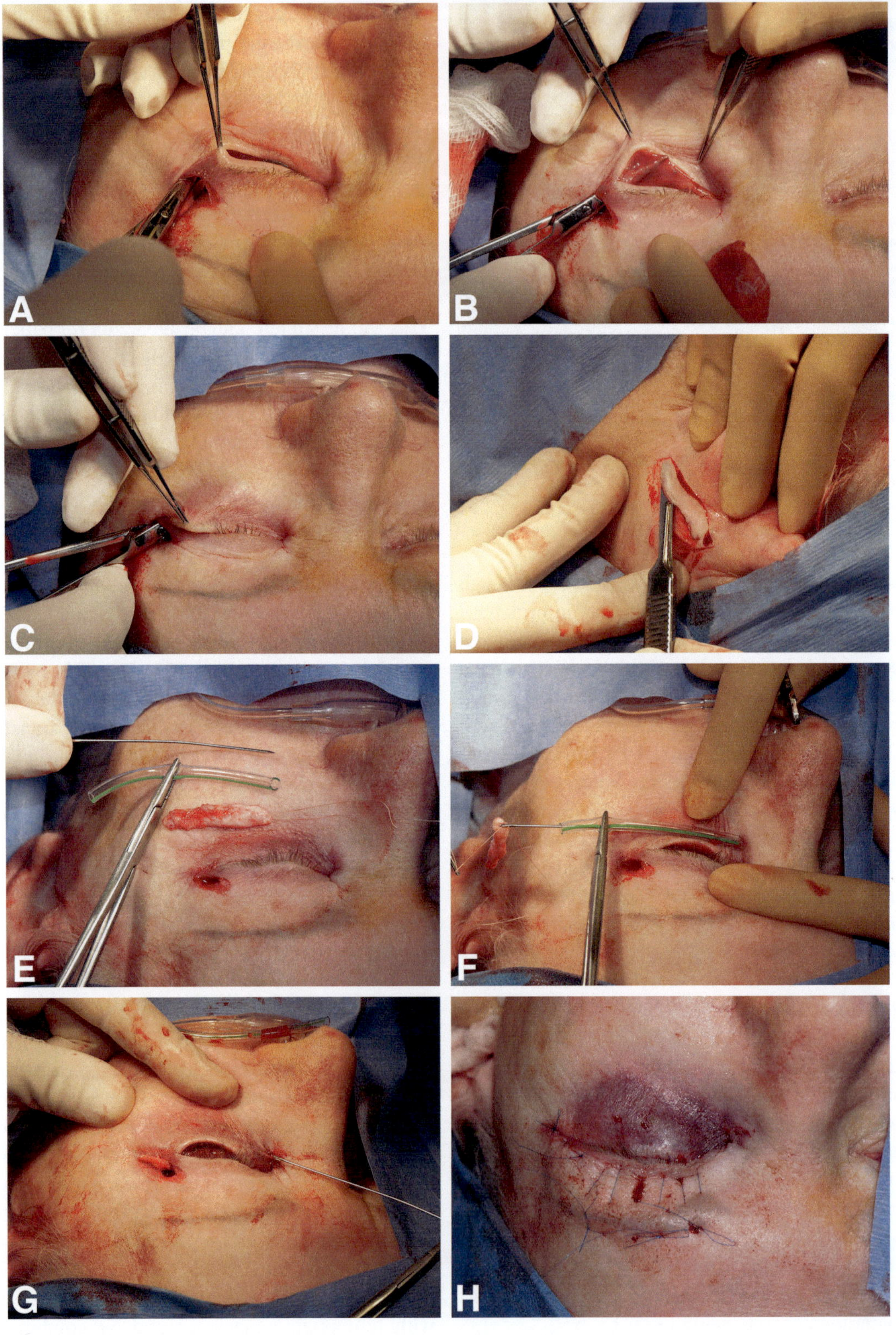
A
B
C
D
E
F
G
H

retraction surgery with other stages of rehabilitation.

There are a few minimally invasive techniques for the management of upper eyelid retraction in active TED. Injecting triamcinolone into the space between Müller's muscle and the conjunctiva has been shown to lower the eyelid and reduce swelling [74, 75]. It is not well established if these injections act like orbital depot injections [76–79] or by some other site-specific mechanism. Their use is limited as the long-term effect is unknown, dosing is not well established, and they carry a small risk of embolic complications.

Similarly, botulinum toxin has been injected into Muller's plane to achieve temporary eyelid lowering [80–84]. This approach has not been widely adopted as the dosing can be variable and rates of temporary ptosis and induced diplopia approach 20 %. Additionally, neither botulinum toxin nor triamcinolone can be used for lower eyelid retraction.

Hyaluronic acid (HA) gels have gained wide popularity for cosmetic applications in filling volume deficit areas [85]. These fillers can be effective in correcting both upper [86] and lower eyelid retraction secondary to TED [87, 88]. This strategy is advantageous in that it is titratable, repeatable, and reversible. These features make their use in TED ideal for active stage disease, when the eyelid position may be changing, and for inactive disease when small amounts of residual asymmetry are evident (existing or postoperative). Some cases may completely avoid surgery altogether. This is considered an off-label use of the medication.

The procedure is performed by first anesthetizing the conjunctiva topically. The upper eyelid is then everted and the conjunctiva just superior to the upper tarsal edge is exposed. Using a 30-gauge needle, a single bolus of HA is placed centrally in the subconjunctival levator-Muller plane. Small volumes (0.1–0.2 mL) of material are injected iteratively with the end point being adequate lid lowering and improved symmetry (Fig. 12.7).

In patients who do require eyelid retraction surgery, it may be advantageous to combine this procedure with decompression. The philosophy here is to usher patients along their course of rehabilitation in a more expedient manner, accepting that small touch up stages of surgery may be required later.

Orbital decompression can lead to small alterations in upper eyelid position [89, 90], and in many cases decompression surgery should be performed prior to eyelid retraction repair. However, patients without any pre-existing motility restriction and mild to moderate eyelid retraction can benefit from combined upper eyelid retraction and decompression surgery [91–93]. Although it is possible that secondary surgeries may be required, such patients tend to have similar final outcomes to staged surgery [91]. The same can be said for combined lower eyelid-decompression surgery [94]. In both cases, small position and contour abnormalities can be managed postoperatively in an office setting with HA fillers.

In terms of surgical technique, a wide range of procedures have been described and most produce acceptable, although periodically unpredictable, results. En glove approaches for both upper and lower eyelid retraction are favored in the case of combined orbital surgery, as this tends to avoid making supplementary incisions. For the upper lid, after lateral decompression, the upper eyelid

Fig. 12.6 Surgical series of en glove lysis for lower eyelid retractors with dermis graft placement. (**a**) A small lateral crows feet or lid crease incision is made. (**b**) The lower eyelid retractors are released from the conjunctiva, creating a window pane thin posterior lamella. (**c**) The orbicularis retaining ligament is released with blunt stretching between the tarsus and the orbital rim. (**d**) A de-epithelialized dermis strip graft is harvested, in this case from the retroauricular area. (**e**) A protective sheath is fashioned from intravenous tubing to match the length of a Keith needle. (**f**) The distance is estimated and the guarded needle is passed through the dissection pocket created earlier. (**g**) The guard is removed and the dermis graft on a suture is passed through the pocket from lateral to medial. (**h**) The eye is placed on stretch with a Frost suture

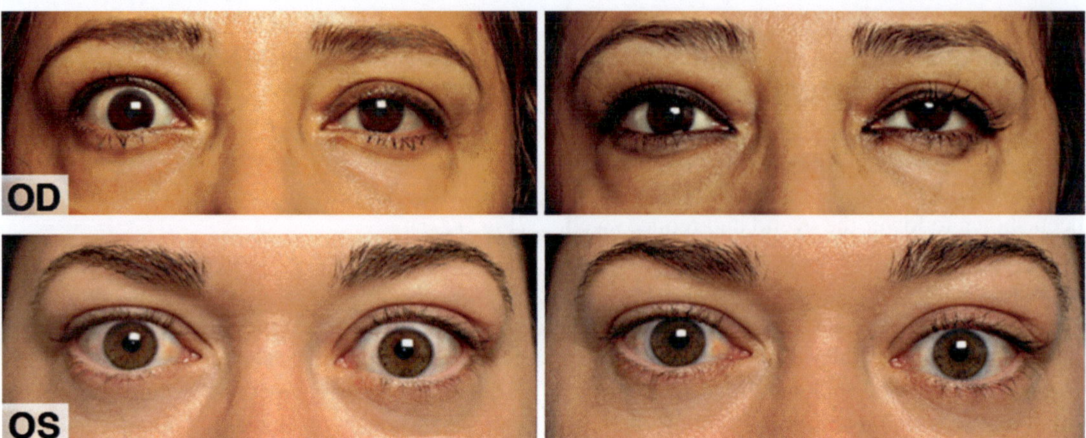

Fig. 12.7 Hyaluronic acid gel injection for upper lid retraction. On the *left* is pre-injection and on the *right* is at 3-month follow-up. The upper series represents active, inflammatory stage disease, while the lower series shows quiescent disease

crease incision can be utilized, or the eyelid can be everted for a posterior approach. A small button hole is made through the lateral horn of the levator aponeurosis and a pocket is dissected between the conjunctiva and levator planes. A blunt dissection stretching maneuver can lengthen the central aponeurosis and sharp dissection of the lateral and medial horns can be graded for contour. Small side cuts into the central pedicle of aponeurosis can increase lid-lengthening effect (Fig. 12.8).

In any upper eyelid retraction surgery, it is important to consider the aesthetic consequences of the brow fat span (BFS)—tarsal platform show (TPS) relationship. Lengthening of the eyelid, without addressing the BFS–TPS ratio can lead to less appealing results with a long TPS, further accentuating the proptotic TED appearance. Further, this can also create the perception of a ptotic and tired eyelid. In cases where there is a short TPS preoperatively (or relatively short compared to the contralateral side), a posterior eyelid lengthening approach may be ideal [91]. However, if there is current or a high risk of late TPS elongation, an anterior approach is preferred, as it allows access to the anterior orbital fat pads and the retro-orbicularis oculus fat in order to contour and manage the BFS. The purpose of this redraping would be to elongate the BFS and the TPS simultaneously in order to maintain the BFS–TPS ratio [95].

In the lower lid, entry through the upper eyelid incision laterally and dissection of the retractors off of the conjunctiva and tarsus can be performed in en glove fashion [72, 73]. If a fat decompression is performed, some small 0.5 mm fat cobblestones can be fashioned from the excised tissue and used as volume augmentation if required.

Periocular Rejuvenation

The stigmata of TED are contextualized within the natural processes of facial aging. Loss of skin elasticity, deepening of glabellar and other furrows, facial volume loss and tissue descent each have aesthetic implications for TED patients as they do for patients without TED. Additional considerations including the coarsening of facial features, expansion of the lateral brow fat and tendency to form fluid pockets in the periorbital region further complicate facial rejuvenation in TED.

Accordingly, treatments to improve facial skin quality including chemical peels, laser treatments,

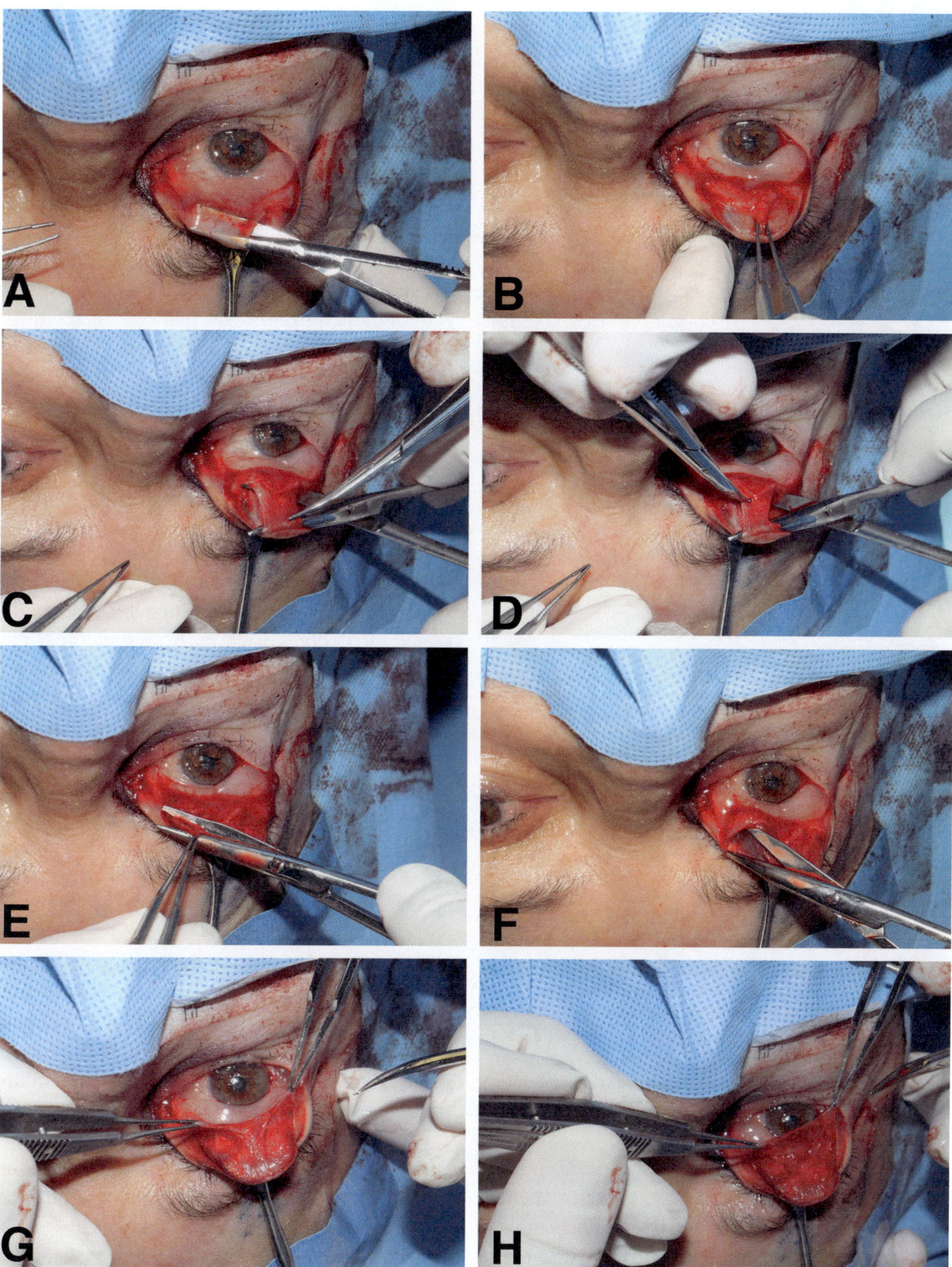

Fig. 12.8 Upper lid retraction stretching sequence. (**a**) The lid is everted and the conjunctiva is incised. (**b**) The levator aponeurosis is grasped. (**c**) A plane between the levator aponeurosis and Muller's muscle is dissected, the levator is stretched and a small myotomy is made laterally adjacent to the tarsus. (**d**) A similar incision medially is made more superiorly. (**e**) The lateral and medial horns of the levator are opened. (**f**) Stretching is performed in these spaces and contour adjusted. (**g**) The conjunctiva is elevated and the Muller's muscle is dissected cleanly off its posterior surface. (**h**) Window pane thin conjunctiva is demonstrated. The iris should be visible through the tissue

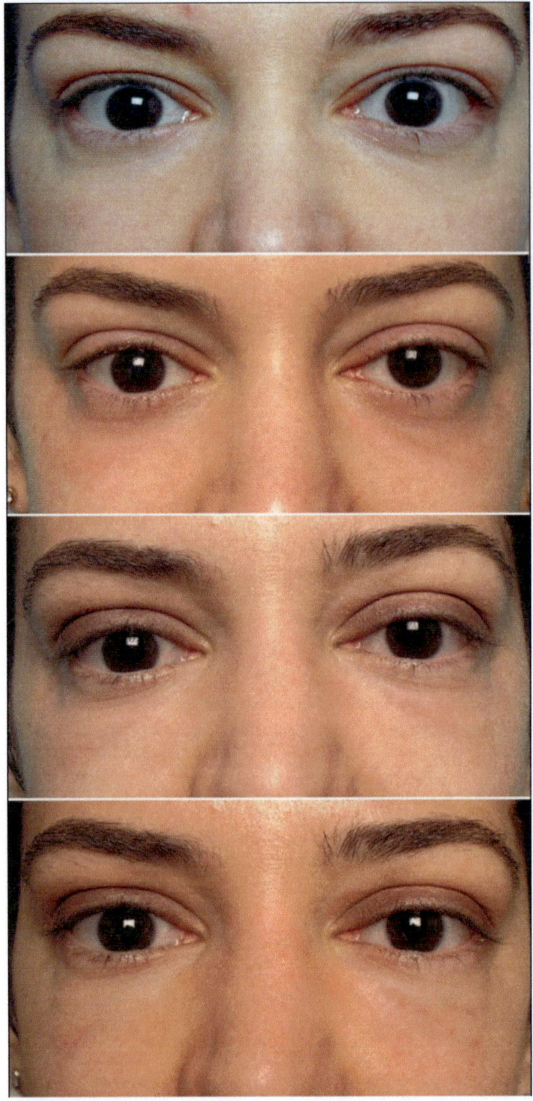

Fig. 12.9 Advanced periocular rejuvenation. The top panel shows preoperative appearance. The second panel is after bilateral decompression. The bottom two panels are after the first and second layer of hyaluronic acid gel filler to the periorbital hollows, respectively

and other skin care regimes can benefit patients with TED. Botulinum toxin can be extremely effective in effacing dynamic and static rhytids over time. Volume augmentation, whether by synthetic fillers [96], fat grafting [97] or transposition and lifting procedures [98] can also benefit appropriately selected patients with periorbital volume collapse (from natural processes or anterior fat decompression) (Fig. 12.9).

The expansion of the lateral brow fat pad [39–41] can be particularly concerning to patients with TED (Fig. 12.10). This is a difficult problem, as no reliable and reproducible techniques for the management of this problem are currently described. In general, during blepharoplasty or eyelid lengthening, this fat pad can be accessed through an eyelid crease incision. Debulking with sharp dissection and/or contouring with electrocautery can be performed.

Concluding Remarks

Smoking cessation, comfort measures and environmental modification can improve the TED experience for patients. Additionally, minimally invasive procedures such as hyaluronic acid gel fillers and botulinum toxin for lid retraction and strabismus can reduce the cosmetic and functional implications of disease while awaiting stabilization for definitive therapy. Surgical rehabilitation that follows can be graded and individualized for the aesthetic and functional needs of each patient. In each phase, the patient and surgeon must consider the aesthetic implications of each surgical approach and weigh them carefully. Surgical approaches to the orbit were discussed that avoid a skin incision or that conceal the incision within the lid crease. The advantages of the lid crease approach to the lateral wall include the excellent access to the deep lateral orbit, avoiding damage to the lateral canthal angle and orbicularis, and minimizing the risk of postoperative diplopia.

The facial metamorphosis in TED can be extensive, and should be contextualized within the natural processes of aging. Taking a holistic view of periorbital rejuvenation during each stage of disease and reconstruction will allow orbital specialists to approach the goal of restoring TED patients to their pre-morbid state.

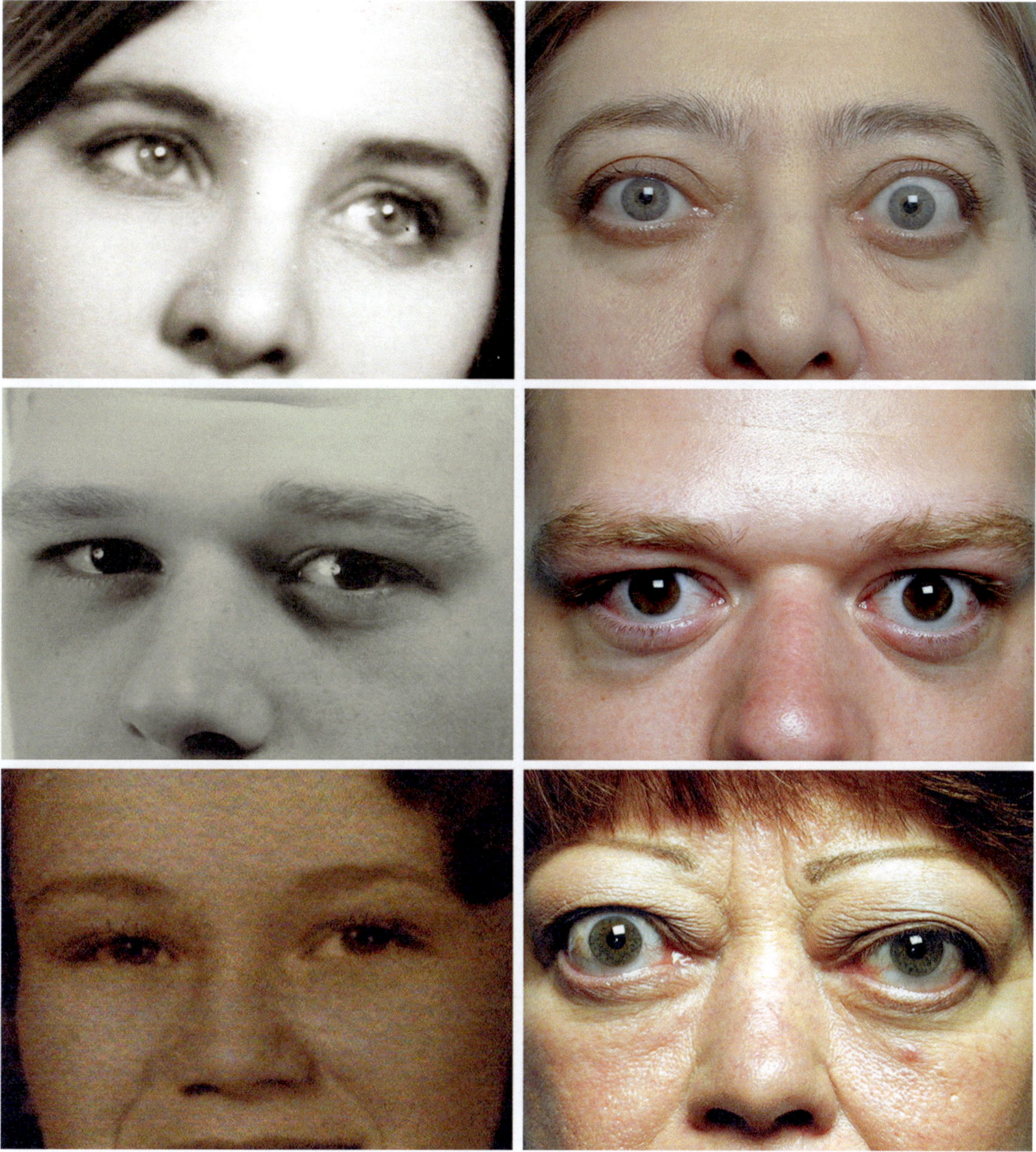

Fig. 12.10 Lateral expansion of the brow fat relative to the pre-thyroid eye disease state

References

1. Elberling TV, Rasmussen AK, Feldt-Rasmussen U, Hørding M, Perrild H, Waldemar G. Impaired health-related quality of life in Graves' disease. A prospective study. Eur J Endocrinol. 2004;151: 549–55.
2. Gerding MN, Terwee CB, Dekker FW, Koornneef L, Prummel MF, Wiersinga WM. Quality of life in patients with Graves' ophthalmopathy is markedly decreased: measurement by the medical outcomes study instrument. Thyroid. 1997;7:885–9.
3. Kahaly GJ, Petrak F, Hardt J, Pitz S, Egle UT. Psychosocial morbidity of Graves' orbitopathy. Clin Endocrinol (Oxf). 2005;63:395–402.

4. Park JJ, Sullivan TJ, Mortimer RH, Wagenaar M, Perry-Keene DA. Assessing quality of life in Australian patients with Graves' ophthalmopathy. Br J Ophthalmol. 2004;88:75–8.
5. Terwee C, Wakelkamp I, Tan S, Dekker F, Prummel MF, Wiersinga W. Long-term effects of Graves' ophthalmopathy on health-related quality of life. Eur J Endocrinol. 2002;146:751–7.
6. Wiersinga W, Prummel M, Terwee C. Effects of Graves' ophthalmopathy on quality of life. J Endocrinol Invest. 2004;27:259–64.
7. Ponto KA, Pitz S, Pfeiffer N, Hommel G, Weber MM, Kahaly GJ. Quality of life and occupational disability in endocrine orbitopathy. Dtsch Arztebl Int. 2009; 106:283–9.
8. Bartley GB, Fatourechi V, Kadrmas EF, et al. Long-term follow-up of Graves ophthalmopathy in an incidence cohort. Ophthalmology. 1996;103:958–62.
9. Coulter I, Frewin S, Krassas GE, Perros P. Psychological implications of Graves' orbitopathy. Eur J Endocrinol. 2007;157:127–31.
10. Jensen AL, Harder I. The impact of bodily change on social behaviour in patients with thyroid-associated ophthalmopathy. Scand J Caring Sci. 2011;25:341–9.
11. Estcourt S, Hickey J, Perros P, Dayan C, Vaidya B. The patient experience of services for thyroid eye disease in the United Kingdom: results of a nationwide survey. Eur J Endocrinol. 2009;161:483–7.
12. Estcourt S, Vaidya B, Quinn A, Shepherd M. The impact of thyroid eye disease upon patients' wellbeing: a qualitative analysis. Clin Endocrinol (Oxf). 2008;68:635–9.
13. Rice G, Ingram J, Mizan J. Enhancing a primary care environment: a case study of effects on patients and staff in a single general practice. Br J Gen Pract. 2008; 58:465–70.
14. Dijkstra K, Pieterse M, Pruyn A. Physical environmental stimuli that turn healthcare facilities into healing environments through psychologically mediated effects: systematic review. J Adv Nurs. 2006;56: 166–81.
15. Drahota A, Ward D, Mackenzie H, et al. Sensory environment on health-related outcomes of hospital patients. Cochrane Database Syst Rev. 2012;3, CD005315.
16. Altiparmak UE, Acar DE, Ozer PA, et al. Topical cyclosporine A for the dry eye findings of thyroid orbitopathy patients. Eye (Lond). 2010;24:1044–50.
17. Sokol JA, Foulks GN, Haider A, Nunery WR. Ocular surface effects of thyroid disease. Ocul Surf. 2010;8:29–39.
18. Lee H, Roh HS, Yoon JS, Lee SY. Assessment of quality of life and depression in Korean patients with Graves' ophthalmopathy. Korean J Ophthalmol. 2010;24:65–72.
19. Shorr N, Seiff SR. The four stages of surgical rehabilitation of the patient with dysthyroid ophthalmopathy. Ophthalmology. 1986;93:476–83.
20. Jackson JL. Nonsurgical management of diplopia after orbital decompression surgery. Am Orthopt J. 2012;62:29–33.
21. Rutstein RP. Use of Bangerter filters with adults having intractable diplopia. Optometry. 2010;81:387–93.
22. Fraine L. Nonsurgical management of diplopia. Am Orthopt J. 2012;62:13–8.
23. Wu X, Lin N, Ai LK, Wang JH, Yan LJ. The application of botulinum toxin A in the treatment of restrictive strabismus in thyroid associated ophthalmopathy. Zhonghua Yan Ke Za Zhi. 2006;42:1063–7.
24. Gair EJ, Lee JP, Khoo BK, Maurino V. What is the role of botulinum toxin in the treatment of dysthyroid strabismus? J AAPOS. 1999;3:272–4.
25. Lyons CJ, Vickers SF, Lee JP. Botulinum toxin therapy in dysthyroid strabismus. Eye (Lond). 1990;4(Pt 4):538–42.
26. Bunevicius R, Velickiene D, Prange Jr AJ. Mood and anxiety disorders in women with treated hyperthyroidism and ophthalmopathy caused by Graves' disease. Gen Hosp Psychiatry. 2005;27:133–9.
27. Farid M, Roch-Levecq AC, Levi L, Brody BL, Granet DB, Kikkawa DO. Psychological disturbance in graves ophthalmopathy. Arch Ophthalmol. 2005;123:491–6.
28. Pfeilschifter J, Ziegler R. Smoking and endocrine ophthalmopathy: impact of smoking severity and current vs lifetime cigarette consumption. Clin Endocrinol (Oxf). 1996;45:477–81.
29. Bartalena L, Marcocci C, Tanda ML, et al. Cigarette smoking and treatment outcomes in Graves ophthalmopathy. Ann Intern Med. 1998;129:632–5.
30. Eckstein A, Quadbeck B, Mueller G, et al. Impact of smoking on the response to treatment of thyroid associated ophthalmopathy. Br J Ophthalmol. 2003;87: 773–6.
31. Stead L, Buitrago D, Preciado N, Sanchez G, Lancaster T. Physician advice for smoking cessation (Review). Cochrane Database Syst Rev. 2013;31.
32. Mills EJ, Wu P, Lockhart IAN, Thorlund K, Puhan M, Ebbert JONO. Comparisons of high-dose and combination nicotine replacement therapy, varenicline, and bupropion for smoking cessation: A systematic review and multiple treatment meta-analysis. Ann Med. 2012;44:588–97.
33. Suls JM, Luger TM, Curry SJ, Mermelstein RJ, Sporer AK, An LC. Efficacy of smoking-cessation interventions for young adults: a meta-analysis. Am J Prev Med. 2012;42:655–62.
34. Tahiri M, Mottillo S, Joseph L, Pilote L, Eisenberg MJ. Alternative smoking cessation aids: a meta-analysis of randomized controlled trials. Am J Med. 2012;125:576–84.
35. Zbikowski SM, Magnusson B, Pockey JR, Tindle HA, Weaver KE. A review of smoking cessation interventions for smokers aged 50 and older. Maturitas. 2012; 71:131–41.
36. Werner SC. Classification of the eye changes of Graves' disease. Am J Ophthalmol. 1969;68:646–8.
37. Mourits MP, Prummel MF, Wiersinga WM, Koornneef L. Clinical activity score as a guide in the management of patients with Graves' ophthalmopathy. Clin Endocrinol (Oxf). 1997;47:9–14.

38. Dolman PJ, Rootman J. VISA classification for Graves orbitopathy. Ophthal Plast Reconstr Surg. 2006;22:319–24.
39. Goldberger S, Sarraf D, Bernstein JM, Hurwitz JJ. Involvement of the eyebrow fat pad in Graves' orbitopathy. Ophthal Plast Reconstr Surg. 1994;10:80–6.
40. Papageorgiou K, Hwang C. Thyroid-associated periorbitopathy eyebrow fat and soft tissue expansion in patients with thyroid-associated orbitopathy. Arch Ophthalmol. 2012;130:319–28.
41. Savar LM, Menghani RM, Chong KK, Garneau HC, Goldberg RA. Eyebrow tissue expansion: an underappreciated entity in thyroid associated orbitopathy. Arch Ophthalmol. 2012;130:1566–9.
42. DeSanto LW, Gorman CA. Selection of patients and choice of operation for orbital decompression in graves ophthalmopathy. Laryngoscope. 1973; 83:945–59.
43. Hurwitz JJ, Birt D. Approach to orbital decompression in Graves' orbitopathy. Arch Ophthalmol. 1985;103(5):660–5.
44. Ogura JH. Surgical results of orbital decompression for malignant exophthalmos. J Laryngol Otol. 1978;92(3):181–95.
45. Borumandi F, Hammer B, Kamer L, von Arx G. How predictable is exophthalmos reduction in Graves' orbitopathy? A review of the literature. Br J Ophthalmol. 2011;95:1625–30.
46. Leong SC, White PS. Outcomes following surgical decompression for dysthyroid orbitopathy (Graves' disease). Curr Opin Otolaryngol Head Neck Surg. 2010;18:37–43.
47. Chong KK, Goldberg RA. Lateral canthal surgery. Facial Plast Surg. 2010;26:193–200.
48. Shorr N, Baylis HI, Goldberg RA, Perry JD. Transcaruncular approach to the medial orbit and orbital apex. Ophthalmology. 2000;107:1459–63.
49. Long JA, Baylis HI. Hypoglobus following orbital decompression for dysthyroid ophthalmopathy. Ophthal Plast Reconstr Surg. 1990;6:185–9.
50. Garrity JA, Fatourechi V, Bergstralh EJ, et al. Results of transantral orbital decompression in 428 patients with severe Graves' ophthalmopathy. Am J Ophthalmol. 1993;116:533–47.
51. Goldberg RA, Shorr N, Cohen MS. The medical orbital strut in the prevention of postdecompression dystopia in dysthyroid ophthalmopathy. Ophthal Plast Reconstr Surg. 1992;8:32–4.
52. Alper MG. Pioneers in the history of orbital decompression for Graves' ophthalmopathy. Doc Ophthalmol. 1995;89:163–71.
53. Moran RE, Letterman GS, Schurter MA. The surgical correction of exophthalmos. History, technique, and long-term follow-up. Plast Reconstr Surg. 1972;49: 595–608.
54. Kroll AJ, Casten VG. Dysthyroid exophthalmos. Palliation by lateral orbital decompression. Arch Ophthalmol. 1966;76:205–10.
55. Fichter N, Krentz H, Guthoff RF. Functional and esthetic outcome after bony lateral wall decompression with orbital rim removal and additional fat resection in graves' orbitopathy with regard to the configuration of the lateral canthal region. Orbit. 2013;32:239–46.
56. Schaaf H, Santo G, Graf M, Howaldt HP. En bloc resection of the lateral orbital rim to reduce exophthalmos in patients with Graves' disease. J Craniomaxillofac Surg. 2010;38:204–10.
57. Fayers T, Barker LE, Verity DH, Rose GE. Oscillopsia after lateral wall orbital decompression. Ophthalmology. 2013;120(9):1920–3.
58. Goldberg RA, Kim AJ, Kerivan KM. The lacrimal keyhole, orbital door jamb, and basin of the inferior orbital fissure. Arch Ophthalmol. 1998;116: 1618–24.
59. Goldberg RA, Perry JD, Hortaleza V, Tong JT. Strabismus after balanced medial plus lateral wall versus lateral wall only orbital decompression for dysthyroid orbitopathy. Ophthal Plast Reconstr Surg. 2000;16:271–7.
60. Ben Simon GJ, Schwarcz RM, Mansury AM, Wang L, McCann JD, Goldberg RA. Minimally invasive orbital decompression: local anesthesia and hand-carved bone. Arch Ophthalmol. 2005;123:1671–5.
61. Chang M, Baek S, Lee TS. Long-term outcomes of unilateral orbital fat decompression for thyroid eye disease. Graefes Arch Clin Exp Ophthalmol. 2013;251:935–9.
62. Richter DF, Stoff A, Olivari N. Transpalpebral decompression of endocrine ophthalmopathy by intraorbital fat removal (Olivari technique): experience and progression after more than 3000 operations over 20 years. Plast Reconstr Surg. 2007;120:109–23.
63. Robert P-YR, Rivas M, Camezind P, Rulfi J-Y, Adenis J-P. Decrease of intraocular pressure after fat-removal orbital decompression in Graves disease. Ophthal Plast Reconstr Surg. 2006;22:92–5.
64. Wu C-H, Chang T-C, Liao S-L. Results and predictability of fat-removal orbital decompression for disfiguring graves exophthalmos in an Asian patient population. Am J Ophthalmol. 2008;145:755–9.
65. Satterfield D, Keltner JL, Morrison TL. Psychosocial aspects of strabismus study. Arch Ophthalmol. 1993;111:1100–5.
66. Hatt SR, Leske DA, Kirgis PA, Bradley EA, Holmes JM. The effects of strabismus on quality of life in adults. Am J Ophthalmol. 2007;144:643–7.
67. Bradley EA, Sloan JA, Novotny PJ, Garrity JA, Woog JJ, West SK. Evaluation of the National Eye Institute visual function questionnaire in Graves' ophthalmopathy. Ophthalmology. 2006;113:1450–4.
68. Kim DB, Meyer DR, Simon JW. Retractor lysis as prophylaxis for lower lid retraction following inferior rectus recession. J Pediatr Ophthalmol Strabismus. 2002;39:198–202.
69. Liao SL, Shih MJ, Lin LL-K. A procedure to minimize lower lid retraction during large inferior rectus recession in graves ophthalmopathy. Am J Ophthalmol. 2006;141:340–5.
70. Meyer DR, Simon JW, Kansora M. Primary infratarsal lower eyelid retractor lysis to prevent eyelid retraction

after inferior rectus muscle recession. Am J Ophthalmol. 1996;122:331–9.
71. Kushner BJ. A surgical procedure to minimize lower-eyelid retraction with inferior rectus recession. Arch Ophthalmol. 1992;110:1011–4.
72. Chang HS, Lee D, Taban M, Douglas RS, Goldberg RA. "En-glove" lysis of lower eyelid retractors with AlloDerm and dermis-fat grafts in lower eyelid retraction surgery. Ophthal Plast Reconstr Surg. 2011; 27:137–41.
73. Holds JB, Anderson RL, Thiese SM. Lower eyelid retraction: a minimal incision surgical approach to retractor lysis. Ophthalmic Surg. 1990;21:767–71.
74. Lee SJ, Rim THT, Jang SY, et al. Treatment of upper eyelid retraction related to thyroid-associated ophthalmopathy using subconjunctival triamcinolone injections. Graefes Arch Clin Exp Ophthalmol. 2013;251(1):261–70.
75. Xu D, Liu Y, Xu H, Li H. Repeated triamcinolone acetonide injection in the treatment of upper-lid retraction in patients with thyroid-associated ophthalmopathy. Can J Ophthalmol. 2012;47:34–41.
76. Aa A, Hussein AM, Ea S. Orbital steroid injection versus oral steroid therapy in management of thyroid-related ophthalmopathy. Clin Experiment Ophthalmol. 2010;38:692–7.
77. Bordaberry M, Marques DL, Pereira-Lima JC, Marcon IM, Schmid H. Repeated peribulbar injections of triamcinolone acetonide: a successful and safe treatment for moderate to severe Graves' ophthalmopathy. Acta Ophthalmol. 2009;87:58–64.
78. Ebner R, Devoto MH, Weil D, et al. Treatment of thyroid associated ophthalmopathy with periocular injections of triamcinolone. Br J Ophthalmol. 2004;88: 1380–6.
79. Goldberg RA. Orbital steroid injections R. Br J Ophthalmol. 2004;88:1359–60.
80. Costa PG, Saraiva FP, Pereira IC, Monteiro MLR, Matayoshi S. Comparative study of Botox (R) injection treatment for upper eyelid retraction with 6-month follow-up in patients with thyroid eye disease in the congestive or fibrotic stage. Eye (Lond). 2009;23:767–73.
81. Morgenstern KE, Evanchan J, Foster JA, et al. Botulinum toxin type A for dysthyroid upper eyelid retraction. Ophthal Plast Reconstr Surg. 2004;20:181–5.
82. Shih MJ, Liao SL, Lu HY. A single transcutaneous injection with Botox (R) for dysthyroid lid retraction. Eye (Lond). 2004;18:466–9.
83. Traisk F, Tallstedt L. Thyroid associated ophthalmopathy: botulinum toxin A in the treatment of upper eyelid retraction—a pilot study. Acta Ophthalmol Scand. 2001;79:585–8.
84. Uddin JM, Davies PD. Treatment of upper eyelid retraction associated with thyroid eye disease with subconjunctival botulinum toxin injection. Ophthalmology. 2002;109:1183–7.
85. Goldberg RA, Fiaschetti D. Filling the periorbital hollows with hyaluronic acid gel: initial experience with 244 injections. Ophthal Plast Reconstr Surg. 2006;22:335–41. discussion 41-3.
86. Mancini R, Khadavi NM, Goldberg RA. Nonsurgical management of upper eyelid margin asymmetry using hyaluronic acid gel filler. Ophthal Plast Reconstr Surg. 2011;27:1–3.
87. Goldberg RA, Lee S, Jayasundera T, Tsirbas A, Douglas RS, McCann JD. Treatment of lower eyelid retraction by expansion of the lower eyelid with hyaluronic acid gel. Ophthal Plast Reconstr Surg. 2007; 23:343–8.
88. Zamani M, Thyagarajan S, Olver JM. Functional use of hyaluronic acid gel in lower eyelid retraction. Arch Ophthalmol. 2008;126:1157–9.
89. Baldeschi L, Wakelkamp IM, Lindeboom R, Prummel MF, Wiersinga WM. Early versus late orbital decompression in Graves' orbitopathy: a retrospective study in 125 patients. Ophthalmology. 2006;113:874–8.
90. Chang EL, Bernardino CR, Rubin PA. Normalization of upper eyelid height and contour after bony decompression in thyroid-related ophthalmopathy: a digital image analysis. Arch Ophthalmol. 2004;122:1882–5.
91. Ben Simon GJ, Mansury AM, Schwarcz RM, Lee S, McCann JD, Goldberg RA. Simultaneous orbital decompression and correction of upper eyelid retraction versus staged procedures in thyroid-related orbitopathy. Ophthalmology. 2005;112:923–32.
92. Morax S, Hurbli T. Choice of surgical treatment for Graves' disease. J Craniomaxillofac Surg. 1987;15: 174–81.
93. Tremolada C, Tremolada MA. The "triple technique" for treating stable Graves' ophthalmopathy. Plast Reconstr Surg. 1997;100:40–8. discussion 9-50.
94. Norris JH, Ross JJ, O'Reilly P, Malhotra R. A review of combined orbital decompression and lower eyelid recession surgery for lower eyelid retraction in thyroid orbitopathy. Br J Ophthalmol. 2011;95:1664–9.
95. Papageorgiou KI, Ang M, Chang SH, Kohn J, Martinez S, Goldberg RA. Aesthetic considerations in upper eyelid retraction surgery. Ophthal Plast Reconstr Surg. 2012;28:419–23.
96. Goldberg RA, Fiaschetti D. Filling the periorbital hollows with hyaluronic acid gel: initial experience with 244 injections. Ophthal Plast Reconstr Surg. 2006;22:335–41. discussion 41-3.
97. Lambros V. Fat injection for the aging midface. Operative Tech Plast Reconstr Surg. 1998;5:129–37.
98. Goldberg RA. Transconjunctival orbital fat repositioning: transposition of orbital fat pedicles into a subperiosteal pocket. Plast Reconstr Surg. 2000;105:743–8. discussion 9-51.

Psychological Disturbances in Thyroid Eye Disease

13

Sally L. Baxter, Richard L. Scawn, Bobby S. Korn, and Don O. Kikkawa

Introduction

In thyroid-associated eye disease (TED), several visual and functional sequelae can affect quality of life, including ocular discomfort, diplopia, keratitis, and visual impairment. Furthermore, the additional burden of physical disfigurement can be devastating. Psychosocial distress is prominent among patients with disfiguring conditions, particularly in the periocular region [1, 2]. In TED, several ocular changes contribute to changes in facial appearance. Exophthalmos and eyelid retraction may cause a frightened, startled, or angry expression, when this may not reflect the patient's internal emotional state [3]. Proptosis may also cause a subconscious depression of the brows in an effort to reduce exposure, resulting in a prolonged frown. Staring due to infrequent blinking can be interpreted as hostile [3]. These changes can cause considerable emotional and psychological distress for the patient due to the misperception of emotional state.

S.L. Baxter, M.D., M.Sc.
D.O. Kikkawa, M.D., F.A.C.S. (✉)
R.L. Scawn, M.B.B.S., F.R.C.Ophth.
B.S. Korn, M.D., Ph.D., F.A.C.S.
Division of Ophthalmic Plastic and Reconstructive Surgery, UCSD Department of Ophthalmology, Shiley Eye Center, University of California San Diego, 9415 Campus Point Drive, La Jolla, CA 92093, USA
e-mail: dkikkawa@ucsd.edu

In recent years, there has been increasing interest in assessing well-being and quality of life from the patient's perspective. More than two decades ago, a joint committee of international thyroid associations recommended that patient-reported outcomes be a key consideration for assessing disease severity and treatment response [4]. Since then, there has been substantial growth in the literature regarding the psychological ramifications of TED.

This chapter reviews several methods of measuring patient-reported outcomes, describes key findings from studies investigating psychological disturbances and changes in quality of life of TED patients, and discusses the implications of these findings.

Measurement Tools for Psychological Disturbances and Health-Related Quality of Life

Several standardized assessment tools have been used in the study of psychological disturbances in TED. They can be categorized into generic, vision specific, and disease specific.

Generic Instruments

Multiple general assessment tools used for investigating psychological effects and health-related quality of life in TED patients are listed in

R.S. Douglas et al. (eds.), *Thyroid Eye Disease*,
DOI 10.1007/978-1-4939-1746-4_13, © Springer Science+Business Media New York 2015

Table 13.1 Generic quality of life measurements that have been used to study patients with thyroid-associated eye disease (TED)

Name of instrument	Number of items	Subscales/categories	Example(s) of use in TED patients
Medical Outcomes Study (MOS)	12, 20, or 36, depending on the form that is used (e.g., Short Form (SF) 12, SF-20, SF-36)	Physical health: physical functioning, role-physical, bodily pain, general health Mental health: vitality, social functioning, role-emotional, mental health	[14, 16, 48–50]
Sickness Impact Profile (SIP)	136	Sleep and rest, eating, work, home management, recreation and pastimes, ambulation, mobility, body care and movement, social interaction, alertness behavior, emotional behavior, and communication	[14]
Profile of Mood States (POMS)	65	Tension-anxiety, anger-hostility, fatigue-inertia, depression-dejection, vigor-activity, confusion-bewilderment	[18, 19]
Hospital Anxiety and Depression Scale (HADS)	14	Anxiety, depression	[17]
Beck Depression Inventory (BDI)	21	Depression	[48]
Middlesex Hospital Questionnaire (MHQ)	48	Free-floating anxiety, phobic anxiety, obsessional traits and symptoms, somatic concomitants of anxiety, neurotic depression, and hysteric personality traits	[20]

Table 13.1. These tools have been used to study the psychological effects of other diseases, so that TED patients can be compared with other patient groups. General health-related quality of life in TED patients has been reported to be worse than in patients with emphysema or heart failure, highlighting the burden of TED [5].

Vision-Specific Instruments

In contrast to general instruments examining a broad health perspective, vision-specific instruments allow greater sensitivity for issues specific to eye disease related quality of life. Scores on the 25-item National Eye Institute Visual Functioning Questionnaire (NEI VFQ-25) show moderate impairment of quality of life for patients with TED, with pronounced effects in the Mental Health and Role Difficulty subscales [6]. However, significant ceiling effects were found in over half of the subscales, and patients with TED felt the questionnaire lacked items addressing important issues including altered physical appearance and ocular discomfort. While the NEI VFQ-25 may have some items that are applicable to TED, it focuses primarily on visual functioning and fails to address changes in appearance, a distinguishing feature of TED.

Disease-Specific Instruments

Disease-specific instruments have been developed to assess quality of life specifically in patients with TED. The most commonly used is the 16-item Graves' Ophthalmopathy Quality of Life (GO-QoL) questionnaire, which addresses visual functioning and altered appearance equally (see Fig. 13.1) [7]. The GO-QoL is valid and reliable, is available in eight languages, and may be considered the current gold standard for measuring patient-reported outcomes in TED [5, 8, 9].

The Thyroid Eye Disease Quality of Life (TED-QoL) questionnaire is the newest instrument [10]. With only three items (measuring global quality of life, the effect of visual function on performing daily activities, and satisfaction with

Fig. 13.1 The Graves' ophthalmopathy quality of life (GO-QoL) questionnaire. This 16-item questionnaire is split into two categories, with one addressing visual functioning and the other addressing altered appearance. From Wiersinga WM. Quality of life in Graves' Ophthalmopathy. Best Practice and Research Clinical Endocrinology and Metabolism. 2012 Jun;26(3):59–70. Reprinted with permission from Elsevier

Appendix 2 **GO-QOL version UK1**

The following questions deal specifically with your thyroid eye disease.
Please focus on the past week while answering these questions
During the past week, to what extent were you limited in carrying out the following activities, because of your thyroid eye disease?
Tick the box that matches your answer. The boxes correspond with the answers above them.
Please tick only one box for each question.

	Yes, seriously limited	Yes, a little limited	No not at all limited
1 Bicycling [never learned to ride a bike ☐]	☐	☐	☐
2 Driving [no driver's licence ☐]	☐	☐	☐
3 Moving around the house	☐	☐	☐
4 Walking outdoors	☐	☐	☐
5 Reading	☐	☐	☐
6 Watching TV	☐	☐	☐
7 Hobby or pastime, i.e..............................	☐	☐	☐

	Yes, severely hindered	Yes a little hindered	No not at all hindered
8 During the past week, did you feel hindered from something that you wanted to do because of your thyroid eye disease?	☐	☐	☐

The following questions deal with your thyroid eye disease in general

	Yes, very much so	Yes, a little	No,not at all
9 Do you feel that your appearane has changed because of your thyroid eye disease?	☐	☐	☐
10 Do you feel that you are stared at in the streets because of your thyroid eye disease?	☐	☐	☐
11 Do you feel that people react unpleasantly because of your thyroid eye disease?	☐	☐	☐
12 Do you feel that your thyroid eye diease has an influnce on your self-confidence?	☐	☐	☐
13 Do you feel socially isolated because of your thyroid eye disease?	☐	☐	☐
14 Do you feel that your thyroid eye disase has an influence on making friends?	☐	☐	☐
15 Do you feel that you appear less often on photos than before you had thyroid eye disease?	☐	☐	☐
16 Do you try to mask changes in appearance caused by your thyroid eye disease?	☐	☐	☐

physical appearance), it has been shown to have similar validity and reproducibility as longer questionnaires, but is faster to complete and touts a higher completion rate, which may make it more practical for everyday clinical use.

Open-Ended Analyses

In addition to standardized questionnaires, several studies have used more open-ended approaches consisting of qualitative analyses of interviews exploring themes [11–13]. While they allow for more flexibility in patient responses and may detect increased subtleties and depth, these sociological analyses take more time and require special training. Their open-ended nature also makes them less practical for quantitative research studies.

Overview of Key Findings in Patient-Reported Outcomes in TED

General Quality of Life

Measurements of general quality of life are significantly lower in patients with TED. Compared to a large published reference group using the

Medical Outcomes Study (MOS-24) and three subscales of the Sickness Impact Profile (SIP), TED patients had lower scores in the categories of physical functioning, social functioning, mental health, health perceptions, and bodily pain [14]. Another study using a 105-item questionnaire combining items from the NEI-VFQ, the Short Form (SF-12), an adapted version of the Dermatology-Specific Quality of Life (DSQL) instrument, and questions specific to TED, found statistically significant lower scores for all measures of quality of life compared to a control group [15]. These included all subscores of the NEI-VFQ (except color vision), both physical and mental components of the SF-12, and the self-perception and social desirability scales. Overall lower quality of life was neither age specific nor gender specific [15].

Psychiatric and Mood Disturbance

The prevalence of psychiatric disturbance is greater among patients with TED compared to controls. TED patients have increased emotional distress, with almost half of patients suffering from symptoms of anxiety and/or depression [16]. Based on the Hospital Anxiety and Depression Scale (HADS), one study estimated the prevalence of psychiatric disorders to be 32 % among a population of TED patients, of which 19 % had depressive disorders and 19 % had current anxiety disorders [17]. Using the Mini-International Neuropsychiatric Interview, Graves' patients were found to have significantly greater prevalence of anxiety disorders, major depression, and total mood disorders even compared to hospitalized patients with other diseases [18].

The increased prevalence of psychiatric disturbances among these patients can be attributed, in part, to the ocular symptoms, functional impairments and changes in appearance produced by TED. Looking at specific subgroups using the Profile of Mood States (POMS) instrument, TED patients for whom proptosis was the predominant feature experienced significantly greater emotional distress than patients for whom strabismus or muscle restriction was the predominant feature [19]. Similarly, on the Middlesex Hospital Questionnaire, patients with proptosis experienced significantly increased anxiety, depression, and phobia when compared to those with TED related muscle restriction [20]. Therefore, not only does proptosis cause functional impairment such as significant dry eye, but it is also associated with psychological distress.

Although this chapter focuses primarily on the effects of TED signs and symptoms, underlying thyroid dysfunction should also be considered when evaluating psychological disturbances in TED patients. Both hyperthyroidism and hypothyroidism have been associated with an increased risk of mood disorders that usually resolve when euthyroidism is achieved [21, 22]. Hypothyroidism results in depressive symptoms due to low production of triiodythyronine (T3, generally considered a "mood-enhancing" hormone), whereas hyperthyroidism causes an increase in free total thyroxine (T4) resulting in a relative decrease in T3 [21]. However, some patients can experience altered mood even after being rendered euthyroid [23–25]. One proposed explanation is that the presence of antithyroid antibodies alone, regardless of the clinical thyroid state, may be linked to a higher prevalence of psychiatric disorders, via a shared underlying immune-mediated neuroendocrine pathway [26, 27]. Other studies have challenged this proposition by showing that the prevalence of antithyroid antibodies does not differ between psychiatric inpatients and controls [28, 29]. Furthermore, some of the studies reporting a linkage between antithyroid antibodies and psychiatric disease failed to control for previous exposure to lithium, which has antithyroid activity and could promote the formation of antibodies, thereby confounding results [21, 30, 31]. Whether or not thyroid autoimmunity ultimately proves to share a common pathogenesis with psychiatric disease, a patient's thyroid hormone state can produce mood changes in patients with TED independent of eye symptoms (Fig. 13.2).

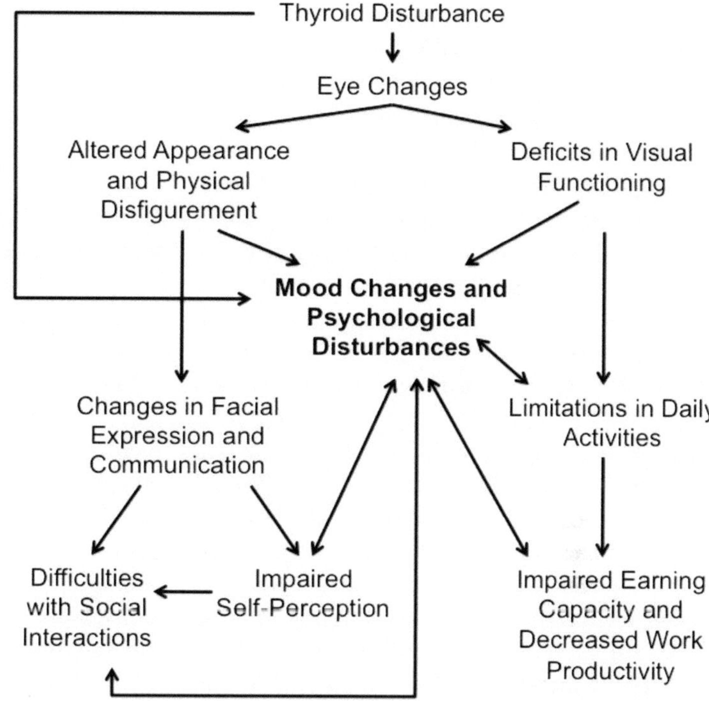

Fig. 13.2 Psychological disturbances in thyroid-associated eye disease (TED). The effects of TED can be divided in two main domains: appearance and visual functioning. Changes in both areas can cause distress and impaired quality of life. Many of the effects are interconnected, with multiple contributing factors to mood changes and psychological disturbances

Dissatisfaction with Appearance and Implications for Identity and Social Relationships

Appearance-related concerns among TED patients have been reported to be as high as 90 %, with greater frequency in younger patients and females [7]. Because physical appearance is closely tied with self-perception, confidence, and identity, the disfiguring changes inflicted by TED can affect these personality traits. In a Dutch study using the GO-QoL, 71 % of patients felt that TED had negatively affected their self-confidence, and more than half felt that they were watched by other people [7]. Similarly, in an Australian cohort assessed using an English language version of the GO-QoL, 33 % of patients reported that their self-confidence had been impaired "a little," while 44 % of patients reported that their self-confidence had been impaired "very much" [32]. Among a German group, 38 % reported impaired self-perception [33]. One of the themes that emerged from an open-ended qualitative analysis of TED patients was the development of an altered identity among TED patients as a result of changes in appearance and abilities [34]. Female gender has also been associated with a greater decline in self-perception [15].

The changes in appearance in TED also affect these patients' social relationships and their interactions with others. The lid retraction, proptosis, and decreased blinking associated with TED can make a patient look hostile, angry, or startled when that is not their intent [3]. Due to a lack of control over facial expression and communication, TED patients may experience altered attitudes and behavior from others, leading to difficult social interactions and strained personal relationships. These patients endorse feeling like they are somebody else, feeling clumsy around others, and feeling cut off from the outside world; they struggle to avoid social withdrawal [12]. Both men and women also report a decline in social desirability [15]. Besides changes in facial appearance, the changes in patients' mood, psychological disturbances, and impaired self-perception may also affect social relationships (Fig. 13.2).

Decreased Visual Function and Limitations in Daily Activities

Functional deficits encountered in TED patients include altered visual acuity, decreased lacrimation, diplopia, and orbital/ocular pain [35]. Pain in particular is a symptom more frequently experienced in TED than in other eye diseases. It may be secondary to exposure keratitis caused by eyelid malposition, or a feeling of elevated pressure associated with periorbital edema, extraocular muscle enlargement, increased orbital fat, and proptosis [15]. One criticism of the GO-QoL is that it does not have any items related to ocular pain and therefore fails to capture an important element of how TED affects quality of life [6].

These functional deficits can limit daily activities. Many patients report impairments in driving, leisure activities, reading, and television viewing [7, 32, 36]. The effects on daily activities may also contribute to mood issues. For example, deficits in visual functioning and the resulting impairment in participating in hobbies may lead to anhedonia and increase the likelihood of developing depression. Quality of life studies in allied conditions of visual impairment, such as dry eye syndrome and ocular surface disease, have also uncovered connections between reduced visual function, interference with activities of leisure and daily living, and a higher prevalence of depression [37–42]. The complex interactions appearance, function, mood, and quality of life in TED are summarized in Fig. 13.2.

Economic Effects

TED incurs considerable direct healthcare expense as well as indirect costs to the individual and society due to impaired productivity. A significant correlation has been found between the costs of TED and the scores on the GO-QoL [43]. In a study of these economic effects in a cohort of TED patients, 36 % were on sick leave, 28 % were disabled, 5 % had retired early, and 3 % had lost their jobs as a result of their disease [33]. Patients with more severe disease were on sick leave for longer periods and more likely to be disabled [33]. A decreased ability to work may also contribute to mood disturbances (Fig. 13.2), incurring considerable emotional and psychological cost in addition to financial losses.

Correlations with Clinical Disease Severity Scores

Several clinical scoring systems have been used in the context of TED, including NO SPECS, Clinical Activity Score (CAS), and the VISA classification. Two groups have found that increased emotional distress correlated with increased clinical severity [19, 36]. The developers of the GO-QoL found a moderate correlation between QoL and visual functioning [7], and similarly, the developers of the TED-QoL found a moderately good correlation between quality of life and clinical disease severity [10]. However, most studies have shown that patient-reported quality of life changes do not necessarily correlate with the duration, severity, or activity of TED as determined by clinicians [7, 15, 16, 31–35]. This reflects the complexity of the relationship between clinical disease severity and quality of life, especially because there is a very high inter-individual variation in the impact of disease on perceived well-being. What some patients view as severe disfigurement may be inconsequential to others. This apparent discrepancy between traditional clinical assessments and patient-reported outcomes underscores the benefit of including quality of life assessments alongside objective disease severity measurements as outcome measures in futures TED studies.

The Effects of Treating TED on Quality of Life

Studies of the effectiveness of treatments have mostly been based on objective clinical disease severity measures. More recently, studies of treatment effects in TED have also incorporated quality of life measures in order to better reflect patients' experience. Quality of life measurements show improvement after treatment with steroids and orbital radiotherapy [32–34, 36–38]. Surgical decompression is associated with a positive change in quality of life measurements, particularly in the appearance division of the GO-QoL [33, 39]. In general, the vast majority (70–80 %) of patients feel that surgical decompression is beneficial, and they are satisfied with the cosmetic result [44]. However, in one study with long-term follow-up (median 9.8 years) in a cohort of 120 patients with TED, more than one-third of patients were still dissatisfied with the ultimate appearance of their eyes, even though few patients had long-term impairment from a functional standpoint [45]. Most treatment techniques appear to have a positive effect by improving quality of life scores, but patients may still have impaired health-related quality of life compared to controls even years after treatment [46]. Therefore, TED should be considered a chronic disease that requires continued support even after the acute phase of immunosuppressive and/or surgical treatments.

Conclusions and Recommendations

Thyroid eye disease (TED) causes changes in the eyes that impact both function and appearance, leading to psychological disturbances and impaired quality of life (Fig. 13.2). Changes in quality of life have not been found to consistently correlate with traditional clinical assessments, and TED patients often have decreased quality of life even after treatment.

These findings have several important implications for clinical practice (summarized in Table 13.2). Including a mental health professional on the multidisciplinary treatment team for TED can help address the range of psychological issues facing these patients. The majority of patients receiving treatment for disfiguring conditions expressed the desire to speak with a professional trained to deal with appearance-related concerns [1, 2]. A system for referrals to psychiatric or psychological care should be standard of care, given that a prior analysis found that approximately half of all TED patients would benefit from psychological intervention [16].

Table 13.2 Key recommendations for addressing psychological disturbances in patients with thyroid eye disease

1.	Include a mental health professional on the multidisciplinary care team and/or set up a referral system for psychological counseling
2.	Build relationships with patient support groups and foundations and refer patients to these organizations for additional support
3.	Consider a lower threshold for surgical intervention—intervene when psychological effects from altered appearance are significant in lieu of intervention only when functional vision impairment is present
4.	Incorporate quality of life scores alongside traditional clinical severity scoring as outcome measures for research studies and clinical practice

Adequate education and counseling are essential for helping patients to cope with their disease [32]. Besides providing psychological care or referring patients for treatment, physicians can also refer patients to local support groups and accept patient referrals from these groups [47]. The Graves' Disease and Thyroid Foundation (www.gdatf.org) is one organization that provides education and support for patients, caregivers, and healthcare professionals. By building relationships with these types of groups, physicians can provide another avenue of support for their TED patients.

Another implication of the significant effects of TED and particularly physical disfigurement in causing psychosocial distress is in surgical planning. Previously, given the complexity of surgical orbital decompression, some practitioners would not operate until vision was actively threatened. However, in the hands of experienced surgeons, surgical decompression is a safe and effective procedure; the distress caused by altered appearance in TED should therefore be factored in when considering surgery [19].

Quality of life considerations and psychological burden assessment may provide more insight into an individual patient's experience of the disease and facilitate discussions regarding medical and surgical treatments. With this information, physicians may be able to better treat their patients and mitigate some of the serious psychological consequences of this disease.

Acknowledgments Generously supported by Steve and Kathleen Flynn, the Bell Charitable Foundation, an unrestricted grant from Research to Prevent Blindness New York, New York, and NIH core grant P30EY022589.

References

1. Clarke A, Rumsey N, Collin JRO, Wyn-Williams M. Psychosocial distress associated with disfiguring eye conditions. Eye (Lond). 2003;17(1):35–40.
2. Rumsey N, Clarke A, White P, Wyn-Williams M, Garlick W. Altered body image: appearance-related concerns of people with visible disfigurement. J Adv Nurs. 2004;48(5):443–53.
3. Davies L. Perceptual problems in thyroid eye disease. Nursing Stand. 1995;9(16):36–9.
4. Classification of eye changes of Graves' disease. Thyroid. 1992;2(3):235–6.
5. Wiersinga WM, Prummel MF, Terwee CB. Effects of Graves' ophthalmopathy on quality of life. J Endocrinol Invest. 2004;27(3):259–64.
6. Bradley EA, Sloan JA, Novotny PJ, Garrity JA, Woog JJ, West SK. Evaluation of the National Eye Institute visual function questionnaire in Graves' ophthalmopathy. Ophthalmology. 2006;113(8):1450–4.
7. Terwee CB, Gerding MN, Dekker FW, Prummel MF, Wiersinga WM. Development of a disease specific quality of life questionnaire for patients with Graves' ophthalmopathy: the GO-QOL. Br J Ophthalmol. 1998;82(7):773–9.
8. Terwee CB, Gerding MN, Dekker FW, Prummel MF, van der Pol JP, Wiersinga WM. Test-retest reliability of the GO-QOL: a disease-specific quality of life questionnaire for patients with Graves' ophthalmopathy. J Clin Epidemiol. 1999;52(9):875–84.
9. Wiersinga WM. Quality of life in Graves' ophthalmopathy. Best Pract Res Clin Endocrinol Metab. 2012;26:359–70.
10. Fayers T, Dolman PJ. Validity and reliability of the TED-QOL: a new three-item questionnaire to assess quality of life in thyroid eye disease. Br J Ophthalmol. 2011;95(12):1670–4.
11. Watt T, Rasmussen AK, Groenvold M, Bjorner JB, Watt SH, Bonnema SJ, et al. Improving a newly developed patient-reported outcome for thyroid patients, using cognitive interviewing. Qual Life Res. 2008;17(7):1009–17.
12. Jensen AL, Harder I. The impact of bodily change on social behaviour in patients with thyroid-associated ophthalmopathy. Scand J Caring Sci. 2011;25(2): 341–9.
13. Estcourt S, Vaidya B, Quinn A, Shepherd M. The impact of thyroid eye disease upon patients' wellbeing: a qualitative analysis. Clin Endocrinol (Oxf). 2008;68(4):635–9.
14. Gerding MN, Terwee CB, Dekker FW, Koornneef L, Prummel MF, Wiersinga WM. Quality of life in patients with Graves' ophthalmopathy is markedly decreased: measurement by the medical outcomes study instrument. Thyroid. 1997;7(6):885–9.
15. Yeatts RP. Quality of life in patients with Graves ophthalmopathy. Trans Am Ophthalmol Soc. 2005; 103:368–411.
16. Egle UT, Kahaly GJ, Petrak F, Hardt J, Batke J, Best J, et al. The relevance of physical and psychosocial factors for the quality of life in patients with thyroid-associated orbitopathy (TAO). Exp Clin Endocrinol Diabetes. 1999;107 Suppl 5:S168–71.
17. Wong VTC, Yu DKH. Usefulness of the Hospital Anxiety and Depression Scale for screening for psychiatric morbidity in Chinese patients with Graves' ophthalmopathy. East Asian Arch Psychiatry. 2013;23(1):6–12.
18. Bunevicius R, Velickiene D, Prange Jr AJ. Mood and anxiety disorders in women with treated hyperthyroidism and ophthalmopathy caused by Graves' disease. Gen Hosp Psychiatry. 2005;27(2):133–9.
19. Farid M, Roch-Levecq AC, Levi L, Brody BL, Granet DB, Kikkawa DO. Psychological disturbance in graves ophthalmopathy. Arch Ophthalmol. 2005;123(4):491–6.
20. Ghanem AA, Amr MA, Araafa LF. Graves opthalmopathy and psychoendocrinopathies. Middle East Afr J Ophthalmol. 2010;17(2):169–74.
21. Hendrick V, Altshuler L, Whybrow P. Psychoneuroendocrinology of mood disorders. The hypothalamic-pituitary-thyroid axis. Psychiatr Clin North Am. 1998;21(2):277–92.
22. Kalra S, Balhara YP. Euthyroid depression: the role of thyroid hormone. Recent Pat Endocr Metab Immune Drug Discov. 2014;8(1):38–41.
23. Fahrenfort JJ, Wilterdink AM, van der Veen EA. Long-term residual complaints and psychosocial sequelae after remission of hyperthyroidism. Psychoneuroendocrinology. 2000;25(2):201–11.
24. Harsch I, Paschke R, Usadel KH. The possible etiological role of psychological disturbances in Graves' disease. Acta Med Austriaca. 1992;19 Suppl 1:62–5.
25. Bunevicius R, Prange Jr AJ. Psychiatric manifestations of Graves' hyperthyroidism: pathophysiology and treatment options. CNS Drugs. 2006;20(11):897–909.
26. Carta MG, Loviselli A, Hardoy MC, Massa S, Cadeddu M, Sardu C, et al. The link between thyroid autoimmunity (antithyroid peroxidase autoantibodies) with anxiety and mood disorders in the community: a field of interest for public health in the future. BMC Psychiatry. 2004;4:25.
27. Nemeroff CB, Simon JS, Haggerty Jr JJ, Evans DL. Antithyroid antibodies in depressed patients. Am J Psychiatry. 1985;142(7):840–3.
28. Joffe RT. Antithyroid antibodies in major depression. Acta Psychiatr Scand. 1987;76(5):598–9.
29. Legros S, Mendlewicz J, Wybran J. Immunoglobulins, autoantibodies and other serum protein fractions in psychiatric disorders. Eur Arch Psychiatry Neurol Sci. 1985;235(1):9–11.
30. Haggerty Jr JJ, Evans DL, Golden RN, Pedersen CA, Simon JS, Nemeroff CB. The presence of antithyroid

antibodies in patients with affective and nonaffective psychiatric disorders. Biol Psychiatry. 1990;27(1): 51–60.
31. Hage MP, Azar ST. The link between thyroid function and depression. J Thyroid Res. 2011;2012:590648.
32. Park JJ, Sullivan TJ, Mortimer RH, Wagenaar M, Perry-Keene DA. Assessing quality of life in Australian patients with Graves' ophthalmopathy. Br J Ophthalmol. 2004;88(1):75–8.
33. Ponto KA, Pitz S, Pfeiffer N, Hommel G, Weber MM, Kahaly GJ. Quality of life and occupational disability in endocrine orbitopathy. Dtsch Arztebl Int. 2009;106(17):283–9.
34. Estcourt S, Quinn AG, Vaidya B. Quality of life in thyroid eye disease: impact of quality of care. Eur J Endocrinol. 2011;164(5):649–55.
35. Coulter I, Frewin S, Krassas GE, Perros P. Psychological implications of Graves' orbitopathy. Eur J Endocrinol. 2007;157(2):127–31.
36. Choi YJ, Lim HT, Lee SJ, Lee SY, Yoon JS. Assessing Graves' ophthalmopathy-specific quality of life in Korean patients. Eye (Lond). 2012;26(4):544–51.
37. Friedman NJ. Impact of dry eye disease and treatment on quality of life. Curr Opin Ophthalmol. 2010; 21(4):310–6.
38. Kim KW, Han SB, Han ER, Woo SJ, Lee JJ, Yoon JC, et al. Association between depression and dry eye disease in an elderly population. Invest Ophthalmol Vis Sci. 2011;52(11):7954–8.
39. Mertzanis P, Abetz L, Rajagopalan K, Espindle D, Chalmers R, Snyder C, et al. The relative burden of dry eye in patients' lives: comparisons to a U.S. normative sample. Invest Ophthalmol Vis Sci. 2005;46(1):46–50.
40. Miljanovic B, Dana R, Sullivan DA, Schaumberg DA. Impact of dry eye syndrome on vision-related quality of life. Am J Ophthalmol. 2007;143(3):409–15.
41. Pouyeh B, Viteri E, Feuer W, Lee DJ, Florez H, Fabian JA, et al. Impact of ocular surface symptoms on quality of life in a United States veterans affairs population. Am J Ophthalmol. 2012;153(6):1061–66.e3.
42. Baudouin C, Creuzot-Garcher C, Hoang-Xuan T, Rigeade MC, Brouquet Y, Bassols A, et al. Severe impairment of health-related quality of life in patients suffering from ocular surface diseases. J Fr Ophtalmol. 2008;31(4):369–78.
43. Ponto KA, Merkesdal S, Hommel G, Pitz S, Pfeiffer N, Kahaly GJ. Public health relevance of Graves' orbitopathy. J Clin Endocrinol Metab. 2013;98(1): 145–52.
44. Tehrani M, Krummenauer F, Mann WJ, Pitz S, Dick HB, Kahaly GJ. Disease-specific assessment of quality of life after decompression surgery for Graves' ophthalmopathy. Eur J Ophthalmol. 2004;14(3): 193–9.
45. Bartley GB, Fatourechi V, Kadrmas EF, Jacobsen SJ, Ilstrup DM, Garrity JA, et al. Long-term follow-up of Graves ophthalmopathy in an incidence cohort. Ophthalmology. 1996;103(6):958–62.
46. Terwee CB, Dekker FW, Prummel MF, Wiersinga WM. Graves' ophthalmopathy through the eyes of the patient: a state of the art on health-related qualify of life assessment. Orbit. 2001;20(4):281–90.
47. Wood LC. Support groups for patients with Graves' disease and other thyroid conditions. Endocrinol Metab Clin North Am. 1998;27(1):101–7.
48. Lee H, Roh HS, Yoon JS, Lee SY. Assessment of quality of life and depression in Korean patients with Graves' ophthalmopathy. Korean J Ophthalmol. 2010;24(2):65–72.
49. Kahaly GJ, Hardt J, Petrak F, Egle UT. Psychosocial factors in subjects with thyroid-associated ophthalmopathy. Thyroid. 2002;12(3):237–9.
50. Elberling TV, Rasmussen AK, Feldt-Rasmussen U, Hørding M, Perrild H, Waldemar G. Impaired health-related quality of life in Graves' disease. A prospective study. Eur J Endocrinol. 2004;151(5):549–55.

Index

R.S. Douglas et al. (eds.), *Thyroid Eye Disease*,
DOI 10.1007/978-1-4939-1746-4, © Springer Science+Business Media New York 2015

MIX
Papier aus verantwortungsvollen Quellen
Paper from responsible sources
FSC® C105338

If you have any concerns about our products,
you can contact us on
ProductSafety@springernature.com

In case Publisher is established outside the EU,
the EU authorized representative is:
Springer Nature Customer Service Center GmbH
Europaplatz 3, 69115 Heidelberg, Germany

Printed by Libri Plureos GmbH
in Hamburg, Germany